Current Topics in Environmental Health and Preventive Medicine

Series editor
T. Otsuki
Kurashiki, Japan

Current Topics in Environmental Health and Preventive Medicine, published in partnership with the Japanese Society of Hygiene, is designed to deliver well written volumes authored by experts from around the globe, covering the prevention and environmental health related to medical, biological, molecular biological, genetic, physical, psychosocial, chemical, and other environmental factors. The series will be a valuable resource to both new and established researchers, as well as students who are seeking comprehensive information on environmental health and health promotion.

More information about this series at http://www.springer.com/series/13556

Takemi Otsuki • Yasuo Yoshioka • Andrij Holian
Editors

Biological Effects of Fibrous and Particulate Substances

Springer

Editors
Takemi Otsuki
Department of Hygiene
Kawasaki Medical School
Kurashiki
Japan

Yasuo Yoshioka
Department of Toxicology and Safety Science
Osaka University
Suita
Japan

Andrij Holian
Center for Environmental Health Sciences
University of Montana
Missoula
USA

ISSN 2364-8333 ISSN 2364-8341 (electronic)
Current Topics in Environmental Health and Preventive Medicine
ISBN 978-4-431-55731-9 ISBN 978-4-431-55732-6 (eBook)
DOI 10.1007/978-4-431-55732-6

Library of Congress Control Number: 2015951622

Springer Tokyo Heidelberg New York Dordrecht London

Printed on acid-free paper

Springer Japan KK is part of Springer Science+Business Media (www.springer.com)

Preface

We have the great pleasure of setting afloat the first volume of *Current Topics in Environmental Health and Preventive Medicine* (*EHPM*), a book series by the Japanese Society for Hygiene (JSH). This first volume, *Biological Effects of Fibrous and Particulate Substances,* is now published. We sincerely appreciate all the authors contributing their wonderful reviews on the theme of this book. All of you who read it can enjoy learning more about the cellular and molecular mechanisms for the biological effects of fibrous and particulate substances including nanomaterials, various effects of nanomaterials, immunological effects of silica and asbestos, and particularly autoimmunity and antitumor immunity. In this eBook, you can learn about biological, especially immunological, effects caused by fibrous and particulate matters such as asbestos fibers and silica particles as well as nanomaterials from the basic cellular and molecular biological aspects and points of view closely related to clinical work.

You—and we too—are learning about recent advances in the study of the immunological effects of fibrous and particulate materials and can imagine and consider how we can translate these findings into therapy. In this respect, we are thinking of the clinical patients who are suffering from diseases due to exposure to these materials as well as people who are in localities that pose higher risks for exposure to these substances and how we can develop preventive and therapeutic methods and tools for these individuals—in short, how scientific achievements can support and cure them.

We truly appreciate your having this book, so that you and we together can proceed hand in hand toward the aims described above.

Kurashiki, Japan
Suita, Japan
Missoula, MT, USA

Takemi Otsuki
Yasuo Yoshioka
Andrij Holian

Acknowledgments

The Japanese Society for Hygiene (JSH) is publishing two journals: the *Japanese Journal of Hygiene* (*JJH*) and *Environmental Health and Preventive Medicine* (*EHPM*). *EHPM* is an international journal with a history of 20 years and is registered in Medline and Journal Citation Report (it will obtain its initial impact factor in 2016). In the year 2014, the editorial board members decided to publish a book series to spread our interests more widely regarding environmental health and preventive medicine and to provide first-rate knowledge to the world by contributing to progress in those fields. I thank Professors Holian and Yoshioka for their skillful editing and organization of this publication.

As the editor in chief of this book series, I will proceed to publish many diverse topics in EHPM fields during the coming 5 years. Readers can look forward to the publication of the next—and the next ones.

I thank the city of Kurashiki, where my medical school is located, surrounded by idyllic scenes and which includes a historical downtown. Furthermore, I should say special thanks to Rie, Riyu, and Yukimi, my family, for their support, making it possible for me to concentrate on my research as well as editing this eBook. I am always glad to see their faces, and I appreciate the communication among us.

Kurashiki, Japan Takemi Otsuki

Contents

Chapter 1
Macrophage and Multinucleated Giant Cell Classification

Kevin L. Trout, Forrest Jessop, and Christopher T. Migliaccio

Abstract The purpose of this chapter is to provide an overview of macrophage subtype and multinucleated giant cell classification with a specific discussion of their role(s) in response to particulates and other foreign bodies. Topics covered for the different subtypes include the following: environmental factors involved in their generation, functional characterization, disease associations, and interactions with particulates. This chapter is separated into three major parts. The first portion describes the normal structure and functions of the macrophage. Second, the currently published macrophage subsets are outlined. The classifications included in the discussion are based on function ("M" polarization) rather than anatomical position (tissue-specific macrophages – Kupffer cells, alveolar macrophages, etc.). As shown in Fig. 1.1, the ontogeny of the various types of macrophages being discussed in this chapter depends on the pathway of activation. The third major section focuses on multinucleated giant cells, which are formed by fusion of individual macrophages. The ontogeny of each subset will be discussed and the current literature regarding particulate/foreign-body interaction will be reviewed.

Keywords Macrophage • Polarization • Multinucleated • Giant cells • Particles

Abbreviations

Arg-1	Arginase-1
CD	Cluster of differentiation
Ch3l3 (Ym1)	Chitinase 3-like 3
CXCL	Chemokine (C-X-C motif) ligand
FcγR	Fc-gamma receptor
GC	Glucocorticoids
GM-CSF	Granulocyte-macrophage colony-stimulating factor
HIV	Human immunodeficiency virus

K.L. Trout • F. Jessop • C.T. Migliaccio (✉)
Center for Environmental Health Sciences, University of Montana, Missoula, MT 59812, USA
e-mail: christopher.migliaccio@umontana.edu

T. Otsuki et al. (eds.), *Biological Effects of Fibrous and Particulate Substances*, Current Topics in Environmental Health and Preventive Medicine,
DOI 10.1007/978-4-431-55732-6_1

IFNγ	Interferon gamma
IL	Interleukin
iNOS	Inducible nitric oxide synthase
LIF	Leukemia inhibitory factor
M-CSF	Macrophage colony-stimulating factor
MGC	Multinucleated giant cell
MHC	Major histocompatibility complex
MMP9	Matrix metalloproteinase 9
RELMα (FIZZ1)	Resistin-like molecule alpha
ROS	Reactive oxygen species
TAM	Tumor-associated macrophage
TGFβ	Transforming growth factor beta
Th1/Th2	Type 1 or type 2 helper T cells
TLR	Toll-like receptor
TNFα	Tumor necrosis factor alpha
VEGF	Vascular endothelial growth factor

1.1 Regulators of Immunity: Macrophages

It is important to note that macrophage behavior in vivo cannot be fully explained by studies in vitro. From all that has been learned, we know that the macrophage is a complex cell in a very complex environment. The environment defines the cell, and the macrophage is altered when the environment is perturbed either by a toxic exposure or by any manipulation to study the tissue. Consequently, our best information always has room for error. In addition, there is much that we do not know about the macrophage response to toxic exposures and the macrophage's role in pathogenesis.

Macrophages are derived from bone marrow stem cells (Fig. 1.1). The monoblasts mature to promonocytes and then to monocytes. Monocytes remain in the bone marrow for a short period and move into the circulatory system where they remain for 36–104 h [1]. From there monocytes enter the tissue and mature into macrophages. Once in the tissue, macrophages are relatively long-lived cells with a lifetime in the order of months [2]. Maturation of monocytes to macrophages is driven by a combination of at least three factors: (1) genetic programming, (2) growth factors/cytokines, and (3) the environment of the tissue. The extent of the effect of the environment on cell maturation is a recent area of research. Current thought is that the environment, growth factors, and cytokines all contribute to the macrophage phenotype.

The term "big eater" was coined by Metchnikoff in 1892 to describe the phagocytic function of the macrophage, which is still considered one of the most important functions of the macrophage. This includes recognition and, if possible, degradation of foreign material. The macrophage is well suited for this activity, as it possesses a large number of receptors functionally linked to phagocytosis, such as

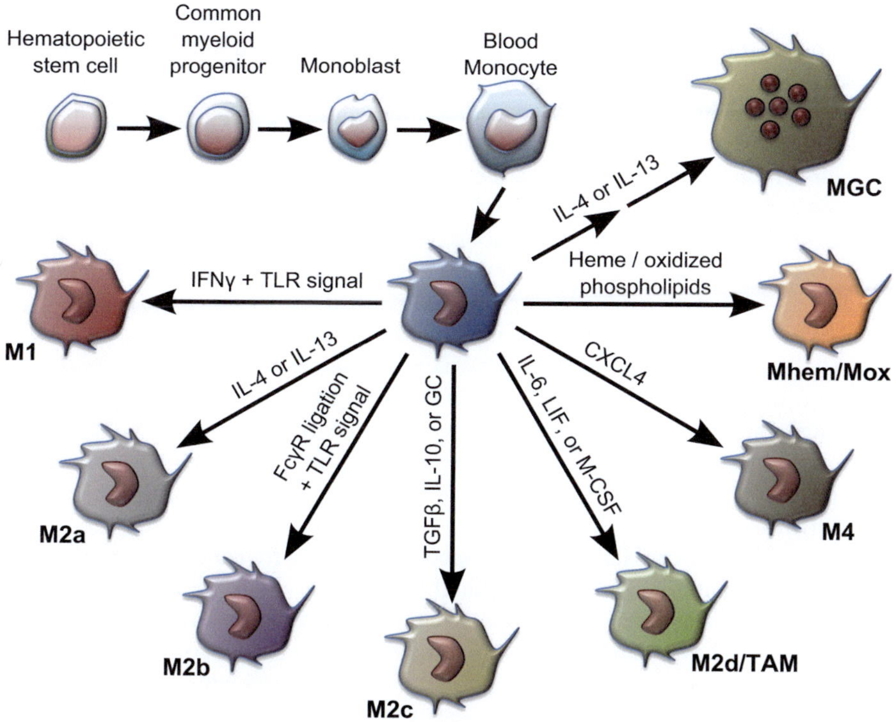

Fig. 1.1 Ontogeny of macrophage subtypes. Tissue macrophages are derived from bone marrow progenitor stem cells. Bone marrow-derived monocytes migrate through the blood, exit into extravascular tissue, and differentiate into macrophages. Once in resident tissue, macrophage differentiation into sub-phenotypes is dependent upon a complex array of microenvironmental stimuli including both endogenous (cytokines, chemokines, and growth factors) and exogenous (TLR-agonists such as pathogens) factors. The deriving factors and resulting subsets depicted are not exhaustive. M1 or "classical" macrophage polarization is often observed during infection or acute inflammation due to particle exposure in which tissue damage is prevalent, and TLR signaling and IFNγ levels are increased to boost phagocytic activity and antimicrobial/viral defenses. These are hallmark characteristics of a Th1 response. M2a and M2c populations are unregulated following the acute inflammatory response and have an important role in wound healing and collagen deposition in response to foreign bodies such as particulates. Other M2 subsets (M2b, M2d), as well as M4 and Mhem/Mox phenotypes, may also be affected by particle exposure, though the link between exposure and macrophage-induced pathology has not been investigated. Multinucleated giant cells (MGC) share common stimulating factors as the M2a subset; however, it is likely that there are additional factors required to induce macrophage fusion into MGC. MGC are observed regularly in granulomas, but their role in the foreign-body response is not well known

immunoglobulin, complement, and scavenger receptors. Since macrophages are relatively large cells, they can accommodate ingested material. Macrophages are mobile cells capable of responding to various chemotactic factors. They can release superoxide anion and proteolytic enzymes to kill and/or digest microbes and can present digested peptide fragments with the major histocompatibility complex

(MHC) to trigger an immune response [3–6]. Finally, they can release various mediators to (1) recruit additional phagocytic cells (polymorphonuclear neutrophils, monocytes, and macrophages); (2) stimulate maturation of phagocytic cells; and (iii) modulate the function of other local cells to respond to the adverse condition. A major function of macrophages is regulatory in nature, in that as a front-line immune responder, it affects the subsequent nature of the response. Therefore, the nature, or phenotype, of the macrophage can have a profound effect on the outcome of an immune response. In the context of exposure to foreign material (i.e., particles), the outcome is dictated by the local macrophage content, which may be dominated by one or several different subsets at any given time.

The term macrophage has occasionally been used to describe monocytes and monocyte-derived cells in culture. This is a misnomer that can create confusion. The term macrophage should be used to describe tissue mononuclear phagocytic cells, and monocytes should be used to describe the circulating mononuclear precursor cells. Since mononuclear-derived cells in vitro may not adequately describe the true macrophage [7, 8] in part for the preceding reasons, they should be clearly distinguished.

Blood monocytes are larger than lymphocytes, have a rounded shape, and have a nuclear/cytoplasmic ratio of approximately one. They often present with a bean-shaped nucleus with considerable margination of heterochromatin. Macrophages are larger cells, have many lamellipodia, many subsurface vacuoles, and an irregularly indented nucleus with little heterochromatin. Macrophages also have more rough endoplasmic reticulum, coated vesicles, lysosomes, and microtubules than monocytes. The macrophage nuclear/cytoplasmic volume ratio is less than one. Consequently, the cells are easily distinguished morphologically.

1.2 "M" Classification of Macrophages

Just a few decades ago macrophages were considered to have a relatively homogeneous phenotype. Macrophages were defined as mediators and regulators of inflammation, and that inflammation was generally considered to be Th1. This is characterized by a response involving classic inflammatory mediators: IFNγ, TNFα, IL-6, and IL-1β. However, recent research has determined that macrophages are subject to their environment and macrophage functions are altered by the local mix of signaling factors. Macrophages are now categorized based on phenotypes that are defined by the expression of surface markers, intracellular pathways, and soluble mediators. These categories are described using an "M" nomenclature system [9–13]. There is no general consensus on macrophage polarization prior to induction of an inflammatory response. Original naming created the M1 and M2 macrophage subsets where the M1 was considered the classic subset and the M2, by default, the alternatively activated. Over time more subsets were defined when the M2 was further divided to account for different phenotypes, mechanisms of activation, and additional pathologies associated with atherosclerosis.

1.2.1 M1: Classic Macrophages

1.2.1.1 Environment/Generation

The "classical" nomenclature, labeled as the M1 subset, refers to the phenotype typically associated with macrophages: inflammatory cytokines, Th1-association, and antigen-presentation capability. This subset is most commonly generated with either IFNγ or TLR-agonists [11, 12]. Recent reports identify GM-CSF stimulation as a partial M1 agonist, specifically through its ability to enhance antigen presentation and many other M1 macrophage functions [14].

1.2.1.2 Function/Phenotype

The M1 subset has a pro-inflammatory phenotype. This manifests in both the types of soluble mediators and surface proteins expressed upon activation. Ex vivo polarization of alveolar macrophages with IFNγ induced changes in approximately 41 genes, specifically including increased expression of toll-like receptors and multiple CXCL chemokines [15]. In addition to the classic cytokines of IFNγ, TNFα, IL-6, and IL-1β, the M1 has been associated with production and release of IL-12p70, reactive oxygen species (ROS), and nitric oxide (NO) [16, 17] (Table 1.1). This subset has also been described to express both MHC II and CD86 on the surface which are key for T lymphocyte activation.

1.2.1.3 Disease Associations

The M1 subset has been found to increase renal cell damage [18], as well as increase disease in the *mdx* mouse model of muscular dystrophy [19]. M1 is the dominant macrophage phenotype in infection (acute and chronic) and is thought to play a critical role in granuloma formation in tuberculosis [17]. In addition, the M1 has been described as the predominant phenotype associated with nonmalignant tumor-associated macrophages (TAM) [20, 21], and aspects of the phenotype have been shown to prevent HIV-1 infection [22].

1.2.1.4 Interaction with Particulates

In animal exposure models to particulates such as silica or nanomaterials, an initial Th1 response has been implicated in the pathology, specifically through IL-1 signaling [23, 24]. In addition, recent studies have described a role of M1 macrophages in the inflammatory response to joint replacement wear debris [25–28]. The usage of replacement joints leads to the generation of particulates that are

Table 1.1 Common markers of M-category subsets

Subset	Markers	References
M1	TNFα	[11, 14, 16, 15, 17, 123]
	IL-1β	
	IL-6	
	IL-12	
	ROS, iNOS	
	CD80/86	
	MHC II	
	CXCL9	
	CXCL10	
	GM-CSF	
M2a	Ch3l3/Ym1 (mouse)	[30, 32, 124–128]
	FIZZ1/RELMα (mouse)	
	IL-1ra	
	Arg-1	
	IL-10	
	CD206	
M2b	IL-1β	[11, 37, 123]
	IL-6	
	IL-10	
	TNFα	
	CD86	
	MHC II	
M2c	TGFβ	[18, 44–49]
	IL-10	
	CD163	
	TLR1	
	TLR8	
M2d/TAM	VEGF	[30, 51, 50, 53, 54, 56]

categorized as wear products. Some have proposed skewing toward an M2a phenotype as a potential treatment for inflammation in worn joint replacement [26, 28].

1.2.2 M2a: Th2-Associated Macrophages

1.2.2.1 Environment/Generation

This subset was originally designated as the M2 or alternatively activated macrophage. However, as more phenotypes were characterized, this subset was given the nomenclature of M2a and was described as being activated by the Th2-associated cytokines IL-4 and IL-13 [10–12, 29, 30]. The dependence of this subset on Th2 immunity was confirmed by studies using IL-4Rα null mice, where this protein is a key functional component of both the IL-4 and IL-13 receptors [31].

1.2.2.2 Function/Phenotype

The M2a subset has a Th2-promoting phenotype. The production of several soluble mediators has been associated with the M2a phenotype and promoting of Th2 type of inflammation. While IL-10 and IL-1ra are more associated with an anti-Th1 inflammation type of activity, the release of Ym1/Chi3l3 has been found to induce Th2 responses [32]. In addition, the surface expression of CD206 is greatly increased in the M2a [30]. The M2a are also associated with increased intracellular expression of Arg-1 and FIZZ1, both of which had been a couple of the original markers used for identification of these cells [9, 33, 34] (Table 1.1).

1.2.2.3 Disease Associations

Both M2a and M2c subsets have been found to increase type VI collagen and fibrosis in an adipocyte model [35]. Furthermore, the M2a phenotype has also been associated with pulmonary and renal fibrosis [18].

1.2.2.4 Interaction with Particulates

Th2 immunity plays a well-accepted role in models of lung fibrosis. This is entirely consistent with the observed function of M2a macrophages in fibrosis and the therapeutic rationale for targeting this subset. In studies comparing wild-type mice and IL-4Rα null mice, a significant increase in the M2a in the wild-type corresponded with the development of silica-induced pulmonary fibrosis. However, IL-4Rα null mice that lack the ability to generate the M2a had a significant decrease in the pathology [31].

1.2.3 M2b: Alternatively Activated Macrophages

1.2.3.1 Environment/Generation

This subset is generated by the presence of antibody-antigen complexes [11, 36, 37]. Because these are also a pro-inflammatory type of macrophages, their activation is via FcγR ligation in conjunction with a TLR signal.

1.2.3.2 Function/Phenotype

The M2b subset has a pro-inflammatory phenotype that is similar to the M1. These macrophages produce the classic inflammatory cytokines IL-1β, TNFα, and IL-6 in addition to the surface proteins MHC II and CD86 [11, 38] (Table 1.1). These markers suggest an ability and propensity to activate nearby immune cells either by contact or within the vicinity. However, a key difference between the M2b and the M1 is the finding that it also produces IL-10 [11, 38].

1.2.3.3 Disease Associations

The M2b subset has been found to play a key role in the pathology in the murine model of lupus, and shifting macrophages to the M2a phenotype was shown to alleviate the disease [39]. M2b have also been found in circulation and peripheral tissues following severe burns, supporting a systemic activity for this subset [40, 41].

1.2.3.4 Interaction with Particulates

Silicosis and asbestosis have been associated with autoimmune comorbidities, including lupus, which involve TLR signaling and FcγR ligation [42, 43]. Though there are no reports on the M2b phenotype in particle exposure and associated disease, their involvement is likely.

1.2.4 M2c: Regulatory Macrophages

1.2.4.1 Environment/Generation

This subset is generated by the presence of classic anti-inflammatory mediators: TGFβ, IL-10, or glucocorticoids [44].

1.2.4.2 Function/Phenotype

The M2c are categorized as regulatory, but have anti-inflammatory or immunosuppressive activity. This subset is a good example of a macrophage being a product of its environment. Because the M2c is activated/generated by known immunosuppressive mediators, it follows that they possess the same qualities. They have been shown to produce TGFβ and IL-10 [45–47]. In addition, surface expression of CD163 is associated with this subset [48] (Table 1.1).

1.2.4.3 Disease Associations

The M2c, or "anti-inflammatory," subset has been shown to be induced by apoptotic cell uptake and promote epithelial and vascular repair [18, 49], as well as play a modulating role to the M1 activity in the *mdx* mouse model [19]. Both M2a and M2c subsets have been found to increase type VI collagen and fibrosis in an adipocyte model [35].

1.2.4.4 Interaction with Particulates

To date there have been no studies focused on the specific interaction between the M2c macrophage subset and particulates. Because the phenotype is considered to be regulatory in activity, the potential role these could play in disease is evident. Some groups have hypothesized (personal communications) that deletion of this subset would result in a loss of regulation, which may be a key event in developing particle-induced pathologies (i.e., nanomaterials, silica). In addition, the use of this subset as a type of cellular therapy could be beneficial in chronic inflammatory pathologies induced by particulates.

1.2.5 M2d: Tumor-Associated Macrophages

1.2.5.1 Environment/Generation

While the M1 subset is considered to be antitumor, the M2d are generated by the local environment and associated with tumor growth [50]. The factors involved in the generation of the M2d include IL-6, leukemia inhibitor factor (LIF), and M-CSF [51].

1.2.5.2 Function/Phenotype

The general definition of the M2d/TAM subset is that it promotes the growth of tumors [52]. It is thought that these cells possess an immunosuppressive phenotype [50, 51]. This activity has been found to be antagonized by the M1 macrophages [53].

1.2.5.3 Disease Associations

This subset is the rare type that is associated with the disease state that generates them.

1.2.5.4 Interaction with Particulates

While such particles as asbestos have been associated with cancer [54, 55], the link between particulates and TAM is not clear. Especially with such cancers as lung or gastrointestinal tumors, where exposures to environmental particulates are relatively consistent, the role of the M2d/TAM as a potential mediator in this process is ripe for investigation. In addition, current research in oncology treatments has started focusing on the use of nanomaterials [56–58]. The use of particulates to treat tumors could take advantage of the phagocytic capacity of macrophages in a targeted therapy.

1.2.6 M4 and Mhem/Mox: Atherosclerotic Associated

1.2.6.1 Environment/Generation

Macrophages and their contribution to atherosclerosis, as an inflammatory disease, have been an area of interest in cardiovascular research [59–61]. There are two to three types of macrophages that have recently been described in association with atherosclerosis: M4 and Mhem/Mox [62–64]. The M4 appear to be generated by activation with the chemokine CXCL4 [63]. The atheroprotective macrophages are generated by the presence of either heme (Mhem) or oxidized phospholipids (Mox) [62, 64].

1.2.6.2 Function/Phenotype

The roles and functions of these subsets are areas of active research. While the M4 appears to fall into a role of promoting atherosclerosis, it is the Mhem/Mox subset (s) that are described as having atheroprotection activities. The M4 is a classical-type macrophage that is pro-inflammatory and, therefore, promotes atherosclerotic pathology through this mechanism. The protective activity of the Mhem/Mox subset(s) involves the stabilization of plaques [64].

1.2.6.3 Disease Associations

As described in the above section regarding the generation of these subsets, they are associated with the environment that is responsible for their generation: atherosclerosis.

1.2.6.4 Interaction with Particulates

To date no studies have investigated, let alone linked, the activities of these subsets with particulate exposures and pathology. However, the association between particulate exposure and cardiovascular disease has been shown [65], as has the effect of air pollution particulates on macrophage functions [66, 67]. With the contradictory functions of these subsets in the pathology, and the known influence of particulates on the disease progression, it is a potential area of research to evaluate a possible connection.

1.3 Multinucleated Giant Cells

Cells with more than two nuclei within a common cytoplasm are described as multinucleated or polykaryotic. Multinucleated cells formed by cell fusion are called syncytia, while multinucleated cells formed by repeated mitoses without cytokinesis are called coenocytes. Multinucleated cells are formed by cell-cell fusion in select human tissues as part of normal physiological processes. These include the fusion of macrophages into osteoclasts, myoblasts into myotubes, cytotrophoblast cells into syncytiotrophoblast, and sperm with oocyte [68]. Additionally, recent discoveries suggest bone marrow stem cells fuse with several cell types as a mechanism of tissue regeneration [69, 70].

Multinucleated giant cells (MGC) are typically defined as macrophage syncytia associated with granulomas. MGC are distinct from osteoclasts, which are associated with bone and are present in normal, noninflammatory conditions. The concept that MGC are formed by macrophages fusing together is supported by fluorescent- and radio-labeling studies [71, 72]. This is in contrast to the mechanism of megakaryocyte formation. Megakaryocytes become polyploid by endomitosis, resulting in a single polylobulated nuclei with a histological appearance similar to MGC [73].

Usage of the phrase "giant cell" is occasionally generalized to include cells of non-monocytic origin that become multinucleated in certain pathological conditions (Box 1.1). These giant cells are less commonly observed than giant cells of monocytic origin and are not necessarily formed by cell fusion in association with granulomas. For the remainder of this chapter, the phrase "multinucleated giant cell" (MGC) will refer to macrophage syncytia associated with granulomas. These macrophage-derived MGC can be classified as Langhans giant cells, foreign-body giant cells, and Touton giant cells.

Box 1.1: Miscellaneous cells that become multinucleated in pathological conditions. These cells may not necessarily be of monocytic origin, associated with granulomas, or formed by fusion

Aschoff cells are formed by fusion of Anitschkow cells (occasionally called caterpillar cells), which are pathognomonic for rheumatic fever [155]. Anitschkow cells are likely to be of macrophage origin, but a potential myocyte origin has been a source of controversy [156, 157].

Balloon cells are pathognomonic for type IIb focal cortical dysplasia (also called Taylor dysplasia) and are found in subependymal giant cell astrocytomas, subependymal nodules, and cortical tubers [158]. These balloon cells (not to be confused with multinucleated melanocytes) have been suggested to be of either neuronal or glial origin [159].

Floret giant cells have been observed in various neoplasms including multinucleate cell angiohistiocytoma, pleomorphic lipoma, giant cell fibroblastoma, giant cell collagenoma [160], neurofibroma [161], pleomorphic fibroma [162], and dermatofibroma [163]. The name "floret" reflects the unique nuclear arrangement around the periphery of the cell, similar to petals on a flower. Although fibroblast or dendritic cell origins have been suggested [161], the etiology of floret giant cells is unknown.

Multinucleated epithelial giant cells are most often observed adjacent to the epithelial surface or lumen in pathological conditions of the epidermis, gastrointestinal tract, vulva, epididymis, and lungs [164–166].

Multinucleated erythroblasts are pathognomonic for congenital dyserythropoietic anemia III and may be formed by incomplete cytokinesis of proerythroblasts [167].

Multinucleated fibroblasts were recently discovered in vitro to form as either syncytia or coenocytes, depending on whether the culture contained cell lines or primary fibroblasts, respectively [168].

Multinucleated hepatocytes are found in neonatal giant cell hepatitis and autoimmune hepatitis [169, 170].

Multinucleated melanocytes found in nevi and melanomas are described as having a balloon appearance due to large vacuoles or a starburst appearance due to nuclear arrangement in lentigo maligna [171, 172].

Reed-Sternberg cells are pathognomonic for Hodgkin's lymphoma and are formed by multinucleation of the B cell-derived Hodgkin cell [173]. They become multinucleated by a unique mechanism: mitosis with incomplete cytokinesis followed by re-fusion of daughter cells [174].

Warthin-Finkeldey cells associated with measles, HIV, and Kimura lymphadenopathies are suggested to be derived from T cells [175] or dendritic cells [176].

1.3.1 Multinucleated Giant Cell (MGC) Morphology

Multinucleated giant cells are classified into three morphological variants. Langhans giant cells and foreign-body giant cells are the most common variants and are observed in a range of granulomatous conditions. Touton giant cells are less common because they are usually only observed lesions with high lipid content.

The eponym of the Langhans giant cell is Theodor Langhans, who was the first to describe their unique nuclear arrangement in 1868 [74, 75]. The nuclei of Langhans giant cells are arranged near the periphery of the cell in a circular pattern or in a semicircular pattern accumulating at one or two pole(s) of the cell (Fig. 1.2). Langhans giant cells usually contain less than 20 nuclei and have a spherical or slightly ovoid shape with a diameter of less than 50 μm. Langhans giant cells should not be confused with Langerhans cells and islets of Langerhans.

The nuclei of foreign-body giant cells are diffuse throughout the cytoplasm with no well-defined spatial pattern (Fig. 1.2). Foreign-body giant cells may have a spherical or irregular shape. The number of nuclei and cell size fluctuates greatly, with some cells containing over 100 nuclei and exceeding one mm in diameter.

The eponym of the Touton giant cell is Karl Touton, who originally called them "xanthelasmatic giant cells" in 1885 [74, 76]. The Touton giant cell size, number of nuclei, and arrangement of nuclei is similar to that of Langhans giant cells, except the nuclei in Touton giant cells are surrounded by a foamy cytoplasm. This suggests that these cells may be formed by fusion of foam cells, which are lipid-laden macrophages.

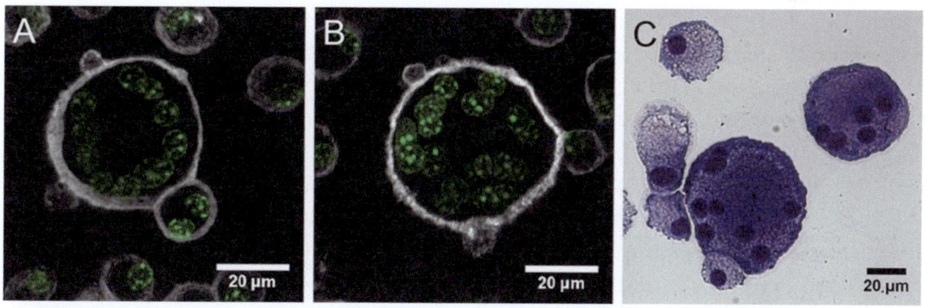

Fig. 1.2 MGC morphology. Two frequently observed morphological variants of MGC are the (**a**) Langhans giant cell and (**b**) foreign-body giant cell. (**c**) MGC with less distinct nuclear patterns can lead to subjectivity or uncertainty when classifications are based upon morphology alone. Not shown is the less common Touton giant cell. Methods: in all three images, MGC were generated in vitro by IL-4 treatment of C57Bl/6 mouse bone marrow-derived macrophages. (**a**, **b**) Fluorescent images were captured using an Olympus FluoView FV1000 IX81 confocal microscope with HCS NuclearMask (*green*) and CellMask Plasma Membrane (*grayscale*) stains (Life Technologies, Gaithersburg, MD). (**c**) Brightfield images were captured using a Zeiss Axioskop with a stain comparable to Wright-Giemsa (Protocol Hema 3, Thermo Fisher Scientific, Waltham, MA). Credit: Kevin Trout – University of Montana, Missoula, MT, USA

The morphology-based classification of these variants can lead to uncertainty in their identification, especially when MGC have relatively few nuclei or unclear patterns of nuclear arrangement. This gray area is augmented because MGC are usually observed at only one timepoint during the continuum of the multinucleation process. For example, it is possible that Langhans giant cells are precursors to foreign-body giant cells or vice versa.

1.3.2 Environment/Generation

One of the environments in which MGC are generated is in granulomas surrounding implanted medical devices or biomaterials. This particular environment provides a useful model system to characterize the dynamics of MGC formation. MGC begin to form within the first three days following biomaterial implantation in rodents, reach a peak population at 2–4 weeks, and slowly decrease in population until reaching a steady state [77, 78]. The relatively short lifespan of an individual MGC is estimated to be approximately one week; at this point the MGC is thought to undergo apoptosis [79]. The MGC population at the implant site is maintained by continuous recruitment and differentiation of monocytes from the circulation until the foreign body has been degraded or removed [80]. These MGC populations have been observed to persist beyond 15 years post-implantation [81].

Well-known stimulators of macrophage fusion into MGC include IL-4 [82], IL-13 [83], and IFNγ [84]. In some in vitro models, MGC formation is increased when these fusion stimulators are combined with macrophage maturation factors: GM-CSF, M-CSF, or IL-3. The macrophage maturation factors alone do not induce fusion [85, 86]. Stimulation with IL-4 or IL-13 in vitro results predominantly in foreign-body giant cell formation, while stimulation with IFNγ results predominantly in Langhans giant cell formation [87]. Other factors suggested to stimulate MGC formation include α-tocopherol (a form of vitamin E) [88], calcitriol (1,25-dihydroxyvitamin D3) [89], phorbol 12-myristate 13-acetate [90], and T-cell mitogenic plant lectins concanavalin A and phytohemagglutinin [91].

Progress in MGC research within the previous two decades has begun to elucidate the mechanism of macrophage fusion. An overview of this mechanism is provided here. For a more comprehensive description of proteins and signaling pathways implicated in MGC formation, excellent summaries have been published as book chapters [81, 92, 93] and reviews [94, 95]. The mechanism of macrophage fusion into MGC can be divided into three major steps [96]:

1. *Competence.* Fusion-stimulating factors such as IL-4 increase macrophage fusogenicity or "fusion-competency." Programming into a fusion-competent state usually involves endogenous or exogenous signals that increase transcription of key proteins such as MMP9 [97], E-cadherin [98], dendritic cell-specific transmembrane protein (DC-STAMP), and osteoclast stimulatory transmembrane protein (OC-STAMP) [99].

2. *Commitment*. The fusion-competent macrophage must migrate into proximity with a fusion partner. A chemokine that induces this migration during MGC formation is chemokine (C-C motif) ligand 2 (CCL2), also called monocyte chemoattractant protein 1 (MCP-1) [100]. Cell-cell and cell-substrate adhesion are part of macrophage commitment to fusion. For example, engagement of β1 and β2 integrins regulates MGC formation [101].
3. *Fusion*. Finally, the membranes merge and the cell undergoes a series of cytoskeletal rearrangements. As an example of a membrane merging event, ATP activation of purinergic receptor P2X7 results in exposure of phosphatidylserine in the plasma membrane [102], which is recognized by class B scavenger receptor CD36 in the fusion partner [103]. Cytoskeletal rearrangements are important during migration as well as post-fusion. A known factor involved in actin polymerization and reorganization during MGC formation is Rac1 [100].

1.3.3 Function/Phenotype

Due to their macrophage origin, it is suspected that MGC share some of the same functions as macrophages. Also, similarly to macrophages, it is likely that MGC possess heterogeneous phenotypes based upon tissue location, pathological association, and stimulating factors (e.g., IL-4 versus IFNγ). Another factor that may affect MGC phenotype is the cell maturation stage. This alteration of activity is evident in MGC capacity for phagocytosis. An MGC is capable of internalizing approximately the same number of particles as a mononuclear macrophage [104, 105], but phagocytosis decreases as the number of MGC nuclei increases [77, 106].

MGC can phagocytose larger particles than macrophages [98]. When a foreign body is too large to be engulfed, MGC attempt to degrade them extracellularly. MGC form adhesive structures called podosomes that are localized to the ventral cell periphery, forming a compartment between the MGC and foreign body [107]. A degradative microenvironment is formed within this sealed compartment, likely as a result of lysosomal exocytosis. This microenvironment contains degradative enzymes, an acidic pH, and reactive oxygen species generated predominantly by NADPH oxidase [95]. In the context of medical implants, MGC can degrade biomaterials through a mechanism similar to osteoclast degradation of bone [108]. Specific enzymes released by MGC that have been implicated in foreign body degradation include MMP9 [97, 109] and cathepsin K [110]. It has been hypothesized that this MGC degradative activity may eventually be down modulated [81]. If this is the case, it is possible that MGC may reach an inactive phase, during which their primary function is to protect the host by sequestering the foreign material or pathogen.

1.3.4 Disease Associations

MGC are most commonly associated with granulomas of diverse etiology (Table 1.2). Multinucleated cells have also been described in giant cell tumor of bone and soft tissues; however, these cells exhibit features more characteristic of osteoclasts [111, 112].

1.3.5 Interaction with Particulates

The most well-known lung conditions associated with MGC include tuberculosis infection [106] and sarcoidosis [71]. There is a growing body of studies that describe MGC formation in response to particle inhalation. MGC are frequently

Table 1.2 Granulomatous conditions in which macrophage-derived multinucleated giant cells are found. This list of example conditions is not exhaustive

Classification	Disease or pathogenic material
Autoimmune/ idiopathic	Annular elastolytic giant cell granuloma or granuloma annulare [129]
	Crohn's disease and ulcerative colitis [130]
	Langerhans cell histiocytosis [131]
	Rheumatoid disease [132]
	Sarcoidosis [71]
	Vasculitides such as giant cell arteritis [133]
Endogenous materials	Keratin [134]
	Lipids [74] and cholesterol crystals [135]
	Monosodium urate crystals [136]
Exogenous materials	Engineered nanomaterials such as silver nanowires [118] and carbon nanotubes [119]
	Medical implants [137]
	Metals such as Al [138], Be [122], Zr [139], and Co/WC alloys [140]
	Minerals such as asbestos [141], silica [141], and talc [142]
	Plant materials [143] such as cactus spines, corn starch used with medical gloves, and wood splinters
Infection – bacteria	Brucellosis [144]
	Cat-scratch disease [145]
	Mycobacteria infection such as leprosy [146] and tuberculosis [106]
	Syphilis [147]
Infection – fungus	African histoplasmosis [148]
	Aspergillosis [149]
	Cryptococcosis [150]
Infection – parasite	Filariasis such as dirofilariasis [151] and onchocerciasis [152]
	Leishmaniasis [153]
	Schistosomiasis [154]

observed in response to inhalation of antigens that cause hypersensitivity pneumonitis [113, 114] and inhalation of other organic materials such as mycobacteria and fungi (Table 1.2). Inhalation of inorganic particles is also known to induce MGC formation. MGC have been observed in the lungs of rodents after exposure to silica [115, 116], asbestos [115, 117], sepiolite nanoclay [116], silver nanowires [118], or multiwalled carbon nanotubes [119]. Giant cell interstitial pneumonitis is a pathological pattern of hard metal lung disease that is characterized by the presence of MGC [120, 121]. This interstitial lung disease is usually observed as a result of occupational exposure tungsten carbide and cobalt alloys. Inhalation of other metals has also been reported to induce formation of MGC, such as beryllium [122].

1.4 Conclusion

The nature of the macrophage as a first-line agent of immunity is to phagocytose foreign material and generate/regulate the subsequent immune response. As this chapter has outlined, there are multiple types of "macrophages" that vary according to morphology and function. While some subsets have already been directly implicated in particulate/foreign-body-induced pathologies, involvement of other subsets may be revealed by further investigation. For example, etiology could be explained if either type of atherosclerotic macrophage (M4, Mhem/Mox) is affected by particulates (i.e., decreased atheroprotective activity or increased atherosclerotic-promoting activity). Although multinucleated giant cell association with granulomas has been known for many years, determining whether or not they significantly contribute to formation of the granuloma requires an increased understanding of their biology. Overall, the implications of various functional subsets illustrate the key role that macrophages play in particulate/foreign-body exposures and their potential in therapeutic development. If a subset is known to have a role in pathology, then it can be targeted or antagonized to treat the disease/pathology.

References

1. van Furth R, Blusse van Oud Alblas A. The current view on the origin of pulmonary macrophages. Pathol Res Pract. 1982;175(1):38–49.
2. Thomas ED, Ramberg RE, Sale GE, Sparkes RS, Golde DW. Direct evidence for a bone marrow origin of the alveolar macrophage in man. Science. 1976;192(4243):1016–18.
3. Byersdorfer CA, Chaplin DD. Visualization of early APC/T cell interactions in the mouse lung following intranasal challenge. J Immunol. 2001;167(12):6756–64.
4. Migliaccio CT, Hamilton Jr RF, Holian A. Increase in a distinct pulmonary macrophage subset possessing an antigen-presenting cell phenotype and *in vitro* APC activity following silica exposure. Toxicol Appl Pharmacol. 2005;205(2):168–76.
5. Toews GB, Vial WC, Dunn MM, Guzzetta P, Nunez G, Stastny P, et al. The accessory cell function of human alveolar macrophages in specific T cell proliferation. J Immunol. 1984;132 (1):181–6.

6. Brodsky FM, Guagliardi LE. The cell biology of antigen processing and presentation. Annu Rev Immunol. 1991;9:707–44. doi:10.1146/annurev.iy.09.040191.003423.
7. Jabbour AJ, Holian A, Scheule RK. Lung lining fluid modification of asbestos bioactivity for the alveolar macrophage. Toxicol Appl Pharmacol. 1991;110(2):283–94.
8. Strieter RM, Remick DG, Lynch 3rd JP, Genord M, Raiford C, Spengler R, et al. Differential regulation of tumor necrosis factor-alpha in human alveolar macrophages and peripheral blood monocytes: a cellular and molecular analysis. Am J Respir Cell Mol Biol. 1989;1 (1):57–63. doi:10.1165/ajrcmb/1.1.57.
9. Gordon S. The macrophage. Bioessays. 1995;17(11):977–86.
10. Gordon S. Alternative activation of macrophages. Nat Rev Immunol. 2003;3(1):23–35.
11. Mosser DM, Edwards JP. Exploring the full spectrum of macrophage activation. Nat Rev Immunol. 2008;8(12):958–69. doi:10.1038/nri2448.
12. Martinez FO, Gordon S. The M1 and M2 paradigm of macrophage activation: time for reassessment. F1000prime reports. 2014;6:13. doi:10.12703/P6-13.
13. Murray PJ, Allen JE, Biswas SK, Fisher EA, Gilroy DW, Goerdt S, et al. Macrophage activation and polarization: nomenclature and experimental guidelines. Immunity. 2014;41 (1):14–20. doi:10.1016/j.immuni.2014.06.008.
14. Verreck FA, de Boer T, Langenberg DM, Hoeve MA, Kramer M, Vaisberg E, et al. Human IL-23-producing type 1 macrophages promote but IL-10-producing type 2 macrophages subvert immunity to (myco)bacteria. Proc Natl Acad Sci U S A. 2004;101(13):4560–5. doi:10.1073/pnas.0400983101.
15. Shaykhiev R, Krause A, Salit J, Strulovici-Barel Y, Harvey BG, O'Connor TP, et al. Smoking-dependent reprogramming of alveolar macrophage polarization: implication for pathogenesis of chronic obstructive pulmonary disease. J Immunol. 2009;183 (4):2867–83. doi:10.4049/jimmunol.0900473.
16. MacMicking J, Xie QW, Nathan C. Nitric oxide and macrophage function. Annu Rev Immunol. 1997;15:323–50. doi:10.1146/annurev.immunol.15.1.323.
17. MacMicking JD, North RJ, LaCourse R, Mudgett JS, Shah SK, Nathan CF. Identification of nitric oxide synthase as a protective locus against tuberculosis. Proc Natl Acad Sci U S A. 1997;94(10):5243–8.
18. Anders HJ, Ryu M. Renal microenvironments and macrophage phenotypes determine progression or resolution of renal inflammation and fibrosis. Kidney Int. 2011;80(9):915–25. doi:10.1038/ki.2011.217.
19. Villalta SA, Rinaldi C, Deng B, Liu G, Fedor B, Tidball JG. Interleukin-10 reduces the pathology of mdx muscular dystrophy by deactivating M1 macrophages and modulating macrophage phenotype. Hum Mol Genet. 2011;20(4):790–805. doi:10.1093/hmg/ddq523.
20. Kaczmarek M, Nowicka A, Kozlowska M, Zurawski J, Batura-Gabryel H, Sikora J. Evaluation of the phenotype pattern of macrophages isolated from malignant and non-malignant pleural effusions. Tumour Biol. 2011;32(6):1123–32. doi:10.1007/s13277-011-0214-1.
21. Sharda DR, Yu S, Ray M, Squadrito ML, De Palma M, Wynn TA, et al. Regulation of macrophage arginase expression and tumor growth by the Ron receptor tyrosine kinase. J Immunol. 2011;187(5):2181–92. doi:10.4049/jimmunol.1003460.
22. Cassol E, Cassetta L, Alfano M, Poli G. Macrophage polarization and HIV-1 infection. J Leukoc Biol. 2010;87(4):599–608. doi:10.1189/jlb.1009673.
23. Guo Z, Wen Z, Qin A, Zhou Y, Liao Z, Liu Z, et al. Antisense oligonucleotide treatment enhances the recovery of acute lung injury through IL-10-secreting M2-like macrophage-induced expansion of CD4+ regulatory T cells. J Immunol. 2013;190(8):4337–48. doi:10.4049/jimmunol.1203233.
24. Dinarello CA. A clinical perspective of IL-1beta as the gatekeeper of inflammation. Eur J Immunol. 2011;41(5):1203–17. doi:10.1002/eji.201141550.
25. Ingham E, Fisher J. The role of macrophages in osteolysis of total joint replacement. Biomaterials. 2005;26(11):1271–86. doi:10.1016/j.biomaterials.2004.04.035.

26. Goodman SB, Gibon E, Pajarinen J, Lin TH, Keeney M, Ren PG, et al. Novel biological strategies for treatment of wear particle-induced periprosthetic osteolysis of orthopaedic implants for joint replacement. J R Soc Interface. 2014;11(93):20130962. doi:10.1098/rsif.2013.0962.
27. Nich C, Takakubo Y, Pajarinen J, Ainola M, Salem A, Sillat T, et al. Macrophages-key cells in the response to wear debris from joint replacements. J Biomed Mater Res A. 2013;101(10):3033–45. doi:10.1002/jbm.a.34599.
28. Antonios JK, Yao Z, Li C, Rao AJ, Goodman SB. Macrophage polarization in response to wear particles *in vitro*. Cell Mol Immunol. 2013;10(6):471–82. doi:10.1038/cmi.2013.39.
29. Webb DC, McKenzie AN, Foster PS. Expression of the Ym2 lectin-binding protein is dependent on interleukin (IL)-4 and IL-13 signal transduction: identification of a novel allergy-associated protein. J Biol Chem. 2001;276(45):41969–76.
30. Ferrante CJ, Pinhal-Enfield G, Elson G, Cronstein BN, Hasko G, Outram S, et al. The adenosine-dependent angiogenic switch of macrophages to an M2-like phenotype is independent of interleukin-4 receptor alpha (IL-4Ralpha) signaling. Inflammation. 2013;36(4):921–31. doi:10.1007/s10753-013-9621-3.
31. Migliaccio CT, Buford MC, Jessop F, Holian A. The IL-4Ralpha pathway in macrophages and its potential role in silica-induced pulmonary fibrosis. J Leukoc Biol. 2008;83(3):630–9. doi:jlb.0807533 [pii] 10.1189/jlb.0807533
32. Arora M, Chen L, Paglia M, Gallagher I, Allen JE, Vyas YM, et al. Simvastatin promotes Th2-type responses through the induction of the chitinase family member Ym1 in dendritic cells. Proc Natl Acad Sci U S A. 2006;103(20):7777–82.
33. Goerdt S, Politz O, Schledzewski K, Birk R, Gratchev A, Guillot P, et al. Alternative versus classical activation of macrophages. Pathobiology. 1999;67(5–6):222–6.
34. Mosser DM. The many faces of macrophage activation. J Leukoc Biol. 2003;73(2):209–12.
35. Spencer M, Yao-Borengasser A, Unal R, Rasouli N, Gurley CM, Zhu B, et al. Adipose tissue macrophages in insulin-resistant subjects are associated with collagen VI and fibrosis and demonstrate alternative activation. Am J Physiol Endocrinol Metab. 2010;299(6):E1016–27. doi:10.1152/ajpendo.00329.2010.
36. Martinez FO, Sica A, Mantovani A, Locati M. Macrophage activation and polarization. Front Biosci. 2008;13:453–61.
37. Luo C, Chen M, Madden A, Xu H. Expression of complement components and regulators by different subtypes of bone marrow-derived macrophages. Inflammation. 2012;35(4):1448–61. doi:10.1007/s10753-012-9458-1.
38. Edwards JP, Zhang X, Frauwirth KA, Mosser DM. Biochemical and functional characterization of three activated macrophage populations. J Leukoc Biol. 2006;80(6):1298–307.
39. Zhang W, Xu W, Xiong S. Macrophage differentiation and polarization via phosphatidylinositol 3-kinase/Akt-ERK signaling pathway conferred by serum amyloid P component. J Immunol. 2011;187(4):1764–77. doi:10.4049/jimmunol.1002315.
40. Asai A, Nakamura K, Kobayashi M, Herndon DN, Suzuki F. CCL1 released from M2b macrophages is essentially required for the maintenance of their properties. J Leukoc Biol. 2012;92(4):859–67. doi:10.1189/jlb.0212107.
41. Kobayashi T, Onodera S, Kondo E, Tohyama H, Fujiki H, Yokoyama A, et al. Impaired fracture healing in macrophage migration inhibitory factor-deficient mice. Osteoporos Int. 2011;22(6):1955–65. doi:10.1007/s00198-010-1385-0.
42. Pradhan V, Patwardhan M, Ghosh K. Fc gamma receptor polymorphisms in systemic lupus erythematosus and their correlation with the clinical severity of the disease. Indian J Hum Genet. 2008;14(3):77–81. doi:10.4103/0971-6866.44998.
43. Urbonaviciute V, Furnrohr BG, Meister S, Munoz L, Heyder P, De Marchis F, et al. Induction of inflammatory and immune responses by HMGB1-nucleosome complexes: implications for the pathogenesis of SLE. J Exp Med. 2008;205(13):3007–18. doi:10.1084/jem.20081165.

44. Lugo-Villarino G, Verollet C, Maridonneau-Parini I, Neyrolles O. Macrophage polarization: convergence point targeted by mycobacterium tuberculosis and HIV. Front Immunol. 2011;2:43. doi:10.3389/fimmu.2011.00043.
45. Li MO, Wan YY, Sanjabi S, Robertson AK, Flavell RA. Transforming growth factor-beta regulation of immune responses. Annu Rev Immunol. 2006;24:99–146. doi:10.1146/annurev.immunol.24.021605.090737.
46. Couper KN, Blount DG, Riley EM. IL-10: the master regulator of immunity to infection. J Immunol. 2008;180(9):5771–7.
47. Couper KN, Blount DG, Wilson MS, Hafalla JC, Belkaid Y, Kamanaka M, et al. IL-10 from CD4CD25Foxp3CD127 adaptive regulatory T cells modulates parasite clearance and pathology during malaria infection. PLoS Pathog. 2008;4(2):e1000004. doi:10.1371/journal.ppat.1000004.
48. Zizzo G, Hilliard BA, Monestier M, Cohen PL. Efficient clearance of early apoptotic cells by human macrophages requires M2c polarization and MerTK induction. J Immunol. 2012;189(7):3508–20. doi:10.4049/jimmunol.1200662.
49. Mantovani A, Sica A, Sozzani S, Allavena P, Vecchi A, Locati M. The chemokine system in diverse forms of macrophage activation and polarization. Trends Immunol. 2004;25(12):677–86.
50. Jeannin P, Duluc D, Delneste Y. IL-6 and leukemia-inhibitory factor are involved in the generation of tumor-associated macrophage: regulation by IFN-gamma. Immunotherapy. 2011;3(4 Suppl):23–6. doi:10.2217/imt.11.30.
51. Duluc D, Delneste Y, Tan F, Moles MP, Grimaud L, Lenoir J, et al. Tumor-associated leukemia inhibitory factor and IL-6 skew monocyte differentiation into tumor-associated macrophage-like cells. Blood. 2007;110(13):4319–30. doi:10.1182/blood-2007-02-072587.
52. Santoni M, Massari F, Amantini C, Nabissi M, Maines F, Burattini L, et al. Emerging role of tumor-associated macrophages as therapeutic targets in patients with metastatic renal cell carcinoma. Cancer Immunol Immunother. 2013;62(12):1757–68. doi:10.1007/s00262-013-1487-6.
53. Duluc D, Corvaisier M, Blanchard S, Catala L, Descamps P, Gamelin E, et al. Interferon-gamma reverses the immunosuppressive and protumoral properties and prevents the generation of human tumor-associated macrophages. Int J Cancer. 2009;125(2):367–73. doi:10.1002/ijc.24401.
54. Birnie KA, Yip YY, Ng DC, Kirschner MB, Reid G, Prele CM et al. Loss of mir-223 and JNK signalling contribute to elevated stathmin in malignant pleural mesothelioma. Mol Cancer Res. 2015;13(7):1106–18. doi:10.1158/1541-7786.MCR-14-0442.
55. Nagai H, Toyokuni S. Biopersistent fiber-induced inflammation and carcinogenesis: lessons learned from asbestos toward safety of fibrous nanomaterials. Arch Biochem Biophys. 2010;502(1):1–7. doi:10.1016/j.abb.2010.06.015.
56. Christie C, Madsen SJ, Peng Q, Hirschberg H. Macrophages as nanoparticle delivery vectors for photothermal therapy of brain tumors. Ther Deliv. 2015;6(3):371–84. doi:10.4155/tde.14.121.
57. Jiang Y, Fei W, Cen X, Tang Y, Liang X. Near-infrared light activatable multimodal gold nanostructures platform: an emerging paradigm for cancer therapy. Current Cancer Drug Targets. 2015;15(5):406–22. doi: 10.2174/1568009615666150407125333.
58. Wang HY, Hua XW, Wu FG, Li B, Liu P, Gu N, et al. Synthesis of ultrastable copper sulfide nanoclusters via trapping the reaction intermediate: potential anticancer and antibacterial applications. ACS Appl Mater Interfaces. 2015;7(13):7082–92. doi:10.1021/acsami.5b01214.
59. Ley K, Miller YI, Hedrick CC. Monocyte and macrophage dynamics during atherogenesis. Arterioscler Thromb Vasc Biol. 2011;31(7):1506–16. doi:10.1161/ATVBAHA.110.221127.
60. Buttari B, Profumo E, Rigano R. Crosstalk between red blood cells and the immune system and its impact on atherosclerosis. BioMed Res Int. 2015;2015:616834. doi:10.1155/2015/616834.

61. Bekkering S, Joosten LA, van der Meer JW, Netea MG, Riksen NP. The epigenetic memory of monocytes and macrophages as a novel drug target in atherosclerosis. Clin Ther. 2015;37 (4):914–23. doi:10.1016/j.clinthera.2015.01.008.
62. Boyle JJ, Johns M, Kampfer T, Nguyen AT, Game L, Schaer DJ, et al. Activating transcription factor 1 directs Mhem atheroprotective macrophages through coordinated iron handling and foam cell protection. Circ Res. 2012;110(1):20–33. doi:10.1161/CIRCRESAHA.111. 247577.
63. Gleissner CA. Macrophage phenotype modulation by CXCL4 in atherosclerosis. Front Physiol. 2012;3:1. doi:10.3389/fphys.2012.00001.
64. Colin S, Chinetti-Gbaguidi G, Staels B. Macrophage phenotypes in atherosclerosis. Immunol Rev. 2014;262(1):153–66. doi:10.1111/imr.12218.
65. Ying Z, Kampfrath T, Thurston G, Farrar B, Lippmann M, Wang A, et al. Ambient particulates alter vascular function through induction of reactive oxygen and nitrogen species. Toxicol Sci. 2009;111(1):80–8. doi:10.1093/toxsci/kfp004.
66. Brook RD, Rajagopalan S, Pope 3rd CA, Brook JR, Bhatnagar A, Diez-Roux AV, et al. Particulate matter air pollution and cardiovascular disease: an update to the scientific statement from the American Heart Association. Circulation. 2010;121(21):2331–78. doi:10. 1161/CIR.0b013e3181dbece1.
67. Rylance J, Fullerton DG, Scriven J, Aljurayyan AN, Mzinza D, Barrett S, et al. Household Air pollution causes dose-dependent inflammation and altered phagocytosis in human macrophages. Am J Respir Cell Mol Biol. 2015;52(5):584–93. doi:10.1165/rcmb.2014-0188OC.
68. Dittmar T, Zanker KS. Cell fusion in health and disease. Volume II: cell fusion in disease. Introduction. Adv Exp Med Biol. 2011;714:1–3. doi:10.1007/978-94-007-0782-5_1.
69. Alvarez-Dolado M, Pardal R, Garcia-Verdugo JM, Fike JR, Lee HO, Pfeffer K, et al. Fusion of bone-marrow-derived cells with Purkinje neurons, cardiomyocytes and hepatocytes. Nature. 2003;425(6961):968–73. doi:10.1038/nature02069.
70. Lluis F, Cosma MP. Cell-fusion-mediated somatic-cell reprogramming: a mechanism for tissue regeneration. J Cell Physiol. 2010;223(1):6–13. doi:10.1002/jcp.22003.
71. van Maarsseveen TC, Vos W, van Diest PJ. Giant cell formation in sarcoidosis: cell fusion or proliferation with non-division? Clin Exp Immunol. 2009;155(3):476–86. doi:10.1111/j. 1365-2249.2008.03841.x.
72. Helming L, Gordon S. Macrophage fusion induced by IL-4 alternative activation is a multistage process involving multiple target molecules. Eur J Immunol. 2007;37(1):33–42. doi:10.1002/eji.200636788.
73. Machlus KR, Italiano Jr JE. The incredible journey: from megakaryocyte development to platelet formation. J Cell Biol. 2013;201(6):785–96. doi:10.1083/jcb.201304054.
74. Aterman K, Remmele W, Smith M. Touton and his "xanthelasmatic giant cell." A selective review of multinucleated giant cells. Am J Dermatopathol. 1988;10(3):257–69.
75. Langhans T. Ueber Riesenzellen mit wandständigen Kernen in Tuberkeln und die fibröse Form des Tuberkels. Archiv für Pathologische Anatomie und Physiologie und für Klinische Medicin. 1868;42(3):382–404. doi:10.1007/bf02006420.
76. Touton K. Ueber das Xanthom, insbesondere dessen Histiologie und Histiogenese. Vierteljahresschrift für Dermatologie und Syphilis. 1885;17(1–4):3–53. doi:10.1007/ bf02199761.
77. Papadimitriou JM, Sforsina D, Papaelias L. Kinetics of multinucleate giant cell formation and their modification by various agents in foreign body reactions. Am J Pathol. 1973;73 (2):349–64.
78. Zhao OH, Anderson JM, Hiltner A, Lodoen GA, Payet CR. Theoretical analysis on cell size distribution and kinetics of foreign-body giant cell formation *in vivo* on polyurethane elastomers. J Biomed Mater Res. 1992;26(8):1019–38. doi:10.1002/jbm.820260805.
79. Honma T, Hamasaki T. Ultrastructure of multinucleated giant cell apoptosis in foreign-body granuloma. Virchows Arch. 1996;428(3):165–76.
80. Anderson JM. Multinucleated giant cells. Curr Opin Hematol. 2000;7(1):40–7.

81. McNally AK, Anderson JM. Macrophage fusion and multinucleated giant cells of inflammation. In: Dittmar T, Zanker KS, editors. Cell fusion in health and disease – I: cell fusion in health. Dordrecht: Springer; 2011. p. 97–111.
82. McInnes A, Rennick DM. Interleukin 4 induces cultured monocytes/macrophages to form giant multinucleated cells. J Exp Med. 1988;167(2):598–611.
83. DeFife KM, Jenney CR, McNally AK, Colton E, Anderson JM. Interleukin-13 induces human monocyte/macrophage fusion and macrophage mannose receptor expression. J Immunol. 1997;158(7):3385–90.
84. Weinberg JB, Hobbs MM, Misukonis MA. Recombinant human gamma-interferon induces human monocyte polykaryon formation. Proc Natl Acad Sci U S A. 1984;81(14):4554–7.
85. McNally AK, Anderson JM. Interleukin-4 induces foreign body giant cells from human monocytes/macrophages. Differential lymphokine regulation of macrophage fusion leads to morphological variants of multinucleated giant cells. Am J Pathol. 1995;147(5):1487–99.
86. Kondo Y, Yasui K, Yashiro M, Tsuge M, Kotani N, Morishima T. Multi-nucleated giant cell formation from human cord blood monocytes *in vitro*, in comparison with adult peripheral blood monocytes. Clin Exp Immunol. 2009;158(1):84–90. doi:10.1111/j.1365-2249.2009.03990.x.
87. Sakai H, Okafuji I, Nishikomori R, Abe J, Izawa K, Kambe N, et al. The CD40-CD40L axis and IFN-gamma play critical roles in Langhans giant cell formation. Int Immunol. 2012;24(1):5–15. doi:10.1093/intimm/dxr088.
88. McNally AK, Anderson JM. Foreign body-type multinucleated giant cell formation is potently induced by alpha-tocopherol and prevented by the diacylglycerol kinase inhibitor R59022. Am J Pathol. 2003;163(3):1147–56.
89. Abe E, Miyaura C, Tanaka H, Shiina Y, Kuribayashi T, Suda S, et al. 1 alpha,25-dihydroxyvitamin D3 promotes fusion of mouse alveolar macrophages both by a direct mechanism and by a spleen cell-mediated indirect mechanism. Proc Natl Acad Sci U S A. 1983;80(18):5583–7.
90. Hassan NF, Kamani N, Meszaros MM, Douglas SD. Induction of multinucleated giant cell formation from human blood-derived monocytes by phorbol myristate acetate in *in vitro* culture. J Immunol. 1989;143(7):2179–84.
91. Takashima T, Ohnishi K, Tsuyuguchi I, Kishimoto S. Differential regulation of formation of multinucleated giant cells from concanavalin A-stimulated human blood monocytes by IFN-gamma and IL-4. J Immunol. 1993;150(7):3002–10.
92. Miyamoto T, Suda T. Molecules regulating macrophage fusions. In: Larsson LI, editor. Cell fusions: regulation and control. Dordrecht: Springer; 2011. p. 233–48. doi:10.1007/978-90-481-9772-9_11.
93. Vignery A. Macrophage fusion: the making of a new cell. In: Larsson LI, editor. Cell fusions: regulation and control. Dordrecht: Springer; 2011. p. 219–31. doi:10.1007/978-90-481-9772-9_10.
94. Helming L, Gordon S. Molecular mediators of macrophage fusion. Trends Cell Biol. 2009;19(10):514–22. doi:10.1016/j.tcb.2009.07.005.
95. Quinn MT, Schepetkin IA. Role of NADPH oxidase in formation and function of multinucleated giant cells. J Innate Immun. 2009;1(6):509–26. doi:10.1159/000228158.
96. Aguilar PS, Baylies MK, Fleissner A, Helming L, Inoue N, Podbilewicz B, et al. Genetic basis of cell-cell fusion mechanisms. Trends Genet TIG. 2013;29(7):427–37. doi:10.1016/j.tig.2013.01.011.
97. MacLauchlan S, Skokos EA, Meznarich N, Zhu DH, Raoof S, Shipley JM, et al. Macrophage fusion, giant cell formation, and the foreign body response require matrix metalloproteinase 9. J Leukoc Biol. 2009;85(4):617–26. doi:10.1189/jlb.1008588.
98. Moreno JL, Mikhailenko I, Tondravi MM, Keegan AD. IL-4 promotes the formation of multinucleated giant cells from macrophage precursors by a STAT6-dependent, homotypic mechanism: contribution of E-cadherin. J Leukoc Biol. 2007;82(6):1542–53. doi:10.1189/jlb.0107058.

99. Miyamoto T. STATs and macrophage fusion. Jakstat. 2013;2(3):e24777. doi:10.4161/jkst.24777.
100. Jay SM, Skokos E, Laiwalla F, Krady MM, Kyriakides TR. Foreign body giant cell formation is preceded by lamellipodia formation and can be attenuated by inhibition of Rac1 activation. Am J Pathol. 2007;171(2):632–40. doi:10.2353/ajpath.2007.061213.
101. McNally AK, Macewan SR, Anderson JM. Alpha subunit partners to beta1 and beta2 integrins during IL-4-induced foreign body giant cell formation. J Biomed Mater Res A. 2007;82(3):568–74. doi:10.1002/jbm.a.31161.
102. Lemaire I, Falzoni S, Adinolfi E. Purinergic signaling in giant cell formation. Front Biosci (Elite Ed). 2012;4:41–55.
103. Helming L, Winter J, Gordon S. The scavenger receptor CD36 plays a role in cytokine-induced macrophage fusion. J Cell Sci. 2009;122(Pt 4):453–9. doi:10.1242/jcs.037200.
104. Enelow RI, Sullivan GW, Carper HT, Mandell GL. Cytokine-induced human multinucleated giant cells have enhanced candidacidal activity and oxidative capacity compared with macrophages. J Infect Dis. 1992;166(3):664–8.
105. Schlesinger L, Musson RA, Johnston Jr RB. Functional and biochemical studies of multinucleated giant cells derived from the culture of human monocytes. J Exp Med. 1984;159(4):1289–94.
106. Lay G, Poquet Y, Salek-Peyron P, Puissegur MP, Botanch C, Bon H, et al. Langhans giant cells from M tuberculosis-induced human granulomas cannot mediate mycobacterial uptake. J Pathol. 2007;211(1):76–85. doi:10.1002/path.2092.
107. DeFife KM, Jenney CR, Colton E, Anderson JM. Cytoskeletal and adhesive structural polarizations accompany IL-13-induced human macrophage fusion. J Histochem Cytochem. 1999;47(1):65–74.
108. Zhao Q, Topham N, Anderson JM, Hiltner A, Lodoen G, Payet CR. Foreign-body giant cells and polyurethane biostability: *in vivo* correlation of cell adhesion and surface cracking. J Biomed Mater Res. 1991;25(2):177–83. doi:10.1002/jbm.820250205.
109. Zhu XW, Price NM, Gilman RH, Recarvarren S, Friedland JS. Multinucleate giant cells release functionally unopposed matrix metalloproteinase-9 *in vitro* and *in vivo*. J Infect Dis. 2007;196(7):1076–9. doi:10.1086/521030.
110. Park JK, Rosen A, Saffitz JE, Asimaki A, Litovsky SH, Mackey-Bojack SM, et al. Expression of cathepsin K and tartrate-resistant acid phosphatase is not confined to osteoclasts but is a general feature of multinucleated giant cells: systematic analysis. Rheumatology. 2013;52(8):1529–33. doi:10.1093/rheumatology/ket184.
111. Cowan RW, Singh G. Giant cell tumor of bone: a basic science perspective. Bone. 2013;52(1):238–46. doi:10.1016/j.bone.2012.10.002.
112. Lau YS, Sabokbar A, Gibbons CL, Giele H, Athanasou N. Phenotypic and molecular studies of giant-cell tumors of bone and soft tissue. Hum Pathol. 2005;36(9):945–54. doi:10.1016/j.humpath.2005.07.005.
113. Castonguay MC, Ryu JH, Yi ES, Tazelaar HD. Granulomas and giant cells in hypersensitivity pneumonitis. Hum Pathol. 2015;46(4):607–13. doi:10.1016/j.humpath.2014.12.017.
114. Kawanami O, Basset F, Barrios R, Lacronique JG, Ferrans VJ, Crystal RG. Hypersensitivity pneumonitis in man. Light- and electron-microscopic studies of 18 lung biopsies. Am J Pathol. 1983;110(3):275–89.
115. Prieditis H, Adamson IY. Alveolar macrophage kinetics and multinucleated giant cell formation after lung injury. J Leukoc Biol. 1996;59(4):534–8.
116. Warheit DB, Sayes CM, Frame SR, Reed KL. Pulmonary exposures to Sepiolite nanoclay particulates in rats: resolution following multinucleate giant cell formation. Toxicol Lett. 2010;192(3):286–93. doi:10.1016/j.toxlet.2009.11.006.
117. Beno M, Hurbankova M, Dusinska M, Cerna S, Volkovova K, Staruchova M, et al. Multinucleate cells (MNC) as sensitive semiquantitative biomarkers of the toxic effect after experimental fibrous dust and cigarette smoke inhalation by rats. Exp Toxicol Pathol. 2005;57(1):77–87.

118. Silva RM, Xu J, Saiki C, Anderson DS, Franzi LM, Vulpe CD, et al. Short versus long silver nanowires: a comparison of *in vivo* pulmonary effects post instillation. Part Fibre Toxicol. 2014;11:52. doi:10.1186/s12989-014-0052-6.
119. Porter DW, Hubbs AF, Mercer RR, Wu N, Wolfarth MG, Sriram K, et al. Mouse pulmonary dose- and time course-responses induced by exposure to multi-walled carbon nanotubes. Toxicology. 2010;269(2–3):136–47. doi:10.1016/j.tox.2009.10.017.
120. Nemery B, Abraham JL. Hard metal lung disease: still hard to understand. Am J Respir Crit Care Med. 2007;176(1):2–3. doi:10.1164/rccm.200704-527ED.
121. Tanaka J, Moriyama H, Terada M, Takada T, Suzuki E, Narita I, et al. An observational study of giant cell interstitial pneumonia and lung fibrosis in hard metal lung disease. BMJ. 2014;4(3):e004407. doi:10.1136/bmjopen-2013-004407.
122. Freiman DG, Hardy HL. Beryllium disease. The relation of pulmonary pathology to clinical course and prognosis based on a study of 130 cases from the U.S. beryllium case registry. Hum Pathol. 1970;1(1):25–44.
123. Martinez VG, Escoda-Ferran C, Tadeu Simoes I, Arai S, Orta Mascaro M, Carreras E, et al. The macrophage soluble receptor AIM/Api6/CD5L displays a broad pathogen recognition spectrum and is involved in early response to microbial aggression. Cell Mol Immunol. 2014;11(4):343–54. doi:10.1038/cmi.2014.12.
124. Chang NC, Hung SI, Hwa KY, Kato I, Chen JE, Liu CH, et al. A macrophage protein, Ym1, transiently expressed during inflammation is a novel mammalian lectin. J Biol Chem. 2001;276(20):17497–506.
125. Giannetti N, Moyse E, Ducray A, Bondier JR, Jourdan F, Propper A, et al. Accumulation of Ym1/2 protein in the mouse olfactory epithelium during regeneration and aging. Neuroscience. 2004;123(4):907–17.
126. Nair MG, Gallagher IJ, Taylor MD, Loke P, Coulson PS, Wilson RA, et al. Chitinase and Fizz family members are a generalized feature of nematode infection with selective upregulation of Ym1 and Fizz1 by antigen-presenting cells. Infect Immun. 2005;73(1):385–94.
127. Raes G, De Baetselier P, Noel W, Beschin A, Brombacher F, Hassanzadeh GG. Differential expression of FIZZ1 and Ym1 in alternatively versus classically activated macrophages. J Leukoc Biol. 2002;71(4):597–602.
128. Welch JS, Escoubet-Lozach L, Sykes DB, Liddiard K, Greaves DR, Glass CK. TH2 cytokines and allergic challenge induce Ym1 expression in macrophages by a STAT6-dependent mechanism. J Biol Chem. 2002;277(45):42821–9.
129. Limas C. The spectrum of primary cutaneous elastolytic granulomas and their distinction from granuloma annulare: a clinicopathological analysis. Histopathology. 2004;44(3):277–82.
130. Mahadeva U, Martin JP, Patel NK, Price AB. Granulomatous ulcerative colitis: a re-appraisal of the mucosal granuloma in the distinction of Crohn's disease from ulcerative colitis. Histopathology. 2002;41(1):50–5.
131. Favara BE, Jaffe R. The histopathology of Langerhans cell histiocytosis. Br J Cancer Suppl. 1994;23:S17–23.
132. Koizumi F, Matsuno H, Wakaki K, Ishii Y, Kurashige Y, Nakamura H. Synovitis in rheumatoid arthritis: scoring of characteristic histopathological features. Pathol Int. 1999;49(4):298–304.
133. Hunder GG, Bloch DA, Michel BA, Stevens MB, Arend WP, Calabrese LH, et al. The American College of Rheumatology 1990 criteria for the classification of giant cell arteritis. Arthritis Rheum. 1990;33(8):1122–8.
134. Kim KR, Scully RE. Peritoneal keratin granulomas with carcinomas of endometrium and ovary and atypical polypoid adenomyoma of endometrium. A clinicopathological analysis of 22 cases. Am J Surg Pathol. 1990;14(10):925–32.
135. Bayliss OB. The giant cell in cholesterol resorption. Br J Exp Pathol. 1976;57(5):610–18.
136. Lai S, Zhou X. Inflammatory cells in tissues of gout patients and their correlations with comorbidities. Open Rheumatol J. 2013;7:26–31. doi:10.2174/1874312901307010026.

137. Anderson JM, Rodriguez A, Chang DT. Foreign body reaction to biomaterials. Semin Immunol. 2008;20(2):86–100. doi:10.1016/j.smim.2007.11.004.
138. Krewski D, Yokel RA, Nieboer E, Borchelt D, Cohen J, Harry J, et al. Human health risk assessment for aluminium, aluminium oxide, and aluminium hydroxide. J Toxicol Environ Health B Critic Rev. 2007;10 Suppl 1:1–269. doi:10.1080/10937400701597766.
139. Black MM, Epstein WL. Formation of multinucleate giant cells in organized epitheloid cell granulomas. Am J Pathol. 1974;74(2):263–74.
140. Nemery B, Verbeken EK, Demedts M. Giant cell interstitial pneumonia (hard metal lung disease, cobalt lung). Semin Respir Critic Care Med. 2001;22(4):435–48. doi:10.1055/s-2001-17386.
141. Takemura T, Rom WN, Ferrans VJ, Crystal RG. Morphologic characterization of alveolar macrophages from subjects with occupational exposure to inorganic particles. Am Rev Respir Dis. 1989;140(6):1674–85. doi:10.1164/ajrccm/140.6.1674.
142. Marchiori E, Lourenco S, Gasparetto TD, Zanetti G, Mano CM, Nobre LF. Pulmonary talcosis: imaging findings. Lung. 2010;188(2):165–71. doi:10.1007/s00408-010-9230-y.
143. Ko CJ, Glusac EJ. Noninfectious granulomas. In: Elder DE, editor. Lever's histopathology of the skin. 11 ed. Philadelphia: Lippincott Williams & Wilkins; 2014. p. 427–57.
144. Hunt AC, Bothwell PW. Histological findings in human brucellosis. J Clin Pathol. 1967;20 (3):267–72.
145. Rosado FG, Stratton CW, Mosse CA. Clinicopathologic correlation of epidemiologic and histopathologic features of pediatric bacterial lymphadenitis. Archiv Pathol Lab Med. 2011;135(11):1490–3. doi:10.5858/arpa.2010-0581-OA.
146. Lockwood DN, Lucas SB, Desikan KV, Ebenezer G, Suneetha S, Nicholls P. The histological diagnosis of leprosy type 1 reactions: identification of key variables and an analysis of the process of histological diagnosis. J Clin Pathol. 2008;61(5):595–600. doi:10.1136/jcp.2007.053389.
147. Barrett AW, Villarroel Dorrego M, Hodgson TA, Porter SR, Hopper C, Argiriadou AS, et al. The histopathology of syphilis of the oral mucosa. J Oral Pathol Med. 2004;33 (5):286–91. doi:10.1111/j.0904-2512.2004.00099.x.
148. Elston DM. Fungal Infections. In: Elston DM, Ferringer T, Peckham S, High WA, DiCaudo DJ, Ko CJ, editors. Dermatopathology. 2 ed. Philadelphia: Elsevier-Saunders; 2014. p. 270–85.
149. Das R, Dey P, Chakrabarti A, Ray P. Fine-needle aspiration biopsy in fungal infections. Diagn Cytopathol. 1997;16(1):31–4.
150. Shibuya K, Hirata A, Omuta J, Sugamata M, Katori S, Saito N, et al. Granuloma and cryptococcosis. J Infect Chemother. 2005;11(3):115–22. doi:10.1007/s10156-005-0387-x.
151. Araya J, Kawabata Y, Tomichi N, Kaneko K, Hayashi K, Iwabuchi K, et al. Allergic inflammatory reaction is involved in necrosis of human pulmonary dirofilariasis. Histopathology. 2007;51(4):484–90. doi:10.1111/j.1365-2559.2007.02822.x.
152. Gatrill AJ, Mackenzie CD, McMahon JE, Williams JF, Guderian RH. A histocytochemical study of the macrophages present in tissue responses to adult Onchocerca volvulus. Histochem J. 1987;19(9):509–19.
153. Mehregan DR, Mehregan AH, Mehregan DA. Histologic diagnosis of cutaneous leishmaniasis. Clin Dermatol. 1999;17(3):297–304.
154. Geboes K, el-Dosoky I, el-Wahab A, Abou Almagd K. The immunopathology of Schistosoma mansoni granulomas in human colonic schistosomiasis. Virchows Archiv. 1990;416(6):527–34.
155. Fraser WJ, Haffejee Z, Cooper K. Rheumatic Aschoff nodules revisited: an immunohistological reappraisal of the cellular component. Histopathology. 1995;27(5):457–61.
156. Chopra P, Wanniang J, Sampath KA. Immunohistochemical and histochemical profile of Aschoff bodies in rheumatic carditis in excised left atrial appendages: an immunoperoxidase study in fresh and paraffin-embedded tissue. Int J Cardiol. 1992;34(2):199–207.

157. Stehbens WE, Zuccollo JM. Anitschkow myocytes or cardiac histiocytes in human hearts. Pathology. 1999;31(2):98–101.
158. Krueger D. Clinical impact of mTOR inhibitors on the management of subependymal Giant cell astrocytomas in tuberous sclerosis complex. Int J Clin Rev. 2011;08:10. doi:10.5275/ijcr.2011.08.10.
159. Rickert CH. Cortical dysplasia: neuropathological aspects. Childs Nerv Syst. 2006;22(8):821–6. doi:10.1007/s00381-006-0126-3.
160. Gomez-Mateo Mdel C, Monteagudo C. Nonepithelial skin tumors with multinucleated giant cells. Semin Diagn Pathol. 2013;30(1):58–72. doi:10.1053/j.semdp.2012.01.004.
161. Magro G, Amico P, Vecchio GM, Caltabiano R, Castaing M, Kacerovska D, et al. Multinucleated floret-like giant cells in sporadic and NF1-associated neurofibromas: a clinicopathologic study of 94 cases. Virchows Arch. 2010;456(1):71–6. doi:10.1007/s00428-009-0859-y.
162. Hassanein A, Telang G, Benedetto E, Spielvogel R. Subungual myxoid pleomorphic fibroma. Am J Dermatopathol. 1998;20(5):502–5.
163. Kim EJ, Park HS, Yoon HS, Cho S. A case of perforating dermatofibroma with floret-like giant cells. Clin Exp Dermatol. 2015;40(3):305–8. doi:10.1111/ced.12539.
164. Zhang L, Peeples ME, Boucher RC, Collins PL, Pickles RJ. Respiratory syncytial virus infection of human airway epithelial cells is polarized, specific to ciliated cells, and without obvious cytopathology. J Virol. 2002;76(11):5654–66.
165. Schoolmeester JK, Smyrk TC. Multinucleated epithelial giant cells in the duodenum. Int J Surg Pathol. 2013;21(2):202–4. doi:10.1177/1066896912452911.
166. Cohen PR, Paravar T, Lee RA. Epidermal multinucleated giant cells are not always a histopathologic clue to a herpes virus infection: multinucleated epithelial giant cells in the epidermis of lesional skin biopsies from patients with acantholytic dermatoses can histologically mimic a herpes virus infection. Dermatol Pract Concept. 2014;4(4):21–7. doi:10.5826/dpc.0404a03.
167. Iolascon A, Heimpel H, Wahlin A, Tamary H. Congenital dyserythropoietic anemias: molecular insights and diagnostic approach. Blood. 2013;122(13):2162–6. doi:10.1182/blood-2013-05-468223.
168. Holt DJ, Grainger DW. Multinucleated giant cells from fibroblast cultures. Biomaterials. 2011;32(16):3977–87. doi:10.1016/j.biomaterials.2011.02.021.
169. Devaney K, Goodman ZD, Ishak KG. Postinfantile giant-cell transformation in hepatitis. Hepatology. 1992;16(2):327–33.
170. Gabor L, Pal K, Zsuzsa S. Giant cell hepatitis in adults. Pathol Oncol Res. 1997;3(3):215–18. doi:10.1007/BF02899924.
171. Cohen LM. The starburst giant cell is useful for distinguishing lentigo maligna from photodamaged skin. J Am Acad Dermatol. 1996;35(6):962–8.
172. Patino WD, Hutchens KA, Kapil J, Chiou Y, Gottlieb GJ. Eosinophilic cytoplasmic inclusion bodies in vesicular multinucleated melanocytes: a clue to the diagnosis of benign melanocytic lesions. Am J Dermatopathol. 2012;34(4):424–7. doi:10.1097/DAD.0b013e318216a822.
173. Kuppers R, Hansmann ML. The Hodgkin and Reed/Sternberg cell. Int J Biochem Cell Biol. 2005;37(3):511–17. doi:10.1016/j.biocel.2003.10.025.
174. Rengstl B, Rieger MA, Newrzela S. On the origin of giant cells in Hodgkin lymphoma. Commun Integr Biol. 2014;7:e28602. doi:10.4161/cib.28602.
175. Kamel OW, LeBrun DP, Berry GJ, Dorfman RF, Warnke RA. Warthin-Finkeldey polykaryocytes demonstrate a T-cell immunophenotype. Am J Clin Pathol. 1992;97(2):179–83.
176. Orenstein JM. The Warthin-Finkeldey-type giant cell in HIV infection, what is it? Ultrastruct Pathol. 1998;22(4):293–303.

Chapter 2
NLRP3 Inflammasome-Mediated Toxicity of Fibrous Particles

Sanae Kanno

Abstract Long airborne fibers such as asbestos and carbon nanotubes (CNTs) are more potent activators of carcinogenesis, inflammation, and genotoxicity than short or tangled fibers. It has recently been reported that fibrous particles trigger the secretion of proinflammatory cytokines such as interleukin (IL)-1β and IL-18 and cause inflammatory diseases through the NOD-like receptor pyrin domain containing 3 (NLRP3) inflammasome. The NLRP3 inflammasome is a major component of the innate immune system in responses to infection and tissue injury in phagocytotic cells. The shape, size, charge, and biopersistence of particulate substances are the most important factors affecting their ability to cause NLRP3 inflammasome-mediated proinflammatory responses. In this review, the current understandings are summarized and discussed regarding the mechanisms of NLRP3 inflammasome induction by various fibrous particles. In addition, the review demonstrates the potential mechanism of IL-1β secretion through the NLRP3 inflammasome, with a focus on the role of the GTPase effector Rho kinases (ROCK1 and 2), which are known to be involved in a wide range of cellular functions including adhesion, regulation of the cytoskeleton, and phagocytosis.

Keywords Rho kinase (ROCK) • NLRP3 inflammasome • Fibrous particles • IL-1β

2.1 Introduction

Epidemiological studies show that exposure to ambient particulate matter (PM) is associated with increased pulmonary and cardiovascular morbidity and mortality [1, 2]. It is well known that inhalation of some types of fibrous particles leads to thoracic diseases including asbestosis, lung cancer, and mesothelioma. Recently, fibrous manufactured nanomaterials (defined as materials designed and produced to have structural features with one or more external dimensions $\leq$100 nm) have been

S. Kanno, Ph.D. (✉)
Department of Legal Medicine, St. Marianna University School of Medicine, 2-16-1 Sugao, Miyamae-ku, Kawasaki 216-8511, Japan
e-mail: sanae@marianna-u.ac.jp

T. Otsuki et al. (eds.), *Biological Effects of Fibrous and Particulate Substances*, Current Topics in Environmental Health and Preventive Medicine,
DOI 10.1007/978-4-431-55732-6_2

widely used for various industrial and medicinal applications; however, concerns have been raised regarding their possible harmful effects. Therefore, the assessments of adverse effects of fibrous particles on human health are imperative for the fields of nanotoxicology and nano-risk.

Inflammation is a tightly regulated response of innate immune systems to infection and tissue injury and is caused by various exogenous and endogenous stimuli [3]. Inflammasomes, which serve a critical role in the innate immune system, are large multimolecular complexes that are composed of a sensor protein, the adaptor apoptosis-associated speck-like protein containing a caspase activation and recruitment domain (CARD) (ASC), and the inflammasome protease caspase-1 [4]. The NOD-like receptor (NLR) pyrin domain containing 3 (NLRP3) inflammasome is activated by a wide range of signals including pathogen-associated molecular patterns (PAMPs) and danger-associated molecular patterns (DAMPs). Activation of the NLRP3 inflammasome triggers activated caspase-1-dependent proteolytic processing of immature proinflammatory cytokine interleukin (IL)-1 family members, such as IL-1β and IL-18, and enhances the secretion of mature proinflammatory cytokines [5]. It has been reported that the production of proinflammatory cytokines initiates immune responses. It has recently been reported that fibrous particles including not only asbestos and silica but also fibrous manufactured nanomaterials act as a danger signal, triggering proinflammatory cytokine secretion and causing inflammatory diseases through the NLRP3 inflammasome in phagocytotic cells [6–10]. NLRP3 inflammasome activation has been reported to be a key factor in the harmful health effects of particulate matter [6].

We recently reported that Rho kinases (ROCKs) are involved in NLRP3 inflammasomes induced by fibrous particles [11]. ROCKs (ROCK1 and ROCK2) are the effectors of Rho GTPase and have a molecular mass of up to 160 kDa [12]. ROCKs are known to be involved in a wide range of fundamental cellular functions [13, 14].

This review briefly describes types of fibrous particles and their toxicity, NLRP3 inflammasomes induced by the particles, the involvement of ROCKs in NLRP3 inflammasomes, and the subsequent pyroptosis.

2.2 Fibrous Materials and Their Toxicity

Inhalation exposure to airborne pollutants is associated with several adverse health effects. It is well known that inhalation of some types of fibrous particles leads to thoracic diseases including asbestosis, lung cancer, and mesothelioma. The bioactivity and toxicity of fibrous particles are dependent not only on fiber dimension but also fiber shape, surface reactivity, chemical composition, the number of fibers, and their biopersistence. Airborne fibrous materials to which people can be exposed to occupationally and environmentally can be divided into two groups based on their origin: naturally occurring and synthetic materials groups.

2.2.1 *Naturally Occurring Materials*

The naturally occurring materials group consists mainly of a variety of asbestos fibers and crystalline silica. Naturally occurring asbestos consists of long thin fibers. Crystalline silica is abundant in nature as granites, quartz, and sands.

2.2.1.1 Asbestos

"Asbestos" is actually composed of six different fiber types: the amphibole types, amosite, crocidolite, tremolite, actinolite, and anthophyllite, and the serpentine type, chrysotile. Although asbestos has been banned in several countries, its use in other countries, especially in third-world countries, is unregulated. It is widely recognized that exposure to asbestos can result in pulmonary fibrotic disease asbestosis, lung cancer, and pleural and peritoneal mesothelioma after a long latency period in humans [15]. The deposition of asbestos fibers in the parietal pleura is an early event of mesothelioma and fibrosis; however, the mechanism of delivery to the parietal pleura remains to be elucidated. Donaldson et al. suggested that retention of long fibers around the parietal pleural stomata due to length-restricted clearance from the pleural space might initiate inflammation and mesothelioma [16]. The critical determinants of fibrogenicity and carcinogenicity of asbestos fibers are dependent on several fiber parameters including fiber dimensions. Wylie et al. reported that there was a good correlation between tumor formation and the number of fibers >8 μm in length and ≤ 0.25 μm in diameter, which are known as Stanton's criteria [17, 18]. There have been some studies of the comparative toxicity of long and short asbestos fibers. Adamson et al. reported that when long fibers (average length, 24.4 μm) or short fibers (average length, 0.6 μm) were administered into mouse lung by intratracheal instillation, long fibers were deposited in the bronchiolar region and induced fibrosis, while short fibers reached the alveoli but did not induce fibrosis [19]. Moreover, mesothelial and subpleural cell proliferation was increased in response to long fibers [20]. On the other hand, Goodglick et al., using mouse peritoneal macrophages, reported that the transition metal ions in crocidolite asbestos fibers generated oxidant stress and caused lung injury, although such toxicity was independent of the length of the crocidolite asbestos fiber [21].

Some studies have investigated and documented the effect of asbestos on the formation of DNA. Both Libby and crocidolite asbestos fibers generate reactive oxygen species (ROS), which is involved in asbestos-related diseases (ARD), in exposed macrophages; but only crocidolite asbestos induces DNA damage [22]. Long amosite asbestos fibers caused more chromosomal aberrations than short fibers in rats exposed to either long or short amosite asbestos fibers [23].

2.2.1.2 Silica

Silica, known as silicon dioxide (SiO_2), is a naturally occurring substance that presents as a crystalline or an amorphous form. Amorphous silica nanoparticles are used in various fields, such as cosmetics, drug delivery, foods, and chemicals. The chronic effects of amorphous silica for human health are regarded to be no more or less than those of crystalline silica [24]. The main exposure routes are considered to be inhalation and dermal contact. Few papers have described the effects of dermal exposure to amorphous silica. Subchronic dermal exposure of rat skin to amorphous silica nanoparticles showed no toxicity and no changes in internal organs [25]. On the other hand, a single intratracheal instillation of ultrafine amorphous silica particles (diameter, 14 nm) into mice elevated mRNA and protein levels of inflammatory cytokines in the lung, indicating that ultrafine amorphous silica particles induced transient lung inflammation [26].

Crystalline silica is classified as a human carcinogen (Group 1) by the International Agency for Research on Cancer (IARC) [24]. Chronic exposure to airborne crystalline silica by occupational inhalation can result not only in progressive pulmonary fibrosis (known as silicosis) and lung cancer but also in immunological disorders [27, 28]. There have been many studies that have examined the details of silica-induced lung fibrosis in mouse or rat experiments. Fibrotic responses are increased by single pharyngeal aspiration of crystalline silica into NMRI mice [29] and into MyD88 knockout mice [30]; however these responses are uncoupled from lung inflammation. Lung fibrosis is caused by the profibrotic activity of anti-inflammatory cytokines such as IL-10 and transforming growth factor (TGF)- β1, rather than by inflammation [31]. Similar results were obtained in rat experiments. Exposure to crystalline silica elevates the generation of reactive nitrogen species (RNS) and ROS. Subsequently, ROS activates nuclear factor-κB (NF-κB), leading to the secretion of proinflammatory cytokines such as tumor necrosis factor (TNF)-α and IL-1 from epithelial cells. These events contribute to the development of fibrosis [32, 33].

In vitro exposure to crystalline silica increased intracellular oxidants such as RNS and ROS as an early event and caused elevation of various signaling pathways in many types of cells. ROS that was induced by crystalline silica activated the activator protein-1 (AP-1) in JB6 cells [34], and in BET-1A human bronchial epithelial cells, it activated NF-κB, subsequently causing IL-8 production [35]. Furthermore, it has been reported that the oxidative stress generated in crystalline silica-exposed rat alveolar macrophages is associated with cytotoxicity and genotoxicity [36].

2.2.2 *Synthetic Materials*

High aspect ratio nanomaterials (HARN), such as nanotubes and nanowires, have considerable beneficial uses in diverse fields. This synthetic materials group consists of single-walled carbon nanotubes (SWCNTs), double-walled carbon nanotubes (DWCNTs), multiwalled carbon nanotubes (MWCNTs), and various metal nanomaterials such as silver (Ag) wires [37], titanium dioxide (TiO_2) [38], or cerium oxide (CeO_2) nanorods [39].

2.2.2.1 Carbon Nanotubes

CNTs are one of the most promising nanomaterials for many industrial and biomedical applications such as electronics, energy, pharmaceuticals, cosmetics, agriculture, biomedical engineering, and gene therapy. There has been considerable concern with the increasing use of CNTs, in view of their environmental and human health effects [9, 10, 40]. Although CNTs display unique physiological properties such as a nanoscale diameter, high aspect ratio and large surface area in comparison with large particles, and biopersistence, their fibrous shape suggests that they may have toxic properties similar to those of asbestos [41, 42].

CNTs are composed of tubular nanoscaled structures rolled up in a graphene sheet. They are classified into two main types, SWCNTs and MWCNTs, based on whether they have one or more layers. The main differences between SWCNTs and MWCNTs are rigidity and physical state, which affect their dispersion, distribution, and pathogenicity. MWCNTs are more rigid, straighter, and discrete than SWCNTs [43]. It is more difficult for SWCNTs to penetrate plasma membranes and boundaries than MWCNTS, due to the low dispersion of SWCNTs in solution. Therefore the distribution of SWCNTs within the lungs differs significantly from that of MWCNTs. SWCNTs inhaled into the lung were present within the interstitial space, with a few being incorporated into alveolar macrophages, whereas MWCNTs readily penetrated cells and were incorporated within alveolar and interstitial macrophages. The differential distribution of SWCNTs and MWCNTs in the lung might be associated with the formation of granuloma [44]. Both SWCNTs and MWCNTs cause genotoxicity in in vivo and in vitro assays [45–49]. Experiments comparing SWCNTs and MWCNTs indicated that MWCNTs and carboxylated, but not plain, short SWCNTs caused in vitro DNA damage [48]. CNTs (SWCNTs >50 %) induced DNA damage assessed by comet assay in BEAS-2B cells [45]. MWCNTs induced mitotic spindle disruption in BEAS-2B cells [49].

Single-Walled Carbon Nanotubes

There have been some studies that documented the toxicological effect of SWCNTs. Single intratracheal exposure of mice to SWCNTs induced peribronchial inflammation and necrosis. The pulmonary toxicity of SWCNTs is higher than that of carbon black and possibly that of quartz, resulting in the possibility that chronic inhalation exposure to SWCNT dust in a work environment might be a serious occupational health hazard [50]. There are several studies that show that SWCNTs induce a strong acute inflammatory reaction through induction of the secretion of proinflammatory cytokines in mice [51, 52]. Pharyngeal aspiration exposure of mice to SWCNTs induced an acute inflammatory reaction with a fibrogenic response and the formation of granulomas [53]. Furthermore, inhalation exposure of mice to SWCNTs was more effective than pharyngeal aspiration exposure in causing an inflammatory response, oxidative stress, collagen deposition, and fibrosis, as well as mutagenesis [51]. It has been reported that repeated intratracheal instillation of SWCNTs in mice exacerbates ovalbumin-induced allergic airway inflammation and increases oxidative stress [52].

It was recently demonstrated that SWCNTs can be biodegraded by the human neutrophil enzyme myeloperoxidase (MPO) in vitro [54]. An in vivo study also showed that, after pharyngeal aspiration exposure to SWCNTs, knockout mice displayed impaired clearance of SWCNTs from the lung and an enhanced pulmonary inflammatory/profibrotic response compared to wild-type mice [55].

Multiwalled Carbon Nanotubes

Experiments regarding the toxicity of MWCNTs have revealed various toxic effects including cytotoxicity, inflammation, fibrosis, genotoxicity, tumorigenesis, and immunotoxicity [43]. Cytotoxicity and a type of cell death caused by MWCNTs have been reported in multiple cell types including macrophages. MWCNTs (diameter, 67 nm) triggered cytotoxic effects in J774.1 mouse macrophages [56], and the effect was higher than that of crocidolite asbestos in BEAS-2B human bronchial epithelial cells [57]. Thin MWCNTs (diameter, <50 nm) with high crystallinity showed cytotoxicity and cell membrane piercing in MeT5A human mesothelial cells without internalization of the MWCNTs [58]. Conversely, in NR8383 rat macrophages, MWCNTs (length, >100 μm; diameter, 10–30 nm) showed no sign of acute toxicity on cell viability as assessed by the WST-1 method and PI staining [59]. Furthermore, the cytotoxicity of CNTs is associated with their functionalization because the functionalization (unpurified > purified > FITC functionalization) of CNTs greatly reduced their toxicity in J774A mouse macrophages [60]. Carboxylated MWCNTs showed increased cytotoxicity compared with pristine MWCNTs in BEAS-2B human bronchial cells, whereas in A549 human alveolar cells, pristine MWCNTs showed higher inflammatory responses than carboxylated MWCNTs [61]. Although the bioactivity of MWCNTs increased with diameter and length, carboxylation of MWCNTs eliminated their bioactive potential regardless of size in an in vitro study [62]. These studies suggested that the toxicity of MWCNTs depends not only on shape and size but also on surface properties, which can alter their surface charge and reactivity.

The cytotoxicity of MWCNTs was due to direct membrane injury or necrosis rather than to apoptosis in J774.1 mouse macrophages [56]. In LE rat lung epithelial cells, MWCNTs activated apoptosis [63]. MWCNTs induce ROS generation in NR8383 rat macrophages in an MWCNT dose-dependent manner [59] and activated oxidative stress-associated signaling pathways such as NF-κB and AP-1 in both A549 human alveolar cells [64] and LE rat lung epithelial cells [63]. Elevated ROS and NF-κB are involved in proinflammatory signaling [65] such as in IL-8 upregulation [64].

Acute pulmonary exposure to inhaled MWCNTs induced dose-dependent inflammation, fibrosis, and rare pleural penetration, indicating that MWCNTs can reach the pleura after inhalation [66]. Acute exposure to a high concentration of MWCNTs caused pleural mononuclear cell accumulation and subpleural fibrosis in mice [67]. Based on in vivo experiments using rats, it was suggested that the administration of large-sized MWCNTs (length, 8 μm; diameter, 150 nm) by transtracheal intrapulmonary spraying has a higher risk of causing asbestos-like pleural lesions relevant to mesothelioma development than small-sized MWCNTs (length, 3 μm; diameter, 15 nm) [68]. A long-term inhalation study of mice exposed to MWCNTs by pharyngeal aspiration demonstrated that MWCNTs (mean dimensions of 3.9 μm × 49 nm) have the potential to produce a progressive, fibrotic response in the alveolar tissues of the lungs [44].

2.3 The NLRP3 Inflammasome

Inflammation is a tightly controlled response of the innate immune system to cell injury and infection. Inflammasomes, which play a key role in inflammation, are large multimolecular complexes composed of a sensor protein, an adaptor protein, ASC, and an effector protein, caspase-1. Four different types of sensor proteins have been identified: NLRP1b, NLRP3, and NLRC4, which belong to the NLR family, and the ALR member absent in melanoma 2 (AIM2) protein [69]. NLRs are characterized by the combined presence of the nucleotide-binding and oligomerization domain (NACHT), a variable number of leucine-rich repeat domains (LRRs), and either a CARD or a pyrin domain (PYD). In general, LRRs found at the carboxyl terminus of most NLRs are thought to survey PAMPs and DAMPs in intracellular compartments [69]. The NLRP3 inflammasome is the most extensively studied receptor.

2.3.1 NLRP3 Inflammasome Activators

It is known that the NLRP3 inflammasome can be activated by diverse triggers including PAMPs and DAMPs. PAMPs include lipopolysaccharide (LPS) and lipoteichoic acid (LTA), which are components of the outer membrane of bacteria, and pneumolysin, nigericin, and maitotoxin, which are pore-forming toxins [70]. DAMPs are classified into two major classes based on their origin: exogenous activators and endogenous activators.

2.3.1.1 Exogenous Activators

The NLRP3 inflammasome is activated by exogenous DAMPs such as crystalline silica [8, 6], asbestos [6, 7, 11, 71, 72], CNTs [11, 10], aluminum salt (alum) [8], and erionite [72] through occupational or environmental exposure. IL-1β, a proinflammatory cytokine, has been reported to be involved in the pathogenesis of asbestos-induced mesothelioma [6]. DWCNT- and needlelike MWCNT-induced IL-1β secretion is linked to NLRP3 inflammasome activation in human monocytes, in a manner similar to the linkage of DAMPs such as asbestos [9, 10]. Ag nanowires or CeO_2 nanorods induce IL-1β secretion in THP-1 human monocytes [39, 73]. Mouse alveolar macrophages exposed to a TiO_2 nanobelt also showed IL-1β secretion via lysosomal rupture and cathepsin B release [38]. Several reports have demonstrated that noncrystalline nanoparticles have the ability to induce the NLRP3 inflammasome. It has been reported that NLRP3 inflammasomes are also induced by nano-sized silica and TiO_2 through adenosine triphosphate (ATP), adenosine diphosphate (ADP), and adenosine in human and murine macrophages [74]. Noncrystalline silica nanoparticles as well as crystalline silica particles induce IL-1β secretion in LPS-primed RAW 264.7 cells and rat primary lung macrophages [75]. Furthermore, diesel exhaust particles have been reported to induce pulmonary inflammation in a manner that depends on IL-1β, but is independent of the classical NLRP3/caspase-1 pathway [76]. Exogenous activators and their mechanisms of action are summarized in Table 2.1.

2.3.1.2 Endogenous Activators

Endogenous fibrous particles include particles such as monosodium urate (MSU) [77, 78], cholesterol crystals [79], β-amyloid fibers [80], and calcium pyrophosphate dehydrate (CPPD) [77]. Hemozoin crystals [81] are also known as endogenous DAMPs, although they are not host derived, but are parasite derived. Many reports indicate that aberrant activation of NLRP3 inflammasomes is observed in autoinflammatory and autoimmune disorders. Inappropriate NLRP3 activation by endogenous DAMPs such as cholesterol crystals and β-amyloid fibers is related to atherosclerosis and Alzheimer's disease, respectively. MSU, which is a well-

Table 2.1 Exogenous activators

Fibrous particles	Size	Cell/animal	Upstream effects of NLRP3	Downstream effects of caspase-1	References
Chrysotile	Length: 21 μm Surface area: 28.83 m^2/g	THP-1 cells, BEAS-2B human bronchial epithelial cells	Lysosomal damage	IL-1β, MAPK activation and induction of IL-6 release in BEAS-2B cells	[7]
Libby six-mix	Length: 7.21 μm Surface area: 5 m^2/g		ROS		
Crocidolite		THP-1 cells (NLRP3, ASC, caspase-1, MyD88, p22phox, TRX (thioredoxin) knock down), human M-CSF-derived macrophages, mouse bone marrow or peritoneal-derived macrophages (NLRP3−/−, ASC−/−), mouse (NLRP3−/−)	NADPH ROS (inhibition by TRX)	IL-1β, inflammation factor in BALF	[6]
Crocidolite	Length: 4.6 μm Diameter: 180 nm	Human monocyte-derived macrophages (NLRP3, P2X7 knockdown)	ROS, cathepsin B, P2X7 receptor, Srk, and Syk tyrosine kinase	IL-1β	[10]
Crocidolite		LP9 human mesothelial cells (hTERT immortalized)	ROS, TXNIP	IL-1β	[71, 72]
Crystalline silica		Mouse peritoneal macrophages (NLRP3, ASC, caspase-1−/−), human alveolar macrophages, mouse (NLRP3−/−, ASC−/−)	ROS, K^+ efflux, cathepsin B	IL-1β, 6 and 18, TNF-α, inflammation, and collagen deposition	[99]
Crystalline silica	Length >15 μm at "polydispersed" preparation	Human peripheral blood mononuclear cells, mouse bone marrow-derived macrophages (NLRP3−/−, ASC−/−, caspase-1−/−, MyD88 + TRIF doubly−/−, IL-1R−/−)	Lysosomal damage, cathepsin B	IL-1β	[8]

(continued)

Table 2.1 (continued)

Fibrous particles	Size	Cell/animal	Upstream effects of NLRP3	Downstream effects of caspase-1	References
DWCNTs	Length: 0.1–100 μm Diameter: 0.5–2.5 nm (inner), 1.2–3.2 nm (outer) Surface area:985 m^2/g	Primary human monocytes (NLRP3 knockdown)	Lysosomal damage, K^+ efflux	IL-1β	[9]
MWCNTs	Length: 0.5–40 μm Diameter: 10–30 nm Surface area: 40–300 m^2/g	HBE human bronchial epithelial cells (NLRP3 knockdown), MRC-5 human lung fibroblasts	ROS	IL-1β, 8, 18, pyroptosis, fibrotic responses in MRC-5 cells	[115]
Long needlelike MWCNTs	OD >50 nm Length: ~13 μm	Human monocyte-derived macrophages (NLRP3, P2X7 knockdown)	ROS, cathepsin B, P2X7 receptor, Srk, and Syk tyrosine kinase	IL-1β	[10]
MWCNTs	Diameter: 67 nm Surface area: 26 m^2/g	THP-1 cells (Rho kinases knockdown)	Rho kinases, cathepsin B	IL-1β	[11]
Aluminum salts		Human peripheral blood mononuclear cells, mouse bone marrow-derived macrophages (NLRP3−/−, ASC−/−, caspase-1−/−, MyD88 + TRIF doubly−/−, IL-1R−/−)	Lysosomal damage, cathepsin B	IL-1β, 6, 18	[8]
Ag wire	274nmX5.3 μm	THP-1 cells	Lysosomal damage, ROS, cathepsin B	IL-1β	[73]
CeO_2 nanorods	Length: 33.2–1000 nm < Diameter: 7–9.5 nm Aspect ratio: 1–100<	THP-1 cells (NLRP3−/−, ASC−/−)	Lysosomal damage, cathepsin B	IL-1β	[39]
TiO_2 nanobelt	Short nanobelt (diameter, 60–300 nm; length, 0.8–4 μm) and long nanobelt (diameter, 60–300 nm; length, 15–30 μm)	Primary mouse alveolar macrophages	Long TiO2 nanobelt → lysosomal damage, ROS, cathepsin B	IL-1β, 18	[38]

studied pathogenic endogenous fiber, or CPPD, deposits in the joints of hyperuricemic humans and can cause acute and chronic inflammatory responses such as gout or pseudo-gout, respectively [77]. Although they do not have a fibrous shape, ATP [82], heat-shock protein hsp72 [83], serum amyloid A, an acute-phase protein in serum [84], and saturated free fatty acids [85] are also known as activators of NLRP3 inflammasomes (Table 2.2).

2.3.2 The Cell Membrane Receptor that Recognizes Fibrous Particles

The deposition rate of ultrafine particles (UFP) with a diameter less than 100 nm or that of the HARN in the peripheral lung is higher than that of larger particles; and these particles are retained more efficiently in exhaustively lavaged lung [86], indicating that the alveolar lining may be affected greatly by nanoparticles or fibrous particles. It is well known that macrophages play an important role in the body's first defense against various environmental particles and microorganisms. Alveolar macrophages bind and ingest environmental particles and bacteria through scavenger receptors [87]. Scavenger receptor class A is known to play a critical role in innate immunity and apoptotic clearance. The macrophage receptor with a collagenous structure (MARCO) was identified as a scavenger receptor class A protein that is expressed on the cell surface of macrophages [88]. MARCO has been reported to play a pivotal role in the phagocytosis of unopsonized environmental particles and in the clearance of bacteria from the lung. The molecular structure of the MARCO resembles that of the scavenger receptor-A1, which contains a triple-helix collagenous domain and a scavenger receptor cysteine-rich domain at the C terminus [89]. Mutagenesis studies with human MARCO have shown that the N-terminal side of the cysteine-rich domain is important for ligand binding [88]. MARCO mediates the binding and ingestion of unopsonized particles such as TiO_2, Fe_2O_3, latex beads [87], silica [90], unopsonized polystyrene nanoparticles [91], and MWCNTs [40]. Recently, there have been a few reports regarding the interaction of MARCO and inflammasomes. Rupa Biswas et al. have reported that silica increased NLRP3 inflammasome activation and the release of IL-1β from $MARCO^{-/-}$ alveolar macrophages compared to wild-type alveolar macrophages [92].

2.3.3 Phagocytosis of Fibrous Particles

Alveolar macrophages play a crucial role in fibrous particle-induced inflammation and pulmonary fibrosis. Macrophages can endocytose small or short fibrous materials and attempt to phagocytose long fibrous materials. However, macrophages

Table 2.2 Endogenous activators

Fibrous particles	Size	Cell/animal	Upstream effects of NLRP3	Downstream effects of caspase-1	References
MSU		Primary human monocytes, THP-1 cells, mouse peritoneal macrophages (NLRP3−/−, ASC−/−, caspase-1−/−, MyD88−/−)		IL-1β, 6, TNF-α, neutrophil influx	[77]
CPPD					
Hemozoin crystals	0.1μmX0.1μmX0.3–0.5 μm	Mouse bone marrow-derived cells (NLRP3−/−, IL-1β −/−), THP-1 cells	ROS, cathepsin B, K^+ efflux, Syk phosphorylation	IL-1β	[78, 81]
Cholesterol crystals		Mouse bone marrow-derived cells and mouse (NLRP3−/−, ASC−/−, IL-1α/β doubly−/−, IL-1R−/−, caspase-1−/−, cathepsin B, L−/−, LDLR−/−), human peripheral blood mononuclear cells	Lysosomal damage, ROS, cathepsin B	IL-1β, 18, peritoneal inflammation, atherosclerosis	[79]
Amyloid-β		Mouse bone marrow-derived macrophages (NLRP3−/−, ASC−/−, IPAF−/−) and microglia (caspase-1−/−, IL-1R−/−), mouse (ASC−/−, caspase-1−/−, IL-1R−/−, MyD88−/−)	Lysosomal damage, ROS, cathepsin B	IL-1β, proinflammatory factors (NO, TNF), chemotactic factors (CCL3, CCL4, CXCL2)	[80]

often cannot enclose such long fibers due to their great length and high potential for aggregation, leading to “frustrated phagocytosis,” which is characterized by prolonged production of ROS. “Frustrated phagocytosis” was observed with silver nanowires $\geq$10–14 μm in length using backscatter scanning electron microscopy in in vivo and in vitro studies [93]. It has been demonstrated that the actin cytoskeleton is necessary for both phagocytosis and “frustrated phagocytosis” [6, 94]. Both phagocytosis and “frustrated phagocytosis” of fibrous particles such as DWCNTs, alum, asbestos, and silica are involved in NLRP3 inflammasome activation [6, 9]. The IL-1β secretion induced by asbestos or MSU was inhibited by cytochalasin D, which disrupts actin filaments, whereas noncrystalline NLRP3 activators were not affected by cytochalasin D [6]. These results indicate that the actin cytoskeleton is necessary for phagocytosis but does not drive mature IL-1β secretion and that phagocytosis is essential for inflammasome activation induced by fibrous particles.

2.4 Activation of the NLRP3 Inflammasome by Fibrous Particles

It has been suggested that NLRP3 responds to certain cellular changes downstream of initial triggering events because it is unlikely that NLRP3 can directly detect many and diverse activating stimuli. The following three possible intermediate activators have been proposed: (1) potassium (K^+) efflux [95], (2) generation of ROS [96], and (3) lysosomal rupture [8]. These intermediates coordinately activate NLRP3 inflammasomes. It has been reported that phagocytosis of fibrous particles is required as an initial step for inflammasome activation [9]. Phagocytosis of fibrous particles leads to lysosomal rupture and K^+ efflux, as well as leakage of the lysosomal cysteine proteases and cathepsins B and L, into the cytoplasm, which is associated with activation of the NLRP3 inflammasome [9]. Activation of the NLRP3 inflammasome triggers activated caspase-1-dependent proteolytic processing of immature proinflammatory cytokine IL-1 family members, such as IL-1β and IL-18, and enhances the secretion of mature proinflammatory cytokines [5]. Mature IL-1β is released from secretory lysosomes through K^+-dependent mechanisms [97] and promotes inflammatory responses [5]. Long aspect ratio materials such as asbestos and CNTs lead to “frustrated phagocytosis,” which generates ROS through an NADH oxidase [6]. This elevated ROS generation activates the NLRP3 inflammasome through two pathways. One pathway is that ROS leads to lysosomal rupture and cathepsin B release and subsequently activates the NLRP3 inflammasome [69]. The other pathway is mediated via the thioredoxin (TRX)-interacting protein (TXNIP). TXNIP dissociates from the TXNIP/TRX-1 complex in a ROS-sensitive manner, acts as an NLRP3 activator, and leads to subsequent IL-1β secretion via the NLRP3 inflammasome [98]. It has been reported that ROS is associated with NLRP3 inflammasome activation by fibrous particles such as MSU [6], Ag nanowires [73], and crystalline silica [99]. DWCNTs activate the NLRP3 inflammasome via K^+ efflux and lysosomal destabilization, but not by ROS generation in primary human monocytes. In addition to NADPH oxidase-induced ROS, recent study demonstrated that mitochondrial damage-induced ROS is implicated in NLRP3 inflammasome activation [100]. The release of mitochondrial ROS leads to subsequent lysosomal and mitochondrial membrane permeabilization and eventual cell death. Such damage may activate the NLRP3 inflammasome [100]. P2X7 receptors, which are extracellular ATP-gated ion channels, are reported to be associated with NLRP3 inflammasome activation [84]. Inflammasome-mediated secretion of IL-1 cytokines is associated with the simultaneous secretion of inflammasome components into the cell culture supernatant [10]. P2X7 receptor inhibition by siRNA clearly decreased IL-1β secretion from primary human macrophages, indicating that the P2X7 receptor is essential for the NLRP3 inflammasome activation that is triggered by needlelike materials [10]. Furthermore, the activation and secretion of proinflammatory cytokines via the NLRP3 inflammasome by needlelike materials is dependent on Src and Syk tyrosine kinases [10].

Activation of the NLRP3 inflammasome by ATP, crystalline silica, or nigericin was recently shown to result in the release of ASC specks that were composed of ASC and a mutant form of NLRP3, as well as the release of mature IL-1β and caspase-1 into extracellular spaces. The ASC speck promoted further activation of caspase-1 extracellularly, as well as intracellularly after phagocytosis by macrophages, and amplified the inflammatory response [101, 102].

2.4.1 ROCKs

There are more than 20 Rho GTPase proteins in humans. Of these proteins, three important Rho GTPase members, Cdc42, Rac1, and Rho, are well characterized in terms of cellular function. The Rho GTPases act as molecular switches that alternate between active GTP-bound forms and inactive GDP-bound forms [103]. Rho GTPases not only have classical roles such as the regulation of cytoskeletal dynamics but more recently have also been shown to have roles in cellular trafficking and tumor invasion [103]. Small GTPases are known to regulate ROCKs (ROCK1 and ROCK2), which have a molecular mass of up to 160 kDa [12]. Activated ROCK1 induces myosin light chain (MLC) phosphorylation and cellular F-actin and activates the actin-myosin contractile system [104], whereas ROCK2 is required for myosin-2-dependent phagocytosis [105]. It has been reported that phagocytosis through the Fcγ receptor (FcγR) or the complement receptor 3 (CR3) requires the actin-organizing complex, Arp2/3. Phagocytosis of opsonized particles via the FcγR is mediated by Rac/Cdc42, and that of C3bi-coated particles is mediated by Rho and ROCKs via CR3 [14]. However, in contrast to opsonized particle phagocytosis, the interaction of unopsonized particles and ROCKs is not well known.

2.4.2 ROCK-Dependent Activation of the NLRP3 Inflammasome by Fibrous Particles

Previous studies have suggested that cytoskeletal proteins such as tubulin and actin are required in the production of fibrous particle-induced IL-1β through the NLRP3 inflammasome [9, 106]. More recently, it has been reported that microtubule-driven transport of mitochondria and the apposition of ASC on mitochondria to NLRP3 on the endoplasmic reticulum are required for NLRP3 inflammasome activation [94]. Inhibitors of tubulin polymerization such as colchicine and nocodazole suppressed NLRP3-dependent IL-1β secretion in response to NLRP3 inflammasome activators such as nigericin, ATP, MSU, or silica, suggesting that microtubules are associated with NLRP3 inflammasome activation by both phagocytosis-dependent and phagocytosis-independent inducers [94]. It has been reported that the guanine nucleotide exchange factor (GEF)-H1/RhoA/ROCK pathway plays an important role in linking microtubule disassembly to remodeling of the actin cytoskeleton [107, 108]. Rho/ROCK signaling has also been reported to be associated with the stability or active role of microtubules [109]. Based on these findings, we considered that ROCKs might possibly contribute to the fibrous particle-induced NLRP3 inflammasome. We examined whether ROCKs are associated with MWCNT-, asbestos-, or LPS-induced IL-1β secretion in human monocytic THP-1 cells using the selective ROCK inhibitor, Y27632, and small interfering RNA targeted against ROCK [11]. These experiments showed that exposure of the cells to MWCNTs or asbestos provoked IL-1β secretion and that this secretion was suppressed by Y27632, whereas LPS-induced IL-1β secretion was not inhibited by Y27632. Consistent with these data, siRNA designed for knockdown of both ROCK1 and ROCK2 suppressed MWCNT- and asbestos-induced IL-1β secretion, but did not change LPS-induced IL-1β secretion. Furthermore, Y27632 suppressed pro-IL-1β protein levels and the release of activated cathepsin B and activated caspase-1 that were induced by MWCNTs or asbestos. In contrast, LPS-induced pro-IL-1β protein was not suppressed by Y27632. These results suggest that ROCKs are involved in fibrous particle-induced NLRP3 inflammasome activation in THP-1 cells. Furthermore, such inhibitory effects were observed not only in THP-1 cells but also in human blood-derived macrophages (our unpublished data). The ROCK inhibitor suppressed only the fibrous particle-induced NLRP3 inflammasome which requires phagocytosis, indicating that ROCKs might be involved in phagocytosis of the fibrous particles. The proposed NLRP3 inflammasome pathway that is activated by fibrous particles is illustrated in Fig. 2.1. Misawa et al. reported that microtubule-driven transport of mitochondria and apposition of ASC on mitochondria to NLRP3 on the endoplasmic reticulum are required for NLRP3 inflammasome activation by both phagocytosis-dependent and phagocytosis-independent inducers [94]. Therefore, there is a possibility that the ROCK inhibitor suppressed the transport of mitochondria and the apposition of ASCs (dotted line shown in Fig. 2.1).

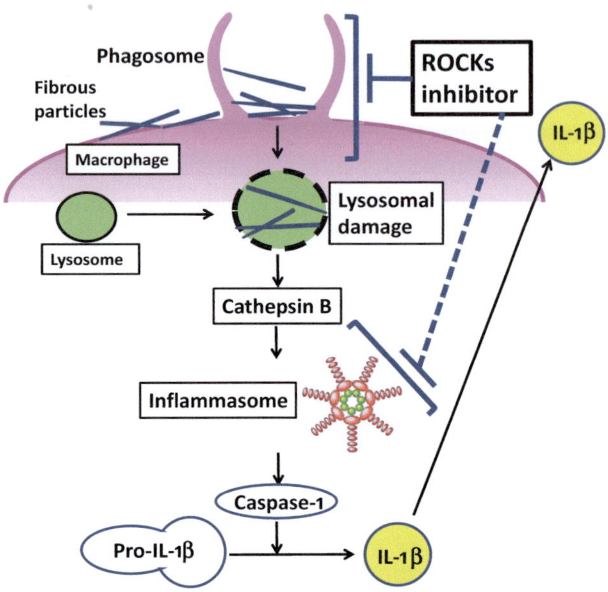

Fig. 2.1 A proposed model for the effect of the inhibitor of ROCKs on fibrous particle-induced NLRP3 inflammasome activation

On the other hand, some studies have reported that nanomaterials can affect ROCK activity. It was reported that crocidolite asbestos lowered the activity of ROCKs in human malignant mesothelioma cells and that the reduced ROCK activity was recovered by the treatment of the cells with antioxidant [110]. Quantum dots inhibit ROCK signaling and impair macrophage morphology and the ability of phagocytosis in J774A.1 cells and in mouse experiments [111].

2.4.3 *Pyroptosis*

Pyroptosis is a recently described programmed and proinflammatory form of cell death. Pyroptosis is dependent on the activation of caspase-1 which is induced through the inflammasome pathway [3]. Unlike apoptosis, the most notable morphological features of pyroptosis are the following: (1) loss of plasma membrane integrity, (2) increase in cell size due to cell swelling and release of cytoplasmic content and membrane vesicles, and (3) rupture of the plasma membrane [112, 113]. However, similar to apoptosis, pyroptosis is also characterized by DNA fragmentation [114]. There have been many studies regarding pyroptosis induced by infection with intracellular pathogens; however pyroptosis induced by DAMPs including fibrous particles has been poorly defined. It has been reported that the exposure to MWCNTs induces NLRP3 inflammasome-dependent pyroptosis in primary human bronchial epithelial cells [115]. Exposure to a high concentration of carbon black nanoparticles induces pyroptosis in RAW264.7 mouse macrophages [116].

2.5 Conclusions

The NLRP3 inflammasome, which serves a critical role in the innate immune system, is activated by a wide range of signals including PAMPs and DAMPs. In addition to endogenous DAMPs, the NLRP3 inflammasome is activated by exogenous DAMPs including naturally occurring materials such as asbestos and crystalline silica and synthetic fibrous nanomaterials such as CNTs. This review summarized the toxicity of fibrous particles including exogenous and endogenous DAMPs that are mediated by the NLRP3 inflammasome. In addition, this review demonstrated that ROCKs are involved in fibrous particle-induced IL-1β secretion via the NLRP3 inflammasome. A proposed pathway of NLRP3 inflammasome induction by fibrous particles is illustrated in Fig. 2.1. Although there have been many studies regarding the mechanisms of NLRP3 inflammasome function, the mechanism of NLRP3 inflammasome induction by fibrous particles remains largely unknown. The application and production of various nanomaterials with a fibrous shape are expanding rapidly due to their unique physical and chemical properties. Therefore, further studies are needed to clarify the mechanism of NLRP3 inflammasome induction by fibrous particles in order to prevent the adverse effects of the use of new fibrous nanomaterials. The understanding of the molecular mechanism(s) that underlie NLRP3 inflammasome activation would make the design and application of new, safe, and useful nanomaterials possible without impairing their benefits. Furthermore, an understanding of these mechanisms would be helpful for the design of therapies targeting inflammasome-related diseases in the future.

Acknowledgments This work was supported in part by JSPS KAKENHI (Grant Number 24590868).

References

1. Graber JM, Stayner LT, Cohen RA, Conroy LM, Attfield MD. Respiratory disease mortality among US coal miners; results after 37 years of follow-up. Occup Environ Med. 2014;71 (1):30–9. doi:10.1136/oemed-2013-101597.
2. Sioutas C, Delfino RJ, Singh M. Exposure assessment for atmospheric ultrafine particles (UFPs) and implications in epidemiologic research. Environ Health Perspect. 2005;113 (8):947–55.
3. Schroder K, Tschopp J. The inflammasomes. Cell. 2010;140(6):821–32. doi:10.1016/j.cell.2010.01.040.
4. Abderrazak A, Syrovets T, Couchie D, El Hadri K, Friguet B, Simmet T, et al. NLRP3 inflammasome: from a danger signal sensor to a regulatory node of oxidative stress and inflammatory diseases. Redox Biol. 2015;4C:296–307. doi:10.1016/j.redox.2015.01.008.
5. Qu Y, Franchi L, Nunez G, Dubyak GR. Nonclassical IL-1 beta secretion stimulated by P2X7 receptors is dependent on inflammasome activation and correlated with exosome release in murine macrophages. J Immunol. 2007;179(3):1913–25. doi:179/3/1913 [pii].

6. Dostert C, Petrilli V, Van Bruggen R, Steele C, Mossman BT, Tschopp J. Innate immune activation through Nalp3 inflammasome sensing of asbestos and silica. Science. 2008;320 (5876):674–7. doi:10.1126/science.1156995 1156995 [pii].
7. Li M, Gunter ME, Fukagawa NK. Differential activation of the inflammasome in THP-1 cells exposed to chrysotile asbestos and Libby "six-mix" amphiboles and subsequent activation of BEAS-2B cells. Cytokine. 2012;60(3):718–30. doi:10.1016/j.cyto.2012.08.025 S1043-4666 (12)00666-7 [pii].
8. Hornung V, Bauernfeind F, Halle A, Samstad EO, Kono H, Rock KL, et al. Silica crystals and aluminum salts activate the NALP3 inflammasome through phagosomal destabilization. Nat Immunol. 2008;9(8):847–56. doi:10.1038/ni.1631.
9. Meunier E, Coste A, Olagnier D, Authier H, Lefevre L, Dardenne C et al. Double-walled carbon nanotubes trigger IL-1beta release in human monocytes through Nlrp3 inflammasome activation. Nanomedicine. 2012;8(6):987–95. doi:S1549-9634(11)00524-7 [pii] 10.1016/j.nano.2011.11.004.
10. Palomaki J, Valimaki E, Sund J, Vippola M, Clausen PA, Jensen KA, et al. Long, needle-like carbon nanotubes and asbestos activate the NLRP3 inflammasome through a similar mechanism. ACS Nano. 2011;5(9):6861–70. doi:10.1021/nn200595c.
11. Kanno S, Hirano S, Chiba S, Takeshita H, Nagai T, Takada M, et al. The role of Rho-kinases in IL-1beta release through phagocytosis of fibrous particles in human monocytes. Arch Toxicol. 2015;89(1):73–85. doi:10.1007/s00204-014-1238-2.
12. Ishizaki T, Maekawa M, Fujisawa K, Okawa K, Iwamatsu A, Fujita A, et al. The small GTP-binding protein Rho binds to and activates a 160 kDa Ser/Thr protein kinase homologous to myotonic dystrophy kinase. EMBO J. 1996;15(8):1885–93.
13. Kanno S, Hirano S, Sagi M, Chiba S, Takeshita H, Ikawa T, et al. Sulfide induces apoptosis and Rho kinase-dependent cell blebbing in Jurkat cells. Arch Toxicol. 2013;87(7):1245–56. doi:10.1007/s00204-013-1027-3.
14. Olazabal IM, Caron E, May RC, Schilling K, Knecht DA, Machesky LM. Rho-kinase and myosin-II control phagocytic cup formation during CR, but not FcgammaR, phagocytosis. Curr Biol. 2002;12(16):1413–18. doi:S0960982202010692 [pii].
15. Mossman BT, Lippmann M, Hesterberg TW, Kelsey KT, Barchowsky A, Bonner JC. Pulmonary endpoints (lung carcinomas and asbestosis) following inhalation exposure to asbestos. J Toxicol Environ Health B Crit Rev. 2011;14(1–4):76–121. doi:10.1080/10937404.2011.556047 936997411 [pii].
16. Donaldson K, Murphy FA, Duffin R, Poland CA. Asbestos, carbon nanotubes and the pleural mesothelium: a review of the hypothesis regarding the role of long fibre retention in the parietal pleura, inflammation and mesothelioma. Part Fibre Toxicol. 2010;7:5. doi:10.1186/1743-8977-7-5.
17. Wylie AG, Virta RL, Segreti JM. Characterization of mineral population by index particle: implication for the Stanton hypothesis. Environ Res. 1987;43(2):427–39.
18. Stanton MF, Layard M, Tegeris A, Miller E, May M, Morgan E, et al. Relation of particle dimension to carcinogenicity in amphibole asbestoses and other fibrous minerals. J Natl Cancer Inst. 1981;67(5):965–75.
19. Adamson IY, Bowden DH. Pulmonary reaction to long and short asbestos fibers is independent of fibroblast growth factor production by alveolar macrophages. Am J Pathol. 1990;137 (3):523–9.
20. Adamson IY, Bakowska J, Bowden DH. Mesothelial cell proliferation after instillation of long or short asbestos fibers into mouse lung. Am J Pathol. 1993;142(4):1209–16.
21. Goodglick LA, Kane AB. Cytotoxicity of long and short crocidolite asbestos fibers *in vitro* and *in vivo*. Cancer Res. 1990;50(16):5153–63.
22. Blake DJ, Bolin CM, Cox DP, Cardozo-Pelaez F, Pfau JC. Internalization of Libby amphibole asbestos and induction of oxidative stress in murine macrophages. Toxicol Sci. 2007;99 (1):277–88. doi:10.1093/toxsci/kfm166.

23. Donaldson K, Golyasnya N. Cytogenetic and pathogenic effects of long and short amosite asbestos. J Pathol. 1995;177(3):303–7. doi:10.1002/path.1711770313.
24. Warheit DB. Inhaled amorphous silica particulates: what do we know about their toxicological profiles? J Environ Pathol Toxicol Oncol. 2001;20 Suppl 1:133–41.
25. Ryu HJ, Seong NW, So BJ, Seo HS, Kim JH, Hong JS, et al. Evaluation of silica nanoparticle toxicity after topical exposure for 90 days. Int J Nanomedicine. 2014;9 Suppl 2:127–36. doi:10.2147/IJN.S57929.
26. Cho WS, Choi M, Han BS, Cho M, Oh J, Park K, et al. Inflammatory mediators induced by intratracheal instillation of ultrafine amorphous silica particles. Toxicol Lett. 2007;175 (1–3):24–33. doi:10.1016/j.toxlet.2007.09.008.
27. Mossman BT, Glenn RE. Bioreactivity of the crystalline silica polymorphs, quartz and cristobalite, and implications for occupational exposure limits (OELs). Crit Rev Toxicol. 2013;43(8):632–60. doi:10.3109/10408444.2013.818617.
28. Otsuki T, Maeda M, Murakami S, Hayashi H, Miura Y, Kusaka M, et al. Immunological effects of silica and asbestos. Cell Mol Immunol. 2007;4(4):261–8.
29. Rabolli V, Lo Re S, Uwambayinema F, Yakoub Y, Lison D, Huaux F. Lung fibrosis induced by crystalline silica particles is uncoupled from lung inflammation in NMRI mice. Toxicol Lett. 2011;203(2):127–34. doi:10.1016/j.toxlet.2011.03.009.
30. Re SL, Yakoub Y, Devosse R, Uwambayinema F, Couillin I, Ryffel B, et al. Uncoupling between inflammatory and fibrotic responses to silica: evidence from MyD88 knockout mice. PLoS One. 2014;9(7):e99383. doi:10.1371/journal.pone.0099383.
31. Barbarin V, Arras M, Misson P, Delos M, McGarry B, Phan SH, et al. Characterization of the effect of interleukin-10 on silica-induced lung fibrosis in mice. Am J Respir Cell Mol Biol. 2004;31(1):78–85. doi:10.1165/rcmb.2003-0299OC.
32. Porter DW, Ye J, Ma J, Barger M, Robinson VA, Ramsey D, et al. Time course of pulmonary response of rats to inhalation of crystalline silica: NF-kappa B activation, inflammation, cytokine production, and damage. Inhal Toxicol. 2002;14(4):349–67. doi:10.1080/08958370252870998.
33. Porter DW, Millecchia L, Robinson VA, Hubbs A, Willard P, Pack D, et al. Enhanced nitric oxide and reactive oxygen species production and damage after inhalation of silica. Am J Physiol Lung Cell Mol Physiol. 2002;283(2):L485–93. doi:10.1152/ajplung.00427.2001.
34. Ding M, Shi X, Lu Y, Huang C, Leonard S, Roberts J, et al. Induction of activator protein-1 through reactive oxygen species by crystalline silica in JB6 cells. J Biol Chem. 2001;276 (12):9108–14. doi:10.1074/jbc.M007666200.
35. Desaki M, Takizawa H, Kasama T, Kobayashi K, Morita Y, Yamamoto K. Nuclear factor-kappa b activation in silica-induced interleukin 8 production by human bronchial epithelial cells. Cytokine. 2000;12(8):1257–60. doi:10.1006/cyto.2000.0704.
36. Zhang Z, Shen HM, Zhang QF, Ong CN. Involvement of oxidative stress in crystalline silica-induced cytotoxicity and genotoxicity in rat alveolar macrophages. Environ Res. 2000;82 (3):245–52. doi:10.1006/enrs.1999.4025.
37. Stoehr LC, Gonzalez E, Stampfl A, Casals E, Duschl A, Puntes V, et al. Shape matters: effects of silver nanospheres and wires on human alveolar epithelial cells. Part Fibre Toxicol. 2011;8:36. doi:10.1186/1743-8977-8-36.
38. Hamilton RF, Wu N, Porter D, Buford M, Wolfarth M, Holian A. Particle length-dependent titanium dioxide nanomaterials toxicity and bioactivity. Part Fibre Toxicol. 2009;6:35. doi:10.1186/1743-8977-6-35.
39. Ji Z, Wang X, Zhang H, Lin S, Meng H, Sun B, et al. Designed synthesis of CeO_2 nanorods and nanowires for studying toxicological effects of high aspect ratio nanomaterials. ACS Nano. 2012;6(6):5366–80. doi:10.1021/nn3012114.
40. Hirano S, Fujitani Y, Furuyama A, Kanno S. Macrophage receptor with collagenous structure (MARCO) is a dynamic adhesive molecule that enhances uptake of carbon nanotubes by CHO-K1 cells. Toxicol Appl Pharmacol. 2012;259(1):96–103. doi:S0041-008X(11)00469-8 [pii] 10.1016/j.taap.2011.12.012.

41. Pacurari M, Castranova V, Vallyathan V. Single- and multi-wall carbon nanotubes versus asbestos: are the carbon nanotubes a new health risk to humans? J Toxicol Environ Health A. 2010;73(5):378–95. doi:919250926 [pii] 10.1080/15287390903486527.
42. Nagai H, Toyokuni S. Biopersistent fiber-induced inflammation and carcinogenesis: lessons learned from asbestos toward safety of fibrous nanomaterials. Arch Biochem Biophys. 2010;502(1):1–7. doi:10.1016/j.abb.2010.06.015 S0003-9861(10)00234-1 [pii].
43. Dong J, Ma Q. Advances in mechanisms and signaling pathways of carbon nanotube toxicity. Nanotoxicology. 2015;13:1–19. doi:10.3109/17435390.2015.1009187.
44. Mercer RR, Hubbs AF, Scabilloni JF, Wang L, Battelli LA, Friend S, et al. Pulmonary fibrotic response to aspiration of multi-walled carbon nanotubes. Part Fibre Toxicol. 2011;8:21. doi:10.1186/1743-8977-8-21.
45. Lindberg HK, Falck GC, Suhonen S, Vippola M, Vanhala E, Catalan J, et al. Genotoxicity of nanomaterials: DNA damage and micronuclei induced by carbon nanotubes and graphite nanofibres in human bronchial epithelial cells *in vitro*. Toxicol Lett. 2009;186(3):166–73. doi:10.1016/j.toxlet.2008.11.019.
46. Ema M, Imamura T, Suzuki H, Kobayashi N, Naya M, Nakanishi J. Genotoxicity evaluation for single-walled carbon nanotubes in a battery of *in vitro* and *in vivo* assays. J Appl Toxicol. 2013;33(9):933–9. doi:10.1002/jat.2772.
47. Kim JS, Song KS, Yu IJ. Evaluation of *in vitro* and *in vivo* genotoxicity of single-walled carbon nanotubes. Toxicol Ind Health. 2013. doi:10.1177/0748233713483201.
48. Mrakovcic M, Meindl C, Leitinger G, Roblegg E, Frohlich E. Carboxylated short single-walled carbon nanotubes but not plain and multi-walled short carbon nanotubes show *in vitro* genotoxicity. Toxicol Sci. 2014. doi:10.1093/toxsci/kfu260.
49. Siegrist KJ, Reynolds SH, Kashon ML, Lowry DT, Dong C, Hubbs AF, et al. Genotoxicity of multi-walled carbon nanotubes at occupationally relevant doses. Part Fibre Toxicol. 2014;11:6. doi:10.1186/1743-8977-11-6.
50. Lam CW, James JT, McCluskey R, Hunter RL. Pulmonary toxicity of single-wall carbon nanotubes in mice 7 and 90 days after intratracheal instillation. Toxicol Sci. 2004;77(1):126–34. doi:10.1093/toxsci/kfg243.
51. Shvedova AA, Kisin E, Murray AR, Johnson VJ, Gorelik O, Arepalli S et al. Inhalation vs. aspiration of single-walled carbon nanotubes in C57BL/6 mice: inflammation, fibrosis, oxidative stress, and mutagenesis. Am J Physiol Lung Cell Mol Physiol. 2008;295(4):L552-65. doi:90287.2008 [pii] 10.1152/ajplung.90287.2008.
52. Inoue K, Yanagisawa R, Koike E, Nishikawa M, Takano H. Repeated pulmonary exposure to single-walled carbon nanotubes exacerbates allergic inflammation of the airway: Possible role of oxidative stress. Free Radic Biol Med. 2010;48(7):924–34. doi:S0891-5849(10)00018-3 [pii] 10.1016/j.freeradbiomed.2010.01.013.
53. Shvedova AA, Kisin ER, Mercer R, Murray AR, Johnson VJ, Potapovich AI et al. Unusual inflammatory and fibrogenic pulmonary responses to single-walled carbon nanotubes in mice. Am J Physiol Lung Cell Mol Physiol. 2005;289(5):L698-708. doi:00084.2005 [pii] 10.1152/ajplung.00084.2005.
54. Andon FT, Kapralov AA, Yanamala N, Feng W, Baygan A, Chambers BJ, et al. Biodegradation of single-walled carbon nanotubes by eosinophil peroxidase. Small. 2013;9(16):2721–9. doi:10.1002/smll.201202508. 16.
55. Shvedova AA, Kapralov AA, Feng WH, Kisin ER, Murray AR, Mercer RR, et al. Impaired clearance and enhanced pulmonary inflammatory/fibrotic response to carbon nanotubes in myeloperoxidase-deficient mice. PLoS One. 2012;7(3):e30923. doi:10.1371/journal.pone.0030923.
56. Hirano S, Kanno S, Furuyama A. Multi-walled carbon nanotubes injure the plasma membrane of macrophages. Toxicol Appl Pharmacol. 2008;232(2):244–51. doi:S0041-008X(08)00271-8 [pii] 10.1016/j.taap.2008.06.016.

57. Hirano S, Fujitani Y, Furuyama A, Kanno S. Uptake and cytotoxic effects of multi-walled carbon nanotubes in human bronchial epithelial cells. Toxicol Appl Pharmacol. 2010;249 (1):8–15. doi:S0041-008X(10)00307-8 [pii] 10.1016/j.taap.2010.08.019.
58. Nagai H, Okazaki Y, Chew SH, Misawa N, Yamashita Y, Akatsuka S, et al. Diameter and rigidity of multiwalled carbon nanotubes are critical factors in mesothelial injury and carcinogenesis. Proc Natl Acad Sci U S A. 2011;108(49):E1330–8. doi:10.1073/pnas.1110013108.
59. Pulskamp K, Diabate S, Krug HF. Carbon nanotubes show no sign of acute toxicity but induce intracellular reactive oxygen species in dependence on contaminants. Toxicol Lett. 2007;168(1):58–74. doi:10.1016/j.toxlet.2006.11.001.
60. Montes-Fonseca SL, Orrantia-Borunda E, Aguilar-Elguezabal A, Gonzalez Horta C, Talamas-Rohana P, Sanchez-Ramirez B. Cytotoxicity of functionalized carbon nanotubes in J774A macrophages. Nanomedicine. 2012;8(6):853–9. doi:10.1016/j.nano.2011.10.002.
61. Ursini CL, Cavallo D, Fresegna AM, Ciervo A, Maiello R, Buresti G, et al. Differences in cytotoxic, genotoxic, and inflammatory response of bronchial and alveolar human lung epithelial cells to pristine and COOH-functionalized multiwalled carbon nanotubes. Biomed Res Int. 2014;2014:359506. doi:10.1155/2014/359506.
62. Hamilton Jr RF, Wu Z, Mitra S, Shaw PK, Holian A. Effect of MWCNT size, carboxylation, and purification on *in vitro* and *in vivo* toxicity, inflammation and lung pathology. Part Fibre Toxicol. 2013;10(1):57. doi:10.1186/1743-8977-10-57.
63. Ravichandran P, Baluchamy S, Sadanandan B, Gopikrishnan R, Biradar S, Ramesh V, et al. Multiwalled carbon nanotubes activate NF-kappaB and AP-1 signaling pathways to induce apoptosis in rat lung epithelial cells. Apoptosis. 2010;15(12):1507–16. doi:10.1007/s10495-010-0532-6.
64. Ye SF, Wu YH, Hou ZQ, Zhang QQ. ROS and NF-kappaB are involved in upregulation of IL-8 in A549 cells exposed to multi-walled carbon nanotubes. Biochem Biophys Res Commun. 2009;379(2):643–8. doi:10.1016/j.bbrc.2008.12.137.
65. Moller P, Christophersen DV, Jensen DM, Kermanizadeh A, Roursgaard M, Jacobsen NR, et al. Role of oxidative stress in carbon nanotube-generated health effects. Arch Toxicol. 2014;88(11):1939–64. doi:10.1007/s00204-014-1356-x.
66. Porter DW, Hubbs AF, Chen BT, McKinney W, Mercer RR, Wolfarth MG, et al. Acute pulmonary dose-responses to inhaled multi-walled carbon nanotubes. Nanotoxicology. 2013;7(7):1179–94. doi:10.3109/17435390.2012.719649.
67. Ryman-Rasmussen JP, Cesta MF, Brody AR, Shipley-Phillips JK, Everitt JI, Tewksbury EW, et al. Inhaled carbon nanotubes reach the subpleural tissue in mice. Nat Nanotechnol. 2009;4 (11):747–51. doi:10.1038/nnano.2009.305.
68. Xu J, Alexander DB, Futakuchi M, Numano T, Fukamachi K, Suzui M, et al. Size- and shape-dependent pleural translocation, deposition, fibrogenesis, and mesothelial proliferation by multiwalled carbon nanotubes. Cancer Sci. 2014;105(7):763–9. doi:10.1111/cas.12437.
69. Lamkanfi M, Dixit VM. Mechanisms and functions of inflammasomes. Cell. 2014;157 (5):1013–22. doi:10.1016/j.cell.2014.04.007.
70. Freche B, Reig N, van der Goot FG. The role of the inflammasome in cellular responses to toxins and bacterial effectors. Semin Immunopathol. 2007;29(3):249–60. doi:10.1007/s00281-007-0085-0.
71. Thompson JK, Westbom CM, MacPherson MB, Mossman BT, Heintz NH, Spiess P, et al. Asbestos modulates thioredoxin-thioredoxin interacting protein interaction to regulate inflammasome activation. Part Fibre Toxicol. 2014;11:24. doi:10.1186/1743-8977-11-24.
72. Hillegass JM, Miller JM, MacPherson MB, Westbom CM, Sayan M, Thompson JK, et al. Asbestos and erionite prime and activate the NLRP3 inflammasome that stimulates autocrine cytokine release in human mesothelial cells. Part Fibre Toxicol. 2013;10:39. doi:10.1186/1743-8977-10-39.

73. Jung HJ, Pak PJ, Park SH, Ju JE, Kim JS, Lee HS, et al. Silver wire amplifies the signaling mechanism for IL-1beta production more than silver submicroparticles in human monocytic THP-1 cells. PLoS One. 2014;9(11):e112256. doi:10.1371/journal.pone.0112256.
74. Baron L, Gombault A, Fanny M, Villeret B, Savigny F, Guillou N, et al. The NLRP3 inflammasome is activated by nanoparticles through ATP, ADP and adenosine. Cell Death Dis. 2015;6:e1629. doi:10.1038/cddis.2014.576.
75. Sandberg WJ, Lag M, Holme JA, Friede B, Gualtieri M, Kruszewski M et al. Comparison of non-crystalline silica nanoparticles in IL-1beta release from macrophages. Part Fibre Toxicol. 2012;9:32. doi:10.1186/1743-8977-9-32 1743-8977-9-32 [pii].
76. Provoost S, Maes T, Pauwels NS, Vanden Berghe T, Vandenabeele P, Lambrecht BN, et al. NLRP3/caspase-1-independent IL-1beta production mediates diesel exhaust particle-induced pulmonary inflammation. J Immunol. 2011;187(6):3331–7. doi:10.4049/jimmunol.1004062.
77. Martinon F, Petrilli V, Mayor A, Tardivel A, Tschopp J. Gout-associated uric acid crystals activate the NALP3 inflammasome. Nature. 2006;440(7081):237–41. doi:nature04516 [pii] 10.1038/nature04516.
78. Tyberghein A, Deroost K, Schwarzer E, Arese P, Van den Steen PE. Immunopathological effects of malaria pigment or hemozoin and other crystals. Biofactors. 2014;40(1):59–78. doi:10.1002/biof.1119.
79. Duewell P, Kono H, Rayner KJ, Sirois CM, Vladimer G, Bauernfeind FG, et al. NLRP3 inflammasomes are required for atherogenesis and activated by cholesterol crystals. Nature. 2010;464(7293):1357–61. doi:10.1038/nature08938.
80. Halle A, Hornung V, Petzold GC, Stewart CR, Monks BG, Reinheckel T, et al. The NALP3 inflammasome is involved in the innate immune response to amyloid-beta. Nat Immunol. 2008;9(8):857–65. doi:10.1038/ni.1636.
81. Shio MT, Eisenbarth SC, Savaria M, Vinet AF, Bellemare MJ, Harder KW, et al. Malarial hemozoin activates the NLRP3 inflammasome through Lyn and Syk kinases. PLoS Pathog. 2009;5(8):e1000559. doi:10.1371/journal.ppat.1000559.
82. Franchi L, Eigenbrod T, Nunez G. Cutting edge: TNF-alpha mediates sensitization to ATP and silica via the NLRP3 inflammasome in the absence of microbial stimulation. J Immunol. 2009;183(2):792–6. doi:10.4049/jimmunol.0900173.
83. Maslanik T, Mahaffey L, Tannura K, Beninson L, Greenwood BN, Fleshner M. The inflammasome and danger associated molecular patterns (DAMPs) are implicated in cytokine and chemokine responses following stressor exposure. Brain Behav Immun. 2013;28:54–62. doi:10.1016/j.bbi.2012.10.014.
84. Niemi K, Teirila L, Lappalainen J, Rajamaki K, Baumann MH, Oorni K et al. Serum amyloid A activates the NLRP3 inflammasome via P2X7 receptor and a cathepsin B-sensitive pathway. J Immunol. 2011;186(11):6119–28. doi:10.4049/jimmunol.1002843 jimmunol.1002843 [pii].
85. Wen H, Gris D, Lei Y, Jha S, Zhang L, Huang MT, et al. Fatty acid-induced NLRP3-ASC inflammasome activation interferes with insulin signaling. Nat Immunol. 2011;12(5):408–15. doi:10.1038/ni.2022.
86. Oberdorster G, Maynard A, Donaldson K, Castranova V, Fitzpatrick J, Ausman K, et al. Principles for characterizing the potential human health effects from exposure to nanomaterials: elements of a screening strategy. Part Fibre Toxicol. 2005;2:8. doi:10.1186/1743-8977-2-8.
87. Palecanda A, Paulauskis J, Al-Mutairi E, Imrich A, Qin G, Suzuki H, et al. Role of the scavenger receptor MARCO in alveolar macrophage binding of unopsonized environmental particles. J Exp Med. 1999;189(9):1497–506.
88. Elomaa O, Sankala M, Pikkarainen T, Bergmann U, Tuuttila A, Raatikainen-Ahokas A, et al. Structure of the human macrophage MARCO receptor and characterization of its bacteria-binding region. J Biol Chem. 1998;273(8):4530–8.

89. van der Laan LJ, Dopp EA, Haworth R, Pikkarainen T, Kangas M, Elomaa O, et al. Regulation and functional involvement of macrophage scavenger receptor MARCO in clearance of bacteria *in vivoin vivo*. J Immunol. 1999;162(2):939–47.
90. Hamilton Jr RF, Thakur SA, Mayfair JK, Holian A. MARCO mediates silica uptake and toxicity in alveolar macrophages from C57BL/6 mice. J Biol Chem. 2006;281(45):34218–26. doi:10.1074/jbc.M605229200.
91. Kanno S, Furuyama A, Hirano S. A murine scavenger receptor MARCO recognizes polystyrene nanoparticles. Toxicol Sci. 2007;97(2):398–406. doi:kfm050 [pii] 10.1093/toxsci/kfm050.
92. Biswas R, Hamilton Jr RF, Holian A. Role of lysosomes in silica-induced inflammasome activation and inflammation in absence of MARCO. J Immunol Res. 2014;2014:304180. doi:10.1155/2014/304180.
93. Schinwald A, Murphy FA, Prina-Mello A, Poland CA, Byrne F, Movia D et al. The threshold length for fiber-induced acute pleural inflammation: shedding light on the early events in asbestos-induced mesothelioma. Toxicol Sci. 2012;128(2):461–70. doi:10.1093/toxsci/kfs171 kfs171 [pii].
94. Misawa T, Takahama M, Kozaki T, Lee H, Zou J, Saitoh T et al. Microtubule-driven spatial arrangement of mitochondria promotes activation of the NLRP3 inflammasome. Nat Immunol. 2013;14(5):454–60. doi:10.1038/ni.2550 ni.2550 [pii].
95. Munoz-Planillo R, Kuffa P, Martinez-Colon G, Smith BL, Rajendiran TM, Nunez G. K(+) efflux is the common trigger of NLRP3 inflammasome activation by bacterial toxins and particulate matter. Immunity. 2013;38(6):1142–53. doi:10.1016/j.immuni.2013.05.016.
96. Tschopp J, Schroder K. NLRP3 inflammasome activation: The convergence of multiple signalling pathways on ROS production? Nat Rev Immunol. 2010;10(3):210–15. doi:10.1038/nri2725.
97. Kahlenberg JM, Dubyak GR. Mechanisms of caspase-1 activation by P2X7 receptor-mediated K+ release. Am J Physiol Cell Physiol. 2004;286(5):C1100-8. doi:10.1152/ajpcell.00494.2003 00494.2003 [pii].
98. Zhou R, Tardivel A, Thorens B, Choi I, Tschopp J. Thioredoxin-interacting protein links oxidative stress to inflammasome activation. Nat Immunol. 2010;11(2):136–40. doi:10.1038/ni.1831.
99. Cassel SL, Eisenbarth SC, Iyer SS, Sadler JJ, Colegio OR, Tephly LA et al. The Nalp3 inflammasome is essential for the development of silicosis. Proc Natl Acad Sci U S A. 2008;105(26):9035–40. doi:0803933105 [pii] 10.1073/pnas.0803933105.
100. Heid ME, Keyel PA, Kamga C, Shiva S, Watkins SC, Salter RD. Mitochondrial reactive oxygen species induces NLRP3-dependent lysosomal damage and inflammasome activation. J Immunol. 2013;191(10):5230–8. doi:10.4049/jimmunol.1301490.
101. Baroja-Mazo A, Martin-Sanchez F, Gomez AI, Martinez CM, Amores-Iniesta J, Compan V, et al. The NLRP3 inflammasome is released as a particulate danger signal that amplifies the inflammatory response. Nat Immunol. 2014;15(8):738–48. doi:10.1038/ni.2919.
102. Franklin BS, Bossaller L, De Nardo D, Ratter JM, Stutz A, Engels G, et al. The adaptor ASC has extracellular and ‘prionoid’ activities that propagate inflammation. Nat Immunol. 2014;15(8):727–37. doi:10.1038/ni.2913.
103. Chi X, Wang S, Huang Y, Stamnes M, Chen JL. Roles of rho GTPases in intracellular transport and cellular transformation. Int J Mol Sci. 2013;14(4):7089–108. doi:10.3390/ijms14047089.
104. Coleman ML, Sahai EA, Yeo M, Bosch M, Dewar A, Olson MF. Membrane blebbing during apoptosis results from caspase-mediated activation of ROCK I. Nat Cell Biol. 2001;3(4):339–45. doi:10.1038/35070009 35070009 [pii].
105. Yoneda A, Multhaupt HA, Couchman JR. The Rho kinases I and II regulate different aspects of myosin II activity. J Cell Biol. 2005;170(3):443–53. doi:jcb.200412043 [pii] 10.1083/jcb.200412043.

106. Martinon F, Mayor A, Tschopp J. The inflammasomes: guardians of the body. Annu Rev Immunol. 2009;27:229–65. doi:10.1146/annurev.immunol.021908.132715.
107. Kitase Y, Shuler CF. Multi-layered hypertrophied MEE formation by microtubule disruption via GEF-H1/RhoA/ROCK signaling pathway. Dev Dyn. 2012;241(7):1169–82. doi:10.1002/dvdy.23800.
108. Etienne-Manneville S, Hall A. Rho GTPases in cell biology. Nature. 2002;420 (6916):629–35. doi:10.1038/nature01148.
109. Takesono A, Heasman SJ, Wojciak-Stothard B, Garg R, Ridley AJ. Microtubules regulate migratory polarity through Rho/ROCK signaling in T cells. PLoS One. 2010;5(1):e8774. doi:10.1371/journal.pone.0008774.
110. Aldieri E, Riganti C, Silvagno F, Orecchia S, Betta PG, Doublier S et al. Antioxidants prevent the RhoA inhibition evoked by crocidolite asbestos in human mesothelial and mesothelioma cells. Am J Respir Cell Mol Biol. 2011;45(3):625–31. doi:2010-0089OC [pii] 10.1165/rcmb.2010-0089OC.
111. Qu G, Zhang C, Yuan L, He J, Wang Z, Wang L, et al. Quantum dots impair macrophagic morphology and the ability of phagocytosis by inhibiting the Rho-associated kinase signaling. Nanoscale. 2012;4(7):2239–44. doi:10.1039/c2nr30243h.
112. Labbe K, Saleh M. Cell death in the host response to infection. Cell Death Differ. 2008;15 (9):1339–49. doi:10.1038/cdd.2008.91.
113. Sollberger G, Strittmatter GE, Garstkiewicz M, Sand J, Beer HD. Caspase-1: the inflammasome and beyond. Innate Immun. 2014;20(2):115–25. doi:10.1177/1753425913484374.
114. Lamkanfi M, Dixit VM. Inflammasomes and their roles in health and disease. Annu Rev Cell Dev Biol. 2012;28:137–61. doi:10.1146/annurev-cellbio-101011-155745.
115. Hussain S, Sangtian S, Anderson SM, Snyder RJ, Marshburn JD, Rice AB, et al. Inflammasome activation in airway epithelial cells after multi-walled carbon nanotube exposure mediates a profibrotic response in lung fibroblasts. Part Fibre Toxicol. 2014;11:28. doi:10.1186/1743-8977-11-28.
116. Reisetter AC, Stebounova LV, Baltrusaitis J, Powers L, Gupta A, Grassian VH et al. Induction of inflammasome-dependent pyroptosis by carbon black nanoparticles. J Biol Chem. 2011;286(24):21844–52. doi:M111.238519 [pii] 10.1074/jbc.M111.238519.

Chapter 3
Approaching a Unified Theory for Particle-Induced Inflammation

Melisa Bunderson-Schelvan, Raymond F. Hamilton, Kevin L. Trout, Forrest Jessop, Mary Gulumian, and Andrij Holian

Abstract Particles such as silica, asbestos, and engineered nanomaterials (ENM) that fall within a relatively small size range (<100 nm in at least one dimension) are known to have serious health consequences following exposure. Studies aimed at determining the mechanisms of toxicity for environmental particles have been ongoing for decades. However, the recent explosion of ENM into the market has resulted in the emergence of many recent studies aimed at determining the mechanisms underlying the pathologies associated with certain forms of ENM. In this chapter, we propose that many of the principles that have guided the toxicity studies of environmental particles may also apply to bioactive ENM. In fact, the initiating event for all downstream pathologies caused by exposure to both bioactive ENM and environmental particles appears to be lysosomal membrane permeabilization (LMP). Therefore, focusing on LMP as the "unifying" principle for particle toxicity studies may allow the field to advance at an increased pace.

Keywords Engineered nanomaterials • Silica • Asbestos • Lysosomal membrane permeabilization • Particle toxicology

3.1 Introduction

The emerging field of engineered nanomaterials (ENM) has gained momentum for its applicability to a wide range of industries and its significant commercial potential. In 2008, total global expenditures for research and development of nanotechnologies were calculated to be US$18.1 billion [1], and global sales of

---

M. Bunderson-Schelvan • R.F. Hamilton • K.L. Trout • F. Jessop • A. Holian (✉)
Center for Environmental Health Sciences, University of Montana, Missoula, MT 59812, USA
e-mail: andrij.holian@umontana.edu

M. Gulumian
Toxicology and Biochemistry Department, National Institute for Occupational Health, Johannesburg, South Africa

Haematology and Molecular Medicine, University of the Witwatersrand, Johannesburg, South Africa

T. Otsuki et al. (eds.), *Biological Effects of Fibrous and Particulate Substances*, Current Topics in Environmental Health and Preventive Medicine,
DOI 10.1007/978-4-431-55732-6_3

engineered nanomedicines were estimated to exceed \$100 billion in 2014 [2]. However, concerns regarding the safety of ENM have resulted in a great deal of scrutiny from the research community. In some cases, biological effects of ENM have been considered to be a new field of research. However, in this chapter, we suggest that the most toxic ENM may share traits with environmental particles that have been extensively studied in the past. Consequently, by incorporating our understanding of the mechanisms of toxicity for environmental particles with recent findings regarding ENM, we are suggesting a unified theory for particle-induced toxicity based on inflammatory pathways.

Prior to recent studies with particulate matter and ENM, particle toxicology included the study of three primary particle types: quartz (silica), asbestos, and carbon-based particles (coal dust, diesel exhaust, urban particulate matter, residual oil fly ash, etc.). Although a link between exposure to environmental particles and disease was mentioned as early as the fifteenth and sixteenth centuries, the modern era of research began around the 1940s when silicosis in rats was initiated following exposures to quartz and mixed dusts [3]. Later, man-made particles known as synthetic vitreous fibers, which were used as industrial alternatives to asbestos, underwent scrutiny for suspected health hazards due to their similarities to environmental particles. Through the formation of the International Agency for Research on Cancer (IARC), it was eventually concluded that particle toxicity is due, in part, to "size" [4] and/or "biopersistence"[5] rather than source (i.e., man-made versus environmental). However, recent focus has shifted from the study of silica, asbestos, coal, and synthetic vitreous fibers to the study of ENM. ENM are widely used in manufacturing processes ranging from medical technologies to cosmetics and can be mass produced under a variety of conditions, elements, and forms [6]. Nanomaterials are often utilized as drug delivery systems with the hope of targeting specific organelles to receive the drug of interest [7]. Many ENM specifically target the lysosome, often through the use of protein modifications, in order to modulate lysosomal function [8]. Other ENM types, such as quantum dots, may naturally accumulate in the lysosomal compartment [9]. A large number of researchers believe the relatively small size (<100 nm in at least one dimension) and resulting unique material physical qualities of ENM have created a new field of particle toxicology that is independent of the mechanisms known to contribute to the health effects following exposure to environmental particles. However, in this chapter, we describe the mechanisms by which particle toxicology is independent of source or type but rather is dependent on the particle's ability to cause lysosomal membrane permeabilization (LMP).

While ENM present new challenges to the field of particle toxicology due to the unlimited methods for manipulation of size, shape, and manufacturing processes, the overall mechanisms for toxicity/bioactivity may remain the same as defined by vintage particle research conducted primarily with asbestos and silica. Specifically, we suggest that LMP is the initiating event that determines whether a particle is "bioactive" and will cause adverse health effects—regardless of the type (i.e., asbestos, silica, ENM, etc.). LMP, as the "unifying" event for downstream particle toxicity, may also provide important insight into the toxicity of endogenous particles that have also been reported to activate the NLRP3 inflammasome, such as amyloid plaques [10], cholesterol crystals [11], and uric acid crystals [12].

There is significant overlap between the properties of "bioactive" natural particles and bioactive ENM (see Table 3.1), suggesting that the mechanisms of toxicity are not dependent on source or type, but on properties contributing to bioactivity (e.g., size, rigidity, and ability to induce LMP). Crystalline silica is generally considered to be a more toxic form than amorphous or colloidal silica particles [13]. Similarly, crocidolite [14, 15] and chrysotile [16] are types of asbestos that have been well documented to cause severe pulmonary disorders and cancer, whereas wollastonite is considered to be a relatively benign form of a crystalline mineral [17, 18]. In fact, wollastonite has been used as a control particle for comparisons to asbestos in toxicity studies [19]. In addition, the degree of bioactivity can be altered through processing methods as described by Sandberg et al. [20], who observed similarities in bioactivity as measured by the release of IL-1β from macrophages treated with both crystalline and noncrystalline silica particles in the nano- and submicron-size range [20]. These differences in toxicity correlate well with the ability of the most toxic forms within the various particle types to increase "bioactive" cellular pathways, resulting in inflammation and/or cell death. This suggests that particle toxicity is due to an initiating event or pathway that is common to all "toxic" particles but absent in the less toxic forms.

3.2 Lysosomal Membrane Permeabilization

Cellular lysosomes are critical organelles that have been affectionately dubbed the "recycling centers" of the cell [21]. The lysosome contains a highly concentrated pool of hydrolases that are capable of degrading macromolecules within the cell. While lysosomes serve an important function in maintaining cellular homeostasis, damage to the lysosomal membrane can result in permeabilization and subsequent "leakage" of the hydrolases into the cytosol. Generally, leakage of the lysosomal contents leads to a phenomenon known as lysosomal cell death, which may oftentimes resemble necrotic or apoptotic pathways. Note that literal usage of the phrase "lysosomal membrane permeabilization" pertains to lysosomes only, but common usage is typically inclusive of both lysosomes and other vesicles formed by fusion with lysosomes (e.g., phagolysosomes). In either scenario, LMP leads to the release of degradative lysosomal contents, which may have significant downstream consequences.

There are a number of environmental agents and/or events that are known to cause LMP, aside from particles. Weak bases that cross through the lysosomal membrane and then become trapped after protonation in the acidic environment of the lysosome can acquire detergent properties that enable them to weaken the lysosomal membrane [22]. These "lysosomotropic detergents" can be potent inducers of LMP. Similarly, viruses that rupture the lysosomal membrane and become active within the acidic environment can cause LMP [23]. Other known

Table 3.1 Evidence for particle-associated lysosomal membrane permeabilization, NLRP3 inflammasome activation, mitochondrial dysfunction, and apoptosis

Particle type		LMP	NLRP3 inflammasome activation	Mitochondrial dysfunction	Apoptosis
Silica	Crystalline	Observed within 1 h in alveolar macrophages [149, 50]	Upregulated components of the NLRP3 inflammasome in BEAS-2B (human bronchial epithelial cell line), normal human bronchial epithelial cells [150], and rat lungs [115]	*In vitro* exposure in MH-S macrophages resulted in significant mitochondrial depolarization within 2 h of exposure [151]	Silica-induced apoptosis in MH-S macrophage cells is preceded by LMP [149]
	Amorphous	Observed within 1 h following exposure in MH-S cells [152]. Nanosized particles are more potent than larger particles in bone marrow-derived macrophages [153]	Effect not observed at micron level. Nanosized particles induce IL-1β in raw 264.7 macrophages [20] and bone marrow-derived macrophages [153]	Effect not observed at micron level. Nanoparticles increased citrate synthase and decreased malate dehydrogenase activity in U87 cells (human astrocytoma) [154]	Effect not observed at micron level. Amorphous silica nanoparticles induce apoptosis in RAW264.7 macrophages [155]
Environmental fibers	Chrysotile	Significant release of lysosomal enzymes in alveolar macrophages [38]	Activates inflammasome in THP-1 macrophage cells [156]	No effects were observed on isolated mitochondria [157]	Low doses induce apoptosis in human alveolar macrophages [19].
	Crocidolite	LMP observed in rat lung cells [158]	Activates the NLRP3 inflammasome in human mesothelial cells [159] and human macrophages [78]	Induces mitochondrial damage in mesothelial cells [160]	Low doses induce apoptosis in human alveolar macrophages [19].
	Wollastonite	No lysosomal damage in alveolar macrophages [38]	Effect not observed	Effect not observed	Effect not observed

ENM	MWCNT	Cause LMP in A549 human lung epithelial cells [161]. LMP is more pronounced in the presence of high nickel contamination [162]	Induce the release of IL-1β in alveolar macrophages [163], which is modified by HMGB1 [109]	Dose-dependent decline in mitochondrial integrity [161]	Enhanced apoptosis was observed with both long and rigid MWCNT in mouse lungs [164]
	Titanium dioxide	Nanosized titanium particles induce LMP in alveolar macrophages [83]	Facilitates the release of IL-1β in macrophages through the active release of ATP into the extracellular space [165, 83]	Decreases mitochondrial membrane potential and release of proapoptotic molecules [166]	Induces apoptotic cell death in Chang (liver), MCF10A (breast epithelial), and WI38 (lung fibroblast) normal human cell lines [166]

inducers of LMP include bacterial toxins that destabilize the lysosomal membrane [24], reactive oxygen species formed from the degradation of iron-containing macromolecules [25], cathepsin proteases [26], apoptotic caspases [27], phospholipase A2 activation [28], and p53 activation [29].

The uptake of both environmental particles [30, 31] and ENM [32] into cellular phagosomes is a well-documented process that has been shown in multiple studies. Subsequent to phagocytosis, the particle-containing phagosomes fuse with the lysosome, resulting in the formation of a phagolysosome. Under normal circumstances, the formation of a phagolysosome allows the degradation of the phagosomal contents via the hydrolytic enzymes within the acidic environment of the lysosome. However, certain bioactive particles cause permeabilization of the phagolysosomal membrane. This phenomenon has been demonstrated with the more toxic environmental particles and ENM tested to date. It is this initial event causing LMP that appears to determine the pathogenic potential of a particle. For example, asbestos fibers are known to cause LMP and have also been demonstrated to be potent pulmonary toxicants [33, 34] and carcinogens [35–37], whereas wollastonite has low toxicity profiles and does not cause LMP [38]. Similarly, titanium dioxide nanoparticles have shown a potent (size-dependent) bioactivity in animal and cell culture studies [39, 40]; carbon nanotubes with long, needlelike properties also display similar bioactivity to that seen with asbestos [41]. Other ENM known to cause pathologies and LMP include zinc oxide nanoparticles [42] and cationic nanoparticles [43].

3.3 Potential Causes of Particle-Induced LMP

3.3.1 Cholesterol Trafficking

It has been suggested that cholesterol trafficking may play a significant role in mediating lysosomal membrane permeability (Fig. 3.1). For example, lysosomal stability is increased by the addition of cholesterol [44–46]; accordingly, reduced lysosomal cholesterol content increases the potential for lysosomal membrane destabilization [47]. In addition, cholesterol cannot be degraded within the lysosome and must be actively transported out of the organelle [48]. Interestingly, crocidolite asbestos has been shown to inhibit the cholesterol synthesis pathway [49], and evidence suggests that exposure to silica reduces lysosomal cholesterol content and subsequent release of pro-inflammatory mediators [50].

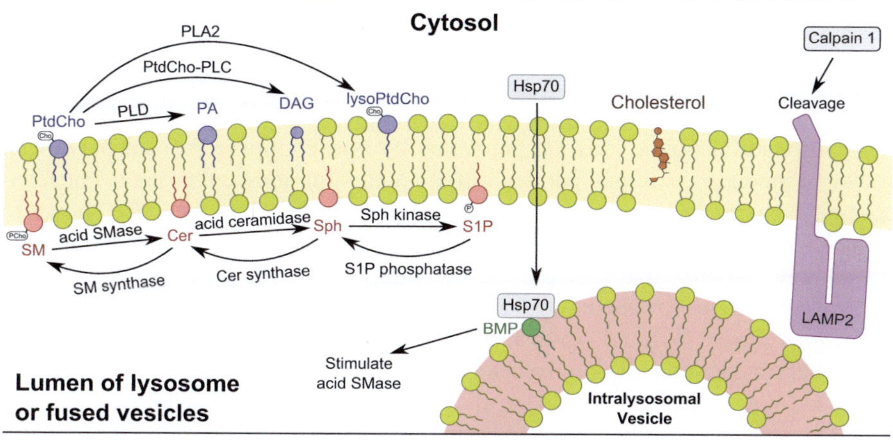

Fig. 3.1 Potential regulators of particle-induced lysosome membrane permeabilization (LMP). Shown in this diagram are membranes of a lysosome and an intralysosomal vesicle. Alterations in lysosomal membrane cholesterol content can contribute to LMP. Similarly, LMP can be caused by a disruption of sphingolipid metabolism at various stages, such as altered acid SMase activity. Hsp70 has been shown to enter the lysosome and bind to the phospholipid BMP, facilitating its activity as an acid SMase cofactor. Activities of phospholipases PLA2, PtdCho-PLC, and PLD have been proposed to contribute to LMP. Finally, LMP can be induced by cleavage of the LAMP2 protein by calpain 1. Abbreviations: *BMP* bis(monoacylglycero)phosphate, *Cer* ceramide, *Cho* choline, *DAG* diacylglycerol, *Hsp70* heat shock protein 70, *LAMP2* lysosome-associated membrane glycoprotein 2, *P* phosphate, *PA* phosphatidic acid, *PL* phospholipase (i.e., phospholipase C=PLC), *PtdCho* phosphatidylcholine, *S1P* sphingosine-1-phosphate, *SM* sphingomyelin, *Sph* sphingosine

3.3.2 Sphingomyelin Pathway

The incorporation of cholesterol into the lysosomal compartment is coordinately regulated by sphingomyelin, which acts as a scaffold within the lysosomal membrane [51]. Proteolytic cleavage of the sterol regulator element-binding proteins also regulates cholesterol and membrane fatty acid profiles within cellular organelles by modifying transcription of their biosynthetic genes [52]. Sphingosine, which is formed due to the activity of either ceramidase or sphingosine-1 phosphate (S1P) phosphatases, promotes apoptosis [53] and contributes to LMP via its detergent-like properties [54]. Heat shock protein (Hsp) 70 binding to the endolysosomal phospholipid BMP leads to increased activity of acid sphingomyelinase, which has been shown to stabilize lysosomal membranes (Fig. 3.1) [55]. Acid sphingomyelinase catalyzes hydrolysis of sphingomyelin to form ceramide and phosphorylcholine and is proposed to promote survival in cancer cells through the stabilization of the lysosomal membrane [56].

3.3.3 Other Membrane Phospholipids

The phospholipid composition of the lysosomal membrane is critical for maintaining membrane integrity. For example, arachidonic acid [57] and lysophosphatidylcholine [58] are generated by phospholipase A2 and have been shown to increase lysosomal permeability to potassium ions and protons. Phosphatidic acid, the hydrolysis product of phosphatidylcholine, has also been shown to destabilize the lysosomal membrane [59]. In addition to the phospholipids themselves, key enzymes that regulate the membrane lipid composition can alter the membrane function, including phospholipase A2, phospholipase C, and sphingomyelinase (Fig. 3.1) [54]. In fact, silica nanoparticles, multiwalled carbon nanotubes, and carbon black have been shown to stimulate the activity of phospholipase C [60]. Similarly, superoxide production caused by exposure to chrysotile asbestos is proposed to be mediated by the phospholipase A2 enzyme [61].

3.3.4 Calpain 1 and LAMP2

The calpains are a family of cysteine proteases that are known to inhibit autophagy [62]. Calpain 1, specifically, has been shown to induce lysosomal membrane permeability through cleavage of the lysosomal-associated membrane protein 2 (LAMP2) (Fig. 3.1)—a process that is inhibited through the use of calpain inhibitors [63, 64]. While there are 25 known lysosomal membrane proteins [65], LAMP2 specifically is a single-spanning transmembrane protein contributing to as much as 50 % of all proteins within the lysosome and late endosome membranes [66]; LAMP2 is also required for maturation of autophagosomes [67].

3.3.5 Autophagy

Autophagy is a highly conserved mechanism by which cells maintain homeostasis through sequestration, degradation, and recycling of damaged cytosolic macromolecules and organelles. Ubiquitinated macromolecular structures are specifically targeted to autophagic vesicles via the sequestosome (p62), which is contained together with the targeted structure inside the forming autophagic vesicle [68]. Autophagosomes are known to take up a variety of nanoparticles within different cell types [69]—a phenomenon that may result in the dysfunction of the autophagy pathway [70]. Disruption of the autophagic pathway has been attributed to increased cytotoxicity and inflammation following exposure to rare earth nanoparticles and CNT. In addition, phagophores—autophagic initiating organelles—have been demonstrated to maintain close proximity with lysosomes and late endosomes [71]; therefore, opportunities exist for the disruption of the lysosomal membrane upon uptake of bioactive particles. Interactions between rare earth oxide nanoparticles and autophagosomes may give some insight into the mechanisms relating autophagy disruption and lysosomal membrane permeabilization. Specifically, rare earth oxide nanoparticles disrupt the autophagic flux and function of the lysosomal phosphoproteins [72]. This, in turn, prevents the acidification necessary for the formation of the autolysosome.

3.4 Consequences of LMP

Downstream events following LMP include mitochondrial damage and reactive oxygen species (ROS) formation, release of cathepsin B, NLRP3 inflammasome activation, and cell death. It is these features that determine whether a particle is labeled as "bioactive" and ultimately allows it to be categorized as safe or hazardous. The initiating event for particle-induced toxicity appears to be LMP. For example, Joshi and Knecht demonstrated that the earliest detectable cellular event following chronic inhalation of crystalline silica was phagolysosomal leakage, which ultimately resulted in macrophage cell death by apoptosis and necrosis [73]. As illustrated in Fig. 3.2, in the presence of a second signaling event such as NF-κB, bioactive particles are taken up by a phagosome, which then fuses with the intracellular lysosomes and effectively causes LMP. Subsequent release of the lysosomal proteases such as cathepsin B causes several downstream events, including 1) the activation of the inflammasome and caspase-1-mediated maturation of IL-1β and IL-18 and 2) mitochondrial damage and production of ROS leading to 3) cell death. Therefore, it is critical to note that the prevention of LMP would, effectively, attenuate the pathological consequences of exposure to bioactive ENM and particles [74].

*3.4.1 NLRP3 Inflammasome Activation and Release of IL-1*β *and IL-18*

Chronic inflammation is gaining recognition as a primary contributing factor to many degenerative and environmentally related diseases such as heart disease [75], cancer [76], and fibrosis [77]. Environmental particles, in particular, are known to contribute to inflammation by activating the NLRP3 inflammasome [78, 79], which results in increased levels of the pro-inflammatory cytokines IL-1β and IL-18 [80–82]. Similarly, titanium nanoparticles have been shown to activate the NLRP3 inflammasome [83]. In addition, some forms of multiwalled carbon nanotubes (MWCNT) also cause lung inflammation and fibrosis. The mechanisms have not been fully elucidated, but it has been shown that lysosomal disruption [69], autophagy [69], and NLRP3 inflammasome activation [84] most likely play a role.

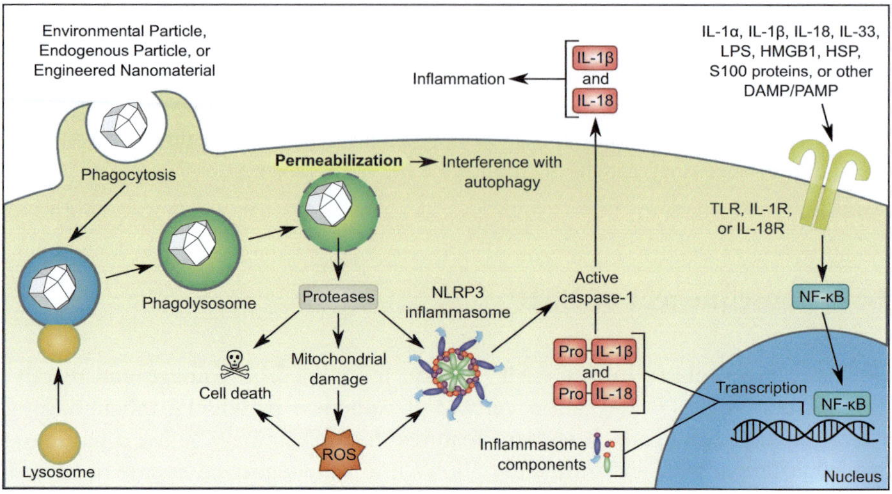

Fig. 3.2 Consequences of lysosome membrane permeabilization. Environmental particles, endogenous particles, or engineered nanomaterials enter the cell by phagocytosis, and then the phagosome fuses with a lysosome to form a phagolysosome. Permeabilization of the phagolysosome leads to the release of proteases into the cytosol, which induces cell death and the activation of the NLRP3 inflammasome, either directly or indirectly through mitochondrial damage. NLRP3 inflammasome assembly leads to the activation of caspase-1, which cleaves the propeptide from IL-1β and IL-18. Secretion of these mature cytokines increases the inflammatory response. A second signal is required to activate NF-κB transcriptional upregulation of pro-IL-1β, pro-IL-18, and inflammasome proteins. This second signal may include various alarmins or IL-1 family cytokines

While mechanisms involved in the activation of the NLRP3 inflammasome have not been entirely elucidated, it is understood that events causing stress or result in "danger" signals promote recruitment of an adaptor protein ASC. The assembly of NLRP3 and ASC facilitates binding of procaspase-1 [85], which is activated by proximity-induced autoproteolysis [86]. In turn, active caspase-1 processes pro-IL-1β and pro-IL-18 to their active forms IL-1β and IL-18, respectively [87]. IL-1β, in particular, has been associated with a wide array of inflammatory conditions [88]. In fact, the activation of the NLRP3 inflammasome and the subsequent release of IL-1β have been linked to pathologies associated with both asbestos and silica [89]; ENM with various physicochemical properties are also known to activate the NLRP3 inflammasome [90, 91]. Lysosomal membrane permeabilization is likely the event that initiates inflammasome activation following particle exposure.

3.4.2 Mitochondrial ROS Production and Cell Death

It is well known that exposure to bioactive ENM and environmental particles results in the generation of ROS. A question that arises is whether the ROS is a cause or consequence of particle-induced bioactivity. While ROS have long been considered a primary player in the toxicity of environmental particles, some evidence suggests their role in determining a particle's bioactivity may be less significant than previously thought. For example, environmental particles causing similar oxidative stress effects *in vitro* are known to cause diverse pathologies *in vivo* [92]. Furthermore, recent evidence suggests that the release of proteases from a compromised lysosome may result in mitochondrial damage and subsequently generate ROS [21, 54] (Fig. 3.2). Consequently, mitochondrial-generated ROS and the release of pro-inflammatory cytokines have attracted attention for their possible role in chronic inflammation and disease [93]. Mitochondrial ROS have also been reported to activate the NLRP3 inflammasome [94], an event that has been well characterized for bioactive nanoparticles. These data provide important insight into the importance of LMP in particle-induced ROS generation and the subsequent initiation of cell death. Moreover, studies have shown that LMP can initiate the intrinsic apoptosis pathway [95], and it is well known that environmental particles and silica can contribute to apoptosis [19, 96–98]. Similarly, the induction of apoptosis has been observed in many types of ENM [83, 99–101]. While LMP has not been confirmed for all types of bioactive ENM, a trend is emerging that could link environmental particle- and ENM-induced apoptosis to the release of lysosomal proteases that lead to mitochondrial damage and initiation of the apoptotic signaling cascades. Exposure to titanium dioxide nanoparticles reduced the stability of the mitochondrial membrane in mouse epidermal JB6 cells, ultimately resulting in apoptosis [102]. The effects of titanium dioxide nanoparticles on the mitochondrial membrane, along with increased ROS generation, were further confirmed in human lung fibroblast WI-38 cells [103]. Similarly, asbestos fibers are known to generate ROS [104, 105] and to cause apoptosis [19, 106, 107]—an effect that is not observed with the nonfibrogenic wollastonite fibers [19].

3.4.3 Role of Cellular "Alarmins"

3.4.3.1 DAMPs

The production of pro-inflammatory cytokines following exposure to bioactive particles is dependent upon the activation of NF-κB, as illustrated in Fig. 3.2. Danger-associated molecular patterns (DAMPs) encompass a broad class of cellular proteins, lipids, and nucleic acids released following sterile injury and are primarily pro-inflammatory or chemotactic in nature. DAMPs play a critical role in regulating the NF-κB pathway during inflammation in acute lung injury caused by trauma or bleomycin and fibrosis that occurs from these conditions. A well-described DAMP involved in particle exposure is high-mobility group box 1 (HMGB1), though others are likely involved such as IL-1α, S100s, and Hsps [108–110]. HMGB1 also plays an important role in autoinflammatory diseases that have been linked to particle exposure [111–113].

Under normal physiological conditions, HMGB1 is an abundant nuclear protein that participates in DNA packaging and transcription regulation. HMGB1 is released from the cell following exposure to particles including silica, asbestos, uric acid crystals, and MWCNT [109, 114–116]. Necrotic cell death is a major source of DAMPs, including HMGB1, and has been implicated in asbestos-induced inflammation [116]. Apoptosis is also elevated following exposure to most bioactive particulates and can also be a source of HMGB1; however, the primary activity of HMGB1, whether pro-inflammatory or chemotactic under these circumstances, is not well defined. Macrophages have been shown to actively secrete HMGB1 through an NLRP3 inflammasome and caspase-1-mediated pathway following exposure to silica, MWCNT, and other nonparticulate NLRP3-activating agents [109, 117]. The mechanism, by which particles induce HMGB1 release, whether it is mediated by cell death or the inflammasome, is likely dependent upon the dose of the particle and the type of cell involved (i.e., whether a lung macrophage or epithelial cell). Many extracellular DAMPs, including HMGB1, bind TLR4 and the receptor for advanced glycation end products (RAGE), resulting in the activation of the NF-κB pathway and MAPK pathways [118]. It is reported that specific redox states of HMGB1 regulate its extracellular activity as a chemotactic DAMP or an activator of TLR4 to promote inflammation [119]. Additionally, extracellular HMGB1 has been shown to complex with other extracellular proteins or nucleic acid and bind to TLR2 and TLR9 [120].

3.4.3.2 PAMPs

Pathogen-associated molecular patterns (PAMPs) and DAMPs act upon similar receptors to activate the NF-κB transcription response. An example of a common PAMP is lipopolysaccharide, which binds TLR4 to activate NF-κB. In addition, exposing rodents to endotoxin exacerbates MWCNT-induced inflammation and pathology [121]. Though PAMPs likely play a role in disease progression in humans, many studies do not account for their potential contribution because the research is typically done in specific-pathogen-free animals.

3.4.3.3 IL-1α

IL-1α is considered to be a cellular alarmin that is released following the activation of caspase-1, -11, and initiation of pyroptosis [122]. Pyroptosis is a caspase-1-dependent inflammatory form of cell death that is characterized by the release of pro-inflammatory cytokines, such as IL-1β, IL-18, and IL-1α. Unlike IL-1β, IL-1α does not require processing into its active form and is available to immediately bind with its receptor to initiate transcription of pro-inflammatory genes via the NF-κB pathway [110]. The cyclical process involving recognition of pyroptotic cells, release of alarmins, inflammasome activation, and further induction of pyroptotic cell death is thought to be a key element of noninfectious inflammatory pathways

[123]. In fact, the early release of IL-1α and IL-33 into the alveolar space following treatment with silica preceded the expression of pro-IL-1β and neutrophilic inflammation in mice [110]. Furthermore, the degree of lung inflammation in mice following exposure to silica correlated with the release of IL-1α in J774 macrophages [110]. The importance of IL-1α in particle-induced toxicity has only recently gained attention, and wide gaps in knowledge still remain to be elucidated. However, the mechanism responsible for IL-1 α secretion in response to particles has not been explained, and the interrelationship between IL-1 α secretion and IL-1β secretion is still unclear.

3.4.3.4 IL-33

IL-33 is a constitutively expressed alarmin that serves to alert the immune system of damage to endothelial or epithelial cells following trauma or infection [124]. Elevated levels of IL-33 have been observed in mice exposed to MWCNT experiencing impaired pulmonary function [125, 126]. Furthermore, the toxicity of MWCNT is attenuated in mice lacking sufficient mast cell populations or mast cells that are unable to respond to the IL-33 danger signals [127].

3.5 Disease Outcomes

While evidence is mounting in support of LMP as the determinant of the pathogenic potential of a particle or fiber and as such the initiating event for the downstream pathologies associated with exposure to bioactive particles and fibers, there are still wide gaps in knowledge. Mechanisms for asbestos, silica, and ENM toxicity may share similar convergent pathways; however, there can be wide differences in actual disease outcomes through divergent pathways (Fig. 3.3). Subsequently, although the prediction of the pathogenic potential of ENM may be achievable through the convergent mechanism of LMP, further investigations will be needed as to the prediction of the disease outcome that may be associated with exposure to ENM.

These differences in divergent pathways produced by environmental particles, fibers, and ENM may be due, in part, to exposure route, duration, location, downstream targets, and/or particle tendency to migrate within the different body compartments. The differences may also be the result of their surface and other properties. For example, transformation of the particles once they have been introduced into a biological system may play a role in the subsequent development of disease. Various rates of diffusion, aggregation, and sedimentation within the bloodstream may modify the way a particle will interact with biomolecules and influence the resulting particle biological outcomes [128] as well as their ability to cross biological barriers. Finally, differential immune responses between the

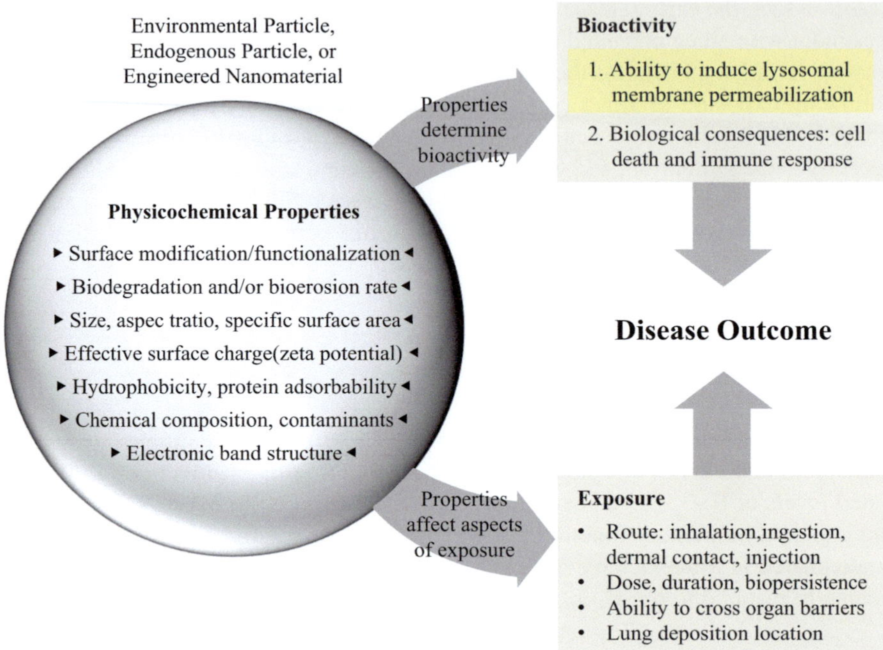

Fig. 3.3 Factors affecting disease outcome. Physicochemical properties of environmental particles, endogenous particles, or engineered nanomaterials determine their bioactivity and affect certain aspects of exposure. For example, particle hydrophobicity will determine the composition of its protein corona, which affects the ability of the particle to cross organ barriers. Exposure and particle bioactivity both contribute to the development of disease

various particles and fibers may also be an important divergent pathway and hence determinant of disease outcome.

3.5.1 ENM Surface Modifications

ENM surface modifications, such as the addition of peptides designed to help penetrate cellular membranes, may affect their ability to move between cells. This transcellular movement has been shown to create temporary holes in the membrane and cause membrane thinning and erosion [129]. Modifications to the ENM surface can also influence whether it is able to penetrate the cell membrane without disrupting the bilayer in order to cross between cells. These modifications may also determine if the ENM will become trapped within the endosomal compartment [130]. The goal of modifying ENM surfaces is to create particles with properties that easily lend them to specific industrial uses. However, disruption of the cellular membrane and facilitation of cell-to-cell translocation can increase particle toxicity [129] and possibly lead to more severe disease outcomes.

3.5.2 Route of Administration

A likely factor for determining the risk of particle-induced pathologies is the route of exposure, including inhalation, ingestion, dermal contact, or direct injection into the circulation. The majority of research has focused on inhalation as the most concerning route. Research has shown that particle size determines whether the particles will be deposited in the nasopharyngeal, tracheobronchial, or alveolar regions of the respiratory tract [128]. These differences in pulmonary deposition may affect outcomes associated with the respiratory tract and the likelihood of translocation to peripheral organs and subsequent disease outcomes. For example, particles entering the body through an inhalation exposure have been observed to translocate to the liver, spleen, kidneys, heart, brain, bone, and soft tissues [131]. Studies analyzing the outcome from ingesting radiolabeled gold nanoparticles also found a differential accumulation of the material depending on size and charge. Specifically, the highest accumulation of the particle in secondary organs occurred with the smaller and positively charged particles. The highest accumulation of gold particles was found in the brain and heart tissues following ingestion [132].

3.5.3 Crossing Organ Barriers

The ability of particles to permeate specific barriers between the different organ systems, such as the blood–brain barrier, the blood–testis barrier, and the placental barrier, may provide powerful clues toward determining disease outcomes. In addition to the route of exposure and size, various physicochemical properties of the nanoparticle may be particularly important for determining their ability to cross organ barriers. For example, it is known that internalized particles may undergo a process of exocytosis [133]. This may, in turn, result in the attachment of various macromolecules that make up a protein coat around the particle known as a "corona." The composition of the particle's corona may then influence its likelihood of undergoing passive or active transport and even subsequent turns of endocytosis in order to cross organ barriers [134]. The formation of a biomolecular corona on the surface of the particles has been described as "conferring a new biological identity" to the particle in question [135], with possible long-term consequences for the development of disease.

3.5.4 Innate and Adaptive Immune Responses

An increased immune response resulting from particle exposure is a hallmark of the bioactivity that results from LMP. However, differential immune responses between the various particles have been observed. For example, the development of silicosis is thought to predominantly involve a T-helper-1-like response in mice that is characterized by lung lymphocytes, primarily CD4+ T cells and natural killer cells [136]. However, silicosis has also been shown to develop in the absence of an adaptive immune response [137]. The transition between innate and adaptive responses and the corresponding release of inflammatory cytokines and transcription factors following particle exposure could have significant consequences for disease development. This phenomenon is being exploited in the development of suitable vaccines against various pathogens. Particle size has been shown to influence the balance of type 1/type 2 cytokines following immunization with nanobeads serving as antigen carriers in mice [138]. While benefits, such as those observed in the development of nanomedicines, may exist, a better understanding of circumstances in which those benefits turn detrimental is warranted.

Finally, it is also important to mention that due to these identified differences, certain but not all bioactive particles and fibers make individuals susceptible to other environmental exposures. For example, asbestosis and silicosis are two well-characterized diseases resulting from exposure to asbestos and silica, respectively, where each disease presents with specific characteristics that are unique to its specific pathology [139]. Although exposure to silica is widely known to increase one's risk of contracting tuberculosis [140, 141], a similar relationship between asbestos and tuberculosis has only recently been investigated [142] and has not been examined for ENM.

3.5.5 Acute Versus Long-Term Effects

Exposure to dissimilar ENM can result in differential effects when comparing acute, local effects to long-term systemic responses [143]; however, the relationship between acute toxicity and long-term progression of disease is not well understood. Evidence suggests that disease outcomes can be variable depending on the number and duration of exposure events. For example, rats exposed to a single dose of cobalt metal dust mixed with tungsten carbide particles experienced acute alveolitis persisting for more than one month, yet no evidence of fibrosis was present four months following the exposure. In contrast, repeated intratracheal instillations of cobalt metal dust mixed with tungsten carbide particles one month apart resulted in interstitial fibrosis that could be differentiated from the fibrotic response following exposure to crystalline silica [144]. Similarly, acute instillations of silver nanoparticles are rapidly cleared by the lung but then enter systemic circulation inducing possible long-term disease outcomes [145]. Size and surface coating may also play an important function in mediating acute versus long-term disease outcomes to ENM, but the details are not well understood [146]. Compounding the issue are unexpected *in vivo* pathological outcomes that differ from those predicted solely from *in vitro* toxicity studies [92]. Clearly there is a very important role for *in vitro* studies that are mechanistically based to screen large numbers of new materials such as ENM. However, due to the infinite number of potential ENM, long-term studies become time and cost prohibitive. Nevertheless, a reliance on *in vitro* studies for assessing risk and disease outcome may be inappropriate.

3.6 Summary

The physicochemical properties of ENM continue to be recognized as important factors in determining the bioactivity or biocompatibility of ENM. Specifically, aspect ratio, dissolution, material bandgap, ROS generation, surface charge, and surface chemistry have been shown to be important factors [147]. Similar conclusions have been reported for natural particles such as silica and asbestos [148]. While these characteristics are undoubtedly important for determining whether or not a particle will be bioactive and therefore cause a pathological response, we propose that these factors either contribute to or are a direct consequence of LMP. As a result, LMP is the most likely defining factor for particle bioactivity and should be used as a routine screening tool for gauging toxicity. However, although the prediction of the pathogenic potential of ENM may be achievable through the convergent mechanism of LMP, further investigations will be needed as to the prediction of the disease outcome that may be associated with exposure to particles. In fact, future research focusing on the divergent mechanisms resulting in variable pathologies following LMP may prove to be critical in the overall risk assessment for particle exposure.

References

1. Delgado GC. Economics and governance of nanomaterials: potential and risks. Technol Soc. 2010;32(2):137–44.
2. Morigi V, Tocchio A, Bellavite Pellegrini C, Sakamoto JH, Arnone M, Tasciotti E. Nanotechnology in medicine: from inception to market domination. J Drug Deliv. 2012;2012:389485. doi:10.1155/2012/389485.
3. Donaldson K, Seaton A. A short history of the toxicology of inhaled particles. Part Fibre Toxicol. 2012;9:13. doi:10.1186/1743-8977-9-13.
4. Stanton MF, Layard M, Tegeris A, Miller E, May M, Morgan E, et al. Relation of particle dimension to carcinogenicity in amphibole asbestoses and other fibrous minerals. J Natl Cancer Inst. 1981;67(5):965–75.
5. Bignon J, Saracci R, Touray JC. Introduction: INSERM-IARC-CNRS workshop on biopersistence of respirable synthetic fibers and minerals. Environ Health Perspect. 1994;102 Suppl 5:3–5.
6. Oberdorster G, Stone V, Donaldson K. Toxicology of nanoparticles: a historical perspective. Nanotoxicology. 2007;1(1):2–25.
7. Yameen B, Choi WI, Vilos C, Swami A, Shi J, Farokhzad OC. Insight into nanoparticle cellular uptake and intracellular targeting. J Control Release. 2014;190:485–99. doi:10.1016/j.jconrel.2014.06.038.

8. Sarrazin S, Wilson B, Sly WS, Tor Y, Esko JD. Guanidinylated neomycin mediates heparan sulfate-dependent transport of active enzymes to lysosomes. Mol Ther. 2010;18(7):1268–74. doi:10.1038/mt.2010.78.
9. Seydoux E, Rothen-Rutishauser B, Nita IM, Balog S, Gazdhar A, Stumbles PA, et al. Size-dependent accumulation of particles in lysosomes modulates dendritic cell function through impaired antigen degradation. Int J Nanomedicine. 2014;9:3885–902. doi:10.2147/IJN.S64353.
10. Niemi K, Teirila L, Lappalainen J, Rajamaki K, Baumann MH, Oorni K, et al. Serum amyloid A activates the NLRP3 inflammasome via P2X7 receptor and a cathepsin B-sensitive pathway. J Immunol. 2011;186(11):6119–28. doi:10.4049/jimmunol.1002843.
11. Samstad EO, Niyonzima N, Nymo S, Aune MH, Ryan L, Bakke SS, et al. Cholesterol crystals induce complement-dependent inflammasome activation and cytokine release. J Immunol. 2014;192(6):2837–45. doi:10.4049/jimmunol.1302484.
12. Gasse P, Riteau N, Charron S, Girre S, Fick L, Petrilli V, et al. Uric acid is a danger signal activating NALP3 inflammasome in lung injury inflammation and fibrosis. Am J Respir Crit Care Med. 2009;179(10):903–13. doi:10.1164/rccm.200808-1274OC.
13. Warheit DB, McHugh TA, Hartsky MA. Differential pulmonary responses in rats inhaling crystalline, colloidal or amorphous silica dusts. Scand J Work Environ Health. 1995;21 Suppl 2:19–21.
14. Luo S, Liu X, Mu S, Tsai SP, Wen CP. Asbestos related diseases from environmental exposure to crocidolite in Da-yao, China. I. Review of exposure and epidemiological data. Occup Environ Med. 2003;60(1):35–41; discussion −2.
15. Gibbs GW, Berry G. Mesothelioma and asbestos. Regul Toxicol Pharmacol. 2008;52 (1 Suppl):S223–31. doi:10.1016/j.yrtph.2007.10.003.
16. Sen D. Working with asbestos and the possible health risks. Occup Med (Lond). 2015;65 (1):6–14. doi:10.1093/occmed/kqu175.
17. Maxim LD, McConnell EE. A review of the toxicology and epidemiology of wollastonite. Inhal Toxicol. 2005;17(9):451–66. doi:10.1080/08958370591002030.
18. Maxim LD, Niebo R, Utell MJ, McConnell EE, Larosa S, Segrave AM. Wollastonite toxicity: an update. Inhal Toxicol. 2014;26(2):95–112. doi:10.3109/08958378.2013.857372.
19. Hamilton RF, Iyer LL, Holian A. Asbestos induces apoptosis in human alveolar macrophages. Am J Physiol. 1996;271(5 Pt 1):L813–19.
20. Sandberg WJ, Lag M, Holme JA, Friede B, Gualtieri M, Kruszewski M, et al. Comparison of non-crystalline silica nanoparticles in IL-1beta release from macrophages. Part Fibre Toxicol. 2012;9:32. doi:10.1186/1743-8977-9-32.
21. Aits S, Jaattela M. Lysosomal cell death at a glance. J Cell Sci. 2013;126(Pt 9):1905–12. doi:10.1242/jcs.091181.
22. de Duve C, de Barsy T, Poole B, Trouet A, Tulkens P, Van Hoof F. Commentary. Lysosomotropic agents. Biochem Pharmacol. 1974;23(18):2495–531.
23. Prchla E, Plank C, Wagner E, Blaas D, Fuchs R. Virus-mediated release of endosomal content *in vitro*: different behavior of adenovirus and rhinovirus serotype 2. J Cell Biol. 1995;131(1):111–23.
24. Sandvig K, van Deurs B. Delivery into cells: lessons learned from plant and bacterial toxins. Gene Ther. 2005;12(11):865–72. doi:10.1038/sj.gt.3302525.
25. Kurz T, Terman A, Gustafsson B, Brunk UT. Lysosomes and oxidative stress in aging and apoptosis. Biochim Biophys Acta. 2008;1780(11):1291–303. doi:10.1016/j.bbagen.2008.01.009.
26. Groth-Pedersen L, Aits S, Corcelle-Termeau E, Petersen NH, Nylandsted J, Jaattela M. Identification of cytoskeleton-associated proteins essential for lysosomal stability and survival of human cancer cells. PLoS ONE. 2012;7(10):e45381. doi:10.1371/journal.pone.0045381.
27. Oberle C, Huai J, Reinheckel T, Tacke M, Rassner M, Ekert PG, et al. Lysosomal membrane permeabilization and cathepsin release is a Bax/Bak-dependent, amplifying event of

apoptosis in fibroblasts and monocytes. Cell Death Differ. 2010;17(7):1167–78. doi:10.1038/cdd.2009.214.
28. Zhao M, Brunk UT, Eaton JW. Delayed oxidant-induced cell death involves activation of phospholipase A2. FEBS Lett. 2001;509(3):399–404.
29. Yuan XM, Li W, Dalen H, Lotem J, Kama R, Sachs L, et al. Lysosomal destabilization in p53-induced apoptosis. Proc Natl Acad Sci U S A. 2002;99(9):6286–91. doi:10.1073/pnas.092135599.
30. Suzuki Y. Interaction of asbestos with alveolar cells. Environ Health Perspect. 1974;9:241–52.
31. Johnson NF, Davies R. Effect of asbestos on the P388D1 macrophagelike cell line: preliminary ultrastructural observations. Environ Health Perspect. 1983;51:109–17.
32. Hamilton RF, Buford M, Xiang C, Wu N, Holian A. NLRP3 inflammasome activation in murine alveolar macrophages and related lung pathology is associated with MWCNT nickel contamination. Inhal Toxicol. 2012;24(14):995–1008.
33. Kopylev L, Christensen KY, Brown JS, Cooper GS. A systematic review of the association between pleural plaques and changes in lung function. Occup Environ Med. 2015;72(8):606–14. doi:10.1136/oemed-2014-102468.
34. Norbet C, Joseph A, Rossi SS, Bhalla S, Gutierrez FR. Asbestos-related lung disease: a pictorial review. Curr Probl Diagn Radiol. 2015;44(4):371–82. doi:10.1067/j.cpradiol.2014.10.002.
35. Markowitz SB, Levin SM, Miller A, Morabia A. Asbestos, asbestosis, smoking, and lung cancer. New findings from the North American insulator cohort. Am J Respir Crit Care Med. 2013;188(1):90–6. doi:10.1164/rccm.201302-0257OC.
36. Bianchi C, Bianchi T. Global mesothelioma epidemic: trend and features. Indian J Occup Environ Med. 2014;18(2):82–8. doi:10.4103/0019-5278.146897.
37. Bounin A, Charbotel B, Fervers B, Bergeret A. Professional risk factors associated with the cancer of the ovary. Lit Rev Bull Cancer. 2014;101(12):1089–108. doi:10.1684/bdc.2014.1978.
38. Pailes WH, Judy DJ, Resnick H, Castranova V. Relative effects of asbestos and wollastonite on alveolar macrophages. J Toxicol Environ Health. 1984;14(4):497–510. doi:10.1080/15287398409530601.
39. Xia T, Hamilton RF, Bonner JC, Crandall ED, Elder A, Fazlollahi F, et al. Interlaboratory evaluation of *in vitro* cytotoxicity and inflammatory responses to engineered nanomaterials: the NIEHS Nano GO Consortium. Environ Health Perspect. 2013;121(6):683–90. doi:10.1289/ehp.1306561.
40. Jin CY, Zhu BS, Wang XF, Lu QH. Cytotoxicity of titanium dioxide nanoparticles in mouse fibroblast cells. Chem Res Toxicol. 2008;21(9):1871–7. doi:10.1021/tx800179f.
41. Palomaki J, Valimaki E, Sund J, Vippola M, Clausen PA, Jensen KA, et al. Long, needle-like carbon nanotubes and asbestos activate the NLRP3 inflammasome through a similar mechanism. ACS Nano. 2011;5(9):6861–70. doi:10.1021/nn200595c.
42. Cho WS, Duffin R, Howie SE, Scotton CJ, Wallace WA, Macnee W, et al. Progressive severe lung injury by zinc oxide nanoparticles; the role of Zn^{2+} dissolution inside lysosomes. Part Fibre Toxicol. 2011;8:27. doi:10.1186/1743-8977-8-27.
43. Bexiga MG, Varela JA, Wang F, Fenaroli F, Salvati A, Lynch I, et al. Cationic nanoparticles induce caspase 3-, 7- and 9-mediated cytotoxicity in a human astrocytoma cell line. Nanotoxicology. 2011;5(4):557–67. doi:10.3109/17435390.2010.539713.
44. Fouchier F, Mego JL, Dang J, Simon C. Thyroid lysosomes: the stability of the lysosomal membrane. Eur J Cell Biol. 1983;30(2):272–8.
45. Appelqvist H, Nilsson C, Garner B, Brown AJ, Kagedal K, Ollinger K. Attenuation of the lysosomal death pathway by lysosomal cholesterol accumulation. Am J Pathol. 2011;178(2):629–39. doi:10.1016/j.ajpath.2010.10.030.

46. Appelqvist H, Sandin L, Bjornstrom K, Saftig P, Garner B, Ollinger K, et al. Sensitivity to lysosome-dependent cell death is directly regulated by lysosomal cholesterol content. PLoS ONE. 2012;7(11):e50262. doi:10.1371/journal.pone.0050262.
47. Deng D, Jiang N, Hao SJ, Sun H, Zhang GJ. Loss of membrane cholesterol influences lysosomal permeability to potassium ions and protons. Biochim Biophys Acta. 2009;1788 (2):470–6. doi:10.1016/j.bbamem.2008.11.018.
48. Schulze H, Kolter T, Sandhoff K. Principles of lysosomal membrane degradation: cellular topology and biochemistry of lysosomal lipid degradation. Biochim Biophys Acta. 2009;1793(4):674–83. doi:10.1016/j.bbamcr.2008.09.020.
49. Riganti C, Orecchia S, Silvagno F, Pescarmona G, Betta PG, Gazzano E, et al. Asbestos induces nitric oxide synthesis in mesothelioma cells via Rho signaling inhibition. Am J Respir Cell Mol Biol. 2007;36(6):746–56. doi:10.1165/rcmb.2006-0011OC.
50. Biswas R, Hamilton Jr RF, Holian A. Role of lysosomes in silica-induced inflammasome activation and inflammation in absence of MARCO. J Immunol Res. 2014;2014:304180. doi:10.1155/2014/304180.
51. Ridgway ND. Interactions between metabolism and intracellular distribution of cholesterol and sphingomyelin. Biochim Biophys Acta. 2000;1484(2–3):129–41.
52. Brown MS, Goldstein JL. A proteolytic pathway that controls the cholesterol content of membranes, cells, and blood. Proc Natl Acad Sci U S A. 1999;96(20):11041–8.
53. Hait NC, Oskeritzian CA, Paugh SW, Milstien S, Spiegel S. Sphingosine kinases, sphingosine 1-phosphate, apoptosis and diseases. Biochim Biophys Acta. 2006;1758(12):2016–26. doi:10.1016/j.bbamem.2006.08.007.
54. Johansson AC, Appelqvist H, Nilsson C, Kagedal K, Roberg K, Ollinger K. Regulation of apoptosis-associated lysosomal membrane permeabilization. Apoptosis. 2010;15(5):527–40. doi:10.1007/s10495-009-0452-5.
55. Zhu H, Yoshimoto T, Yamashima T. Heat shock protein 70.1 (Hsp70.1) affects neuronal cell fate by regulating lysosomal acid sphingomyelinase. J Biol Chem. 2014;289(40):27432–43. doi:10.1074/jbc.M114.560334.
56. Kirkegaard T, Roth AG, Petersen NH, Mahalka AK, Olsen OD, Moilanen I, et al. Hsp70 stabilizes lysosomes and reverts Niemann-Pick disease-associated lysosomal pathology. Nature. 2010;463(7280):549–53. doi:10.1038/nature08710.
57. Zhang G, Yi YP, Zhang GJ. Effects of arachidonic acid on the lysosomal ion permeability and osmotic stability. J Bioenerg Biomembr. 2006;38(1):75–82. doi:10.1007/s10863-006-9008-3.
58. Hu JS, Li YB, Wang JW, Sun L, Zhang GJ. Mechanism of lysophosphatidylcholine-induced lysosome destabilization. J Membr Biol. 2007;215(1):27–35. doi:10.1007/s00232-007-9002-7.
59. Yi YP, Wang X, Zhang G, Fu TS, Zhang GJ. Phosphatidic acid osmotically destabilizes lysosomes through increased permeability to K+ and H+. Gen Physiol Biophys. 2006;25 (2):149–60.
60. Guidetti GF, Consonni A, Cipolla L, Mustarelli P, Balduini C, Torti M. Nanoparticles induce platelet activation *in vitro* through stimulation of canonical signalling pathways. Nanomedicine. 2012;8(8):1329–36. doi:10.1016/j.nano.2012.04.001.
61. Nakajima T, Ito M, Tchoua U, Tojo H, Hashimoto M. Phospholipase A2-mediated superoxide production of murine peritoneal macrophages induced by chrysotile stimulation. Int J Biochem Cell Biol. 2000;32(7):779–87.
62. Ono Y, Sorimachi H. Calpains: an elaborate proteolytic system. Biochim Biophys Acta. 2012;1824(1):224–36. doi:10.1016/j.bbapap.2011.08.005.
63. Villalpando Rodriguez GE, Torriglia A. Calpain 1 induce lysosomal permeabilization by cleavage of lysosomal associated membrane protein 2. Biochim Biophys Acta. 2013;1833 (10):2244–53. doi:10.1016/j.bbamcr.2013.05.019.
64. Arnandis T, Ferrer-Vicens I, Garcia-Trevijano ER, Miralles VJ, Garcia C, Torres L, et al. Calpains mediate epithelial-cell death during mammary gland involution: mitochondria

and lysosomal destabilization. Cell Death Differ. 2012;19(9):1536–48. doi:10.1038/cdd.2012.46.

65. Lubke T, Lobel P, Sleat DE. Proteomics of the lysosome. Biochim Biophys Acta. 2009;1793(4):625–35. doi:10.1016/j.bbamcr.2008.09.018.
66. Eskelinen EL. Roles of LAMP-1 and LAMP-2 in lysosome biogenesis and autophagy. Mol Aspects Med. 2006;27(5–6):495–502. doi:10.1016/j.mam.2006.08.005.
67. Endo Y, Furuta A, Nishino I. Danon disease: a phenotypic expression of LAMP-2 deficiency. Acta Neuropathol. 2015;129(3):391–8. doi:10.1007/s00401-015-1385-4.
68. Cherra 3rd SJ, Chu CT. Autophagy in neuroprotection and neurodegeneration: a question of balance. Future Neurol. 2008;3(3):309–23. doi:10.2217/14796708.3.3.309.
69. Stern ST, Adiseshaiah PP, Crist RM. Autophagy and lysosomal dysfunction as emerging mechanisms of nanomaterial toxicity. Part Fibre Toxicol. 2012;9:20. doi:10.1186/1743-8977-9-20.
70. Johnson-Lyles DN, Peifley K, Lockett S, Neun BW, Hansen M, Clogston J, et al. Fullerenol cytotoxicity in kidney cells is associated with cytoskeleton disruption, autophagic vacuole accumulation, and mitochondrial dysfunction. Toxicol Appl Pharmacol. 2010;248(3):249–58. doi:10.1016/j.taap.2010.08.008.
71. Biazik J, Yla-Anttila P, Vihinen H, Jokitalo E, Eskelinen EL. Ultrastructural relationship of the phagophore with surrounding organelles. Autophagy. 2015;11(3):439–51. doi:10.1080/15548627.2015.1017178.
72. Li R, Ji Z, Qin H, Kang X, Sun B, Wang M, et al. Interference in autophagosome fusion by rare earth nanoparticles disrupts autophagic flux and regulation of an interleukin-1beta producing inflammasome. ACS Nano. 2014;8(10):10280–92. doi:10.1021/nn505002w.
73. Joshi GN, Knecht DA. Silica phagocytosis causes apoptosis and necrosis by different temporal and molecular pathways in alveolar macrophages. Apoptosis. 2013;18(3):271–85. doi:10.1007/s10495-012-0798-y.
74. Yang M, Zhang M, Tahara Y, Chechetka S, Miyako E, Iijima S, et al. Lysosomal membrane permeabilization: carbon nanohorn-induced reactive oxygen species generation and toxicity by this neglected mechanism. Toxicol Appl Pharmacol. 2014;280(1):117–26. doi:10.1016/j.taap.2014.07.022.
75. Fenyo IM, Gafencu AV. The involvement of the monocytes/macrophages in chronic inflammation associated with atherosclerosis. Immunobiology. 2013;218(11):1376–84. doi:10.1016/j.imbio.2013.06.005.
76. Bartsch H, Nair J. Chronic inflammation and oxidative stress in the genesis and perpetuation of cancer: role of lipid peroxidation, DNA damage, and repair. Langenbecks Arch Surg. 2006;391(5):499–510. doi:10.1007/s00423-006-0073-1.
77. Ather JL, Martin RA, Ckless K, Poynter ME. Inflammasome activity in non-microbial lung inflammation. J Environ Immunol Toxicol. 2014;1(3):108–17.
78. Dostert C, Petrilli V, Van Bruggen R, Steele C, Mossman BT, Tschopp J. Innate immune activation through Nalp3 inflammasome sensing of asbestos and silica. Science. 2008;320(5876):674–7. doi:10.1126/science.1156995.
79. Sun B, Wang X, Ji Z, Li R, Xia T. NLRP3 inflammasome activation induced by engineered nanomaterials. Small. 2013;9(9–10):1595–607. doi:10.1002/smll.201201962.
80. Tschopp J, Schroder K. NLRP3 inflammasome activation: the convergence of multiple signalling pathways on ROS production? Nat Rev Immunol. 2010;10(3):210–15. doi:10.1038/nri2725.
81. Cassel SL, Joly S, Sutterwala FS. The NLRP3 inflammasome: a sensor of immune danger signals. Semin Immunol. 2009;21(4):194–8. doi:10.1016/j.smim.2009.05.002.
82. Ozaki E, Campbell M, Doyle SL. Targeting the NLRP3 inflammasome in chronic inflammatory diseases: current perspectives. J Inflamm Res. 2015;8:15–27. doi:10.2147/JIR.S51250.

83. Hamilton RF, Wu N, Porter D, Buford M, Wolfarth M, Holian A. Particle length-dependent titanium dioxide nanomaterials toxicity and bioactivity. Part Fibre Toxicol. 2009;6:35. doi:10.1186/1743-8977-6-35.
84. Sun B, Wang X, Ji Z, Wang M, Liao YP, Chang CH, et al. NADPH oxidase-dependent NLRP3 inflammasome activation and its important role in lung fibrosis by multiwalled carbon nanotubes. Small. 2015;11(17):2087–97. doi:10.1002/smll.201402859.
85. Mariathasan S, Monack DM. Inflammasome adaptors and sensors: intracellular regulators of infection and inflammation. Nat Rev Immunol. 2007;7(1):31–40. doi:10.1038/nri1997.
86. Guey B, Bodnar M, Manie SN, Tardivel A, Petrilli V. Caspase-1 autoproteolysis is differentially required for NLRP1b and NLRP3 inflammasome function. Proc Natl Acad Sci U S A. 2014;111(48):17254–9. doi:10.1073/pnas.1415756111.
87. Franchi L, Eigenbrod T, Munoz-Planillo R, Nunez G. The inflammasome: a caspase-1-activation platform that regulates immune responses and disease pathogenesis. Nat Immunol. 2009;10(3):241–7. doi:10.1038/ni.1703.
88. Dinarello CA. Biologic basis for interleukin-1 in disease. Blood. 1996;87(6):2095–147.
89. Cassel SL, Eisenbarth SC, Iyer SS, Sadler JJ, Colegio OR, Tephly LA, et al. The Nalp3 inflammasome is essential for the development of silicosis. Proc Natl Acad Sci U S A. 2008;105(26):9035–40. doi:10.1073/pnas.0803933105.
90. Ji Z, Wang X, Zhang H, Lin S, Meng H, Sun B, et al. Designed synthesis of CeO_2 nanorods and nanowires for studying toxicological effects of high aspect ratio nanomaterials. ACS Nano. 2012;6(6):5366–80. doi:10.1021/nn3012114.
91. Lunov O, Syrovets T, Loos C, Nienhaus GU, Mailander V, Landfester K, et al. Amino-functionalized polystyrene nanoparticles activate the NLRP3 inflammasome in human macrophages. ACS Nano. 2011;5(12):9648–57. doi:10.1021/nn203596e.
92. Donaldson K, Borm PJ, Castranova V, Gulumian M. The limits of testing particle-mediated oxidative stress *in vitro* in predicting diverse pathologies; relevance for testing of nanoparticles. Part Fibre Toxicol. 2009;6:13. doi:10.1186/1743-8977-6-13.
93. West AP, Shadel GS, Ghosh S. Mitochondria in innate immune responses. Nat Rev Immunol. 2011;11(6):389–402. doi:10.1038/nri2975.
94. Zhou R, Yazdi AS, Menu P, Tschopp J. A role for mitochondria in NLRP3 inflammasome activation. Nature. 2011;469(7329):221–5. doi:10.1038/nature09663.
95. Blomgran R, Zheng L, Stendahl O. Cathepsin-cleaved Bid promotes apoptosis in human neutrophils via oxidative stress-induced lysosomal membrane permeabilization. J Leukoc Biol. 2007;81(5):1213–23. doi:10.1189/jlb.0506359.
96. Holian A, Hamilton Jr RF, Morandi MT, Brown SD, Li L. Urban particle-induced apoptosis and phenotype shifts in human alveolar macrophages. Environ Health Perspect. 1998;106 (3):127–32.
97. Iyer R, Hamilton RF, Li L, Holian A. Silica-induced apoptosis mediated via scavenger receptor in human alveolar macrophages. Toxicol Appl Pharmacol. 1996;141(1):84–92. doi:10.1006/taap.1996.0263.
98. Hamilton Jr RF, Thakur SA, Holian A. Silica binding and toxicity in alveolar macrophages. Free Radic Biol Med. 2008;44(7):1246–58. doi:10.1016/j.freeradbiomed.2007.12.027.
99. Soderstjerna E, Bauer P, Cedervall T, Abdshill H, Johansson F, Johansson UE. Silver and gold nanoparticles exposure to in vitro cultured retina–studies on nanoparticle internalization, apoptosis, oxidative stress, glial- and microglial activity. PLoS ONE. 2014;9(8):e105359. doi:10.1371/journal.pone.0105359.
100. Wahab R, Dwivedi S, Khan F, Mishra YK, Hwang IH, Shin HS, et al. Statistical analysis of gold nanoparticle-induced oxidative stress and apoptosis in myoblast (C2C12) cells. Colloids Surf B: Biointerfaces. 2014;123:664–72. doi:10.1016/j.colsurfb.2014.10.012.
101. Schaeublin NM, Braydich-Stolle LK, Schrand AM, Miller JM, Hutchison J, Schlager JJ, et al. Surface charge of gold nanoparticles mediates mechanism of toxicity. Nanoscale. 2011;3(2):410–20. doi:10.1039/c0nr00478b.

102. Zhao J, Bowman L, Zhang X, Vallyathan V, Young SH, Castranova V, et al. Titanium dioxide (TiO_2) nanoparticles induce JB6 cell apoptosis through activation of the caspase-8/Bid and mitochondrial pathways. J Toxicol Environ Health A. 2009;72(19):1141–9. doi:10.1080/15287390903091764.
103. Periasamy VS, Athinarayanan J, Al-Hadi AM, Juhaimi FA, Alshatwi AA. Effects of titanium dioxide nanoparticles isolated from confectionery products on the metabolic stress pathway in human lung fibroblast cells. Arch Environ Contam Toxicol. 2015;68(3):521–33. doi:10.1007/s00244-014-0109-4.
104. Kopnin PB, Kravchenko IV, Furalyov VA, Pylev LN, Kopnin BP. Cell type-specific effects of asbestos on intracellular ROS levels, DNA oxidation and G1 cell cycle checkpoint. Oncogene. 2004;23(54):8834–40. doi:10.1038/sj.onc.1208108.
105. Valavanidis A, Vlachogianni T, Fiotakis K, Loridas S. Pulmonary oxidative stress, inflammation and cancer: respirable particulate matter, fibrous dusts and ozone as major causes of lung carcinogenesis through reactive oxygen species mechanisms. Int J Environ Res Public Health. 2013;10(9):3886–907. doi:10.3390/ijerph10093886.
106. Li P, Liu T, Kamp DW, Lin Z, Wang Y, Li D, et al. The c-Jun N-terminal kinase signaling pathway mediates chrysotile asbestos-induced alveolar epithelial cell apoptosis. Mol Med Rep. 2015;11(5):3626–34. doi:10.3892/mmr.2014.3119.
107. Nishimura Y, Maeda M, Kumagai-Takei N, Lee S, Matsuzaki H, Wada Y, et al. Altered functions of alveolar macrophages and NK cells involved in asbestos-related diseases. Environ Health Prev Med. 2013;18(3):198–204. doi:10.1007/s12199-013-0333-y.
108. Archimandriti DT, Dalavanga YA, Cianti R, Bianchi L, Manda-Stachouli C, Armini A, et al. Proteome analysis of bronchoalveolar lavage in individuals from Metsovo, nonoccupationally exposed to asbestos. J Proteome Res. 2009;8(2):860–9. doi:10.1021/pr800370n.
109. Jessop F, Holian A. Extracellular HMGB1 regulates multi-walled carbon nanotube-induced inflammation *in vivo*. Nanotoxicology. 2015;9(3):365–72. doi:10.3109/17435390.2014.933904.
110. Rabolli V, Badissi A, Devosse R, Uwambayinema F, Yakoub Y, Palmai-Pallag M, et al. The alarmin IL-1 inverted question mark is a master cytokine in acute lung inflammation induced by silica micro- and nanoparticles. Part Fibre Toxicol. 2014;11(1):69. doi:10.1186/s12989-014-0069-x.
111. Magna M, Pisetsky DS. The role of HMGB1 in the pathogenesis of inflammatory and autoimmune diseases. Mol Med. 2014;20:138–46. doi:10.2119/molmed.2013.00164.
112. Miller FW, Alfredsson L, Costenbader KH, Kamen DL, Nelson LM, Norris JM, et al. Epidemiology of environmental exposures and human autoimmune diseases: findings from a National Institute of Environmental Health Sciences Expert Panel Workshop. J Autoimmun. 2012;39(4):259–71. doi:10.1016/j.jaut.2012.05.002.
113. Pfau JC, Serve KM, Noonan CW. Autoimmunity and asbestos exposure. Autoimmun Dis. 2014;2014:782045. doi:10.1155/2014/782045.
114. Lu B, Nakamura T, Inouye K, Li J, Tang Y, Lundback P, et al. Novel role of PKR in inflammasome activation and HMGB1 release. Nature. 2012;488(7413):670–4. doi:10.1038/nature11290.
115. Peeters PM, Eurlings IM, Perkins TN, Wouters EF, Schins RP, Borm PJ, et al. Silica-induced NLRP3 inflammasome activation *in vitro* and in rat lungs. Part Fibre Toxicol. 2014;11(1):58. doi:10.1186/s12989-014-0058-0.
116. Yang H, Rivera Z, Jube S, Nasu M, Bertino P, Goparaju C, et al. Programmed necrosis induced by asbestos in human mesothelial cells causes high-mobility group box 1 protein release and resultant inflammation. Proc Natl Acad Sci U S A. 2010;107(28):12611–16. doi:10.1073/pnas.1006542107.
117. Willingham SB, Allen IC, Bergstralh DT, Brickey WJ, Huang MT, Taxman DJ, et al. NLRP3 (NALP3, Cryopyrin) facilitates *in vivo* caspase-1 activation, necrosis, and HMGB1 release via inflammasome-dependent and -independent pathways. J Immunol. 2009;183(3):2008–15. doi:10.4049/jimmunol.0900138.

118. Sims GP, Rowe DC, Rietdijk ST, Herbst R, Coyle AJ. HMGB1 and RAGE in inflammation and cancer. Annu Rev Immunol. 2010;28:367–88. doi:10.1146/annurev.immunol.021908.132603.
119. Venereau E, Casalgrandi M, Schiraldi M, Antoine DJ, Cattaneo A, De Marchis F, et al. Mutually exclusive redox forms of HMGB1 promote cell recruitment or proinflammatory cytokine release. J Exp Med. 2012;209(9):1519–28. doi:10.1084/jem.20120189.
120. Hreggvidsdottir HS, Lundberg AM, Aveberger AC, Klevenvall L, Andersson U, Harris HE. High mobility group box protein 1 (HMGB1)-partner molecule complexes enhance cytokine production by signaling through the partner molecule receptor. Mol Med. 2012;18:224–30. doi:10.2119/molmed.2011.00327.
121. Cesta MF, Ryman-Rasmussen JP, Wallace DG, Masinde T, Hurlburt G, Taylor AJ, et al. Bacterial lipopolysaccharide enhances PDGF signaling and pulmonary fibrosis in rats exposed to carbon nanotubes. Am J Respir Cell Mol Biol. 2010;43(2):142–51. doi:10.1165/rcmb.2009-0113OC.
122. Kono H, Kimura Y, Latz E. Inflammasome activation in response to dead cells and their metabolites. Curr Opin Immunol. 2014;30:91–8. doi:10.1016/j.coi.2014.09.001.
123. Zheng F, Xing S, Gong Z, Mu W, Xing Q. Silence of NLRP3 suppresses atherosclerosis and stabilizes plaques in apolipoprotein E-deficient mice. Mediat Inflamm. 2014;2014:507208. doi:10.1155/2014/507208.
124. Moussion C, Ortega N, Girard JP. The IL-1-like cytokine IL-33 is constitutively expressed in the nucleus of endothelial cells and epithelial cells *in vivo*: a novel 'alarmin'? PLoS ONE. 2008;3(10):e3331. doi:10.1371/journal.pone.0003331.
125. Beamer CA, Girtsman TA, Seaver BP, Finsaas KJ, Migliaccio CT, Perry VK, et al. IL-33 mediates multi-walled carbon nanotube (MWCNT)-induced airway hyper-reactivity via the mobilization of innate helper cells in the lung. Nanotoxicology. 2013;7(6):1070–81. doi:10.3109/17435390.2012.702230.
126. Wang X, Katwa P, Podila R, Chen P, Ke PC, Rao AM, et al. Multi-walled carbon nanotube instillation impairs pulmonary function in C57BL/6 mice. Part Fibre Toxicol. 2011;8:24. doi:10.1186/1743-8977-8-24.
127. Katwa P, Wang X, Urankar RN, Podila R, Hilderbrand SC, Fick RB, et al. A carbon nanotube toxicity paradigm driven by mast cells and the IL-(3)(3)/ST(2) axis. Small. 2012;8(18):2904–12. doi:10.1002/smll.201200873.
128. Zhu M, Perrett S, Nie G. Understanding the particokinetics of engineered nanomaterials for safe and effective therapeutic applications. Small. 2013;9(9–10):1619–34. doi:10.1002/smll.201201630.
129. Berry G, Gibbs GW. An overview of the risk of lung cancer in relation to exposure to asbestos and of taconite miners. Regul Toxicol Pharmacol. 2008;52(1 Suppl):S218–22. doi:10.1016/j.yrtph.2007.09.012.
130. Verma A, Uzun O, Hu Y, Han HS, Watson N, Chen S, et al. Surface-structure-regulated cell-membrane penetration by monolayer-protected nanoparticles. Nat Mater. 2008;7(7):588–95. doi:10.1038/nmat2202.
131. Kreyling WG, Semmler-Behnke M, Seitz J, Scymczak W, Wenk A, Mayer P, et al. Size dependence of the translocation of inhaled iridium and carbon nanoparticle aggregates from the lung of rats to the blood and secondary target organs. Inhal Toxicol. 2009;21 Suppl 1:55–60. doi:10.1080/08958370902942517.
132. Schleh C, Semmler-Behnke M, Lipka J, Wenk A, Hirn S, Schaffler M, et al. Size and surface charge of gold nanoparticles determine absorption across intestinal barriers and accumulation in secondary target organs after oral administration. Nanotoxicology. 2012;6(1):36–46. doi:10.3109/17435390.2011.552811.
133. Jin H, Heller DA, Sharma R, Strano MS. Size-dependent cellular uptake and expulsion of single-walled carbon nanotubes: single particle tracking and a generic uptake model for nanoparticles. ACS Nano. 2009;3(1):149–58. doi:10.1021/nn800532m.

134. Pietroiusti A, Campagnolo L, Fadeel B. Interactions of engineered nanoparticles with organs protected by internal biological barriers. Small. 2013;9(9–10):1557–72. doi:10.1002/smll.201201463.
135. Mahon E, Salvati A, Baldelli Bombelli F, Lynch I, Dawson KA. Designing the nanoparticle-biomolecule interface for "targeting and therapeutic delivery". J Control Release. 2012;161(2):164–74. doi:10.1016/j.jconrel.2012.04.009.
136. Davis GS, Holmes CE, Pfeiffer LM, Hemenway DR. Lymphocytes, lymphokines, and silicosis. J Environ Pathol Toxicol Oncol. 2001;20 Suppl 1:53–65.
137. Beamer CA, Migliaccio CT, Jessop F, Trapkus M, Yuan D, Holian A. Innate immune processes are sufficient for driving silicosis in mice. J Leukoc Biol. 2010;88(3):547–57. doi:10.1189/jlb.0210108.
138. Mottram PL, Leong D, Crimeen-Irwin B, Gloster S, Xiang SD, Meanger J, et al. Type 1 and 2 immunity following vaccination is influenced by nanoparticle size: formulation of a model vaccine for respiratory syncytial virus. Mol Pharm. 2007;4(1):73–84. doi:10.1021/mp060096p.
139. Perkins TN, Peeters PM, Shukla A, Arijs I, Dragon J, Wouters EF, et al. Indications for distinct pathogenic mechanisms of asbestos and silica through gene expression profiling of the response of lung epithelial cells. Hum Mol Genet. 2015;24(5):1374–89. doi:10.1093/hmg/ddu551.
140. teWaternaude JM, Ehrlich RI, Churchyard GJ, Pemba L, Dekker K, Vermeis M, et al. Tuberculosis and silica exposure in South African gold miners. Occup Environ Med. 2006;63(3):187–92. doi:10.1136/oem.2004.018614.
141. Cowie RL. The epidemiology of tuberculosis in gold miners with silicosis. Am J Respir Crit Care Med. 1994;150(5 Pt 1):1460–2. doi:10.1164/ajrccm.150.5.7952577.
142. Tse LA, Chen MH, Au RK, Wang F, Wang XR, Yu IT. Pulmonary tuberculosis and lung cancer mortality in a historical cohort of workers with asbestosis. Pub Health. 2012;126(12):1013–16. doi:10.1016/j.puhe.2012.09.012.
143. Armstead AL, Minarchick VC, Porter DW, Nurkiewicz TR, Li B. Acute inflammatory responses of nanoparticles in an intra-tracheal instillation rat model. PLoS ONE. 2015;10(3):e0118778. doi:10.1371/journal.pone.0118778.
144. Lasfargues G, Lardot C, Delos M, Lauwerys R, Lison D. The delayed lung responses to single and repeated intratracheal administration of pure cobalt and hard metal powder in the rat. Environ Res. 1995;69(2):108–21. doi:10.1006/enrs.1995.1032.
145. Takenaka S, Karg E, Roth C, Schulz H, Ziesenis A, Heinzmann U, et al. Pulmonary and systemic distribution of inhaled ultrafine silver particles in rats. Environ Health Perspect. 2001;109 Suppl 4:547–51.
146. Sung JH, Ji JH, Yoon JU, Kim DS, Song MY, Jeong J, et al. Lung function changes in Sprague–Dawley rats after prolonged inhalation exposure to silver nanoparticles. Inhal Toxicol. 2008;20(6):567–74. doi:10.1080/08958370701874671.
147. Zhu M, Nie G, Meng H, Xia T, Nel A, Zhao Y. Physicochemical properties determine nanomaterial cellular uptake, transport, and fate. Acc Chem Res. 2013;46(3):622–31. doi:10.1021/ar300031y.
148. Sporn TA. Mineralogy of asbestos. Recent Results Cancer Res. 2011;189:1–11. doi:10.1007/978-3-642-10862-4_1.
149. Thibodeau MS, Giardina C, Knecht DA, Helble J, Hubbard AK. Silica-induced apoptosis in mouse alveolar macrophages is initiated by lysosomal enzyme activity. Toxicol Sci. 2004;80(1):34–48. doi:10.1093/toxsci/kfh121.
150. Peeters PM, Perkins TN, Wouters EF, Mossman BT, Reynaert NL. Silica induces NLRP3 inflammasome activation in human lung epithelial cells. Part Fibre Toxicol. 2013;10:3. doi:10.1186/1743-8977-10-3.
151. Thibodeau M, Giardina C, Hubbard AK. Silica-induced caspase activation in mouse alveolar macrophages is dependent upon mitochondrial integrity and aspartic proteolysis. Toxicol Sci. 2003;76(1):91–101. doi:10.1093/toxsci/kfg178.

152. Costantini LM, Gilberti RM, Knecht DA. The phagocytosis and toxicity of amorphous silica. PLoS ONE. 2011;6(2):e14647. doi:10.1371/journal.pone.0014647.
153. Kusaka T, Nakayama M, Nakamura K, Ishimiya M, Furusawa E, Ogasawara K. Effect of silica particle size on macrophage inflammatory responses. PLoS ONE. 2014;9(3):e92634. doi:10.1371/journal.pone.0092634.
154. Lai JC, Ananthakrishnan G, Jandhyam S, Dukhande VV, Bhushan A, Gokhale M, et al. Treatment of human astrocytoma U87 cells with silicon dioxide nanoparticles lowers their survival and alters their expression of mitochondrial and cell signaling proteins. Int J Nanomedicine. 2010;5:715–23. doi:10.2147/IJN.S5238.
155. Hashimoto M, Imazato S. Cytotoxic and genotoxic characterization of aluminum and silicon oxide nanoparticles in macrophages. Dent Mater. 2015;31(5):556–64. doi:10.1016/j.dental.2015.02.009.
156. Li M, Gunter ME, Fukagawa NK. Differential activation of the inflammasome in THP-1 cells exposed to chrysotile asbestos and Libby "six-mix" amphiboles and subsequent activation of BEAS-2B cells. Cytokine. 2012;60(3):718–30. doi:10.1016/j.cyto.2012.08.025.
157. Bergamini C, Fato R, Biagini G, Pugnaloni A, Giantomassi F, Foresti E, et al. Mitochondrial changes induced by natural and synthetic asbestos fibers: studies on isolated mitochondria. Cell Mol Biol (Noisy-le-grand). 2006;52(Suppl):OL905–13.
158. Jajte J, Lao I, Wisniewska-Knypl JM. Enhanced lipid peroxidation and lysosomal enzyme activity in the lungs of rats with prolonged pulmonary deposition of crocidolite asbestos. Br J Ind Med. 1987;44(3):180–6.
159. Thompson JK, Westbom CM, MacPherson MB, Mossman BT, Heintz NH, Spiess P, et al. Asbestos modulates thioredoxin-thioredoxin interacting protein interaction to regulate inflammasome activation. Part Fibre Toxicol. 2014;11:24. doi:10.1186/1743-8977-11-24.
160. Shukla A, Jung M, Stern M, Fukagawa NK, Taatjes DJ, Sawyer D, et al. Asbestos induces mitochondrial DNA damage and dysfunction linked to the development of apoptosis. Am J Physiol Lung Cell Mol Physiol. 2003;285(5):L1018–25. doi:10.1152/ajplung.00038.2003.
161. Visalli G, Bertuccio MP, Iannazzo D, Piperno A, Pistone A, Di Pietro A. Toxicological assessment of multi-walled carbon nanotubes on A549 human lung epithelial cells. Toxicol In vitro. 2015;29(2):352–62. doi:10.1016/j.tiv.2014.12.004.
162. Hamilton RF, Girtsman TA, Xiang C, Wu N, Holian A. Nickel contamination on MWCNT is related to particle bioactivity but not toxicity in the THP-1 transformed macrophage model. Int J Biomed Nanosci Nanotechnol. 2013;3(1/2):107–26.
163. Xia T, Hamilton RF, Bonner JC, Crandall ED, Elder E, Fazlollahi F et al. Interlaboratory evaluation of in vitro cytotoxicity and inflammatory responses to engineered nanomaterials: the NIEHS Nano Go Consortium. Environ Health Perspect. 2013;121(6):683–90.
164. van Berlo D, Wilhelmi V, Boots AW, Hullmann M, Kuhlbusch TA, Bast A, et al. Apoptotic, inflammatory, and fibrogenic effects of two different types of multi-walled carbon nanotubes in mouse lung. Arch Toxicol. 2014;88(9):1725–37. doi:10.1007/s00204-014-1220-z.
165. Baron L, Gombault A, Fanny M, Villeret B, Savigny F, Guillou N, et al. The NLRP3 inflammasome is activated by nanoparticles through ATP, ADP and adenosine. Cell Death Dis. 2015;6:e1629. doi:10.1038/cddis.2014.576.
166. Yoo KC, Yoon CH, Kwon D, Hyun KH, Woo SJ, Kim RK, et al. Titanium dioxide induces apoptotic cell death through reactive oxygen species-mediated Fas upregulation and Bax activation. Int J Nanomedicine. 2012;7:1203–14. doi:10.2147/IJN.S28647.

Chapter 4
Reproductive and Developmental Effects of Nanomaterials

Yuki Morishita, Yasuo Yoshioka, Kazuma Higashisaka, and Yasuo Tsutsumi

Abstract Reproductive and developmental toxicity are among the most important factors for evaluating the safety of chemical substances. Some critical organs for reproduction are protected by biological barriers: the fetus is protected by the blood–placental barrier and the testes by the blood–testis barrier. The small size of nanomaterials affords them unique biodistribution characteristics and thus biological effects that differ from those of larger materials. Their small size might allow nanoparticles to penetrate barriers and cause unexpected reproductive and developmental toxicity. In this chapter, the reproductive and developmental toxicity of nanomaterials, including biodistribution within and biological effects on reproductive tissues, fetuses, and offspring, are reviewed. Investigations show that nanomaterials can penetrate biological barriers and can be distributed to the ovaries, testes, and fetuses of rodents. Nanomaterials thus have the potential to affect both male and female reproductive functions. Maternal exposure to nanomaterials during gestation or lactation could also adversely affect the fetus

Y. Morishita • K. Higashisaka
Laboratory of Toxicology and Safety Science, Graduate School of Pharmaceutical Sciences, Osaka University, 1-6 Yamadaoka, Suita, Osaka 565-0871, Japan

Y. Yoshioka (✉)
Laboratory of Toxicology and Safety Science, Graduate School of Pharmaceutical Sciences, Osaka University, 1-6 Yamadaoka, Suita, Osaka 565-0871, Japan

Vaccine Creation Project, BIKEN Innovative Vaccine Research Alliance Laboratories, Research Institute for Microbial Diseases, Osaka University, 3-1 Yamadaoka, Suita, 565-0871 Osaka, Japan

BIKEN Center for Innovative Vaccine Research and Development, The Research Foundation for Microbial Diseases of Osaka University, 3-1 Yamadaoka, Suita, 565-0871 Osaka, Japan
e-mail: y-yoshioka@biken.osaka-u.ac.jp

Y. Tsutsumi
Laboratory of Toxicology and Safety Science, Graduate School of Pharmaceutical Sciences, Osaka University, 1-6 Yamadaoka, Suita, Osaka 565-0871, Japan

Laboratory of Innovative Antibody Engineering and Design, Center for Drug Innovation and Screening, National Institute of Biomedical Innovation, Health and Nutrition, 7-6-8 Saitoasagi, Ibaragi, 567-0085 Osaka, Japan

T. Otsuki et al. (eds.), *Biological Effects of Fibrous and Particulate Substances*, Current Topics in Environmental Health and Preventive Medicine,
DOI 10.1007/978-4-431-55732-6_4

or offspring. This review compiles current knowledge and highlights remaining open questions in evaluating the reproductive and developmental toxicity of nanomaterials.

Keywords Nanomaterials • Nanoparticles • Blood–placental barrier • Blood–testis barrier • Reproductive and developmental toxicity

4.1 Introduction

Fetuses and infants are more sensitive than adults to environmental toxins [1, 2]. Therefore, some chemicals transmitted through the placenta or through breast milk could adversely affect fetuses or infants, even if the dose is low enough not to induce adverse effects in mothers [2–4]. In addition, adverse effects that are induced in offspring during the fetal or infant period of development could affect the offspring's subsequent growth [5]. Ensuring the safety of these susceptible populations is one of the most important issues in chemical safety. In addition, when evaluating the safety of chemicals for progeny, effects on reproductive functions of parents should also be considered. Rates of male and female infertility continue to increase, and infertility has been a difficult problem to solve [6, 7]. Unlike toxicity-induced problems such as congenital abnormalities, infertility is less visibly apparent. Nevertheless, the damaging effect of infertility is severe when one considers the potential lives lost. Therefore, the reproductive and developmental toxicity of chemicals are very important points to be evaluated.

There is increasing concern regarding the safety of fine particles. For example, exposure to particulate matter less than 2.5 μm in diameter (PM2.5) is well known to increase cardiovascular or respiratory mortality [8]. In addition, effects of PM2.5 on fetuses, infants, or reproductive functions of parents have also been reported [9, 10]. Collection of more detailed information about reproductive and developmental toxicity of fine particles is still urgently needed. Importantly, recent epidemiological studies have shown that exposure to nanoparticles, rather than microparticles, highly relates to relate health risks caused by fine particles [11, 12]. In addition, there is an increasing use of engineered nanomaterials, including nanoparticles, nanofibers, and nanosheets, in various applications such as foods, cosmetics, and medicines [13–15]. Consequently, opportunities for humans to be exposed to nanoparticles are increasing rapidly. Some health risks of these engineered nanoparticles on humans have been reported [16–18]. Thus, further collection and understanding of safety information of nanomaterials should be regarded as an urgent need.

In this chapter, we summarize the current body of knowledge regarding the reproductive and developmental toxicity of nanomaterials, focusing mainly on *in vivo* and *ex vivo* studies of nanoparticle toxicity in mammals.

4.2 Reproductive and Developmental Toxicity of Nanomaterials in Females

4.2.1 Effects of Nanomaterials on Female Reproductive Functions

Compared to the amount of safety information focused on gestational and lactational exposure (described in Sects. 4.2.2 and 4.2.3), relatively little information has been collected regarding the effects of nanomaterials on female reproductive functions. Gao G. et al. showed that, after oral administration for 90 days at 10 mg/kg in mice, titanium oxide nanoparticles could be distributed to the ovaries and could induce ovarian damage, altered gene expression in the ovaries, an imbalance of sex hormones, and decreased fertility [19]. Distribution to ovaries and an imbalance of sex hormones after oral administration of titanium dioxide nanoparticles (1 or 2 mg/kg for 5 days) were demonstrated also by Tassinari et al. [20]. At the moment, it is difficult to judge whether these results can be generalized to multiple types of nanomaterials or whether they are specific to titanium dioxide. Therefore, the effects of nanomaterials on female reproductive functions should be investigated more thoroughly through the use of various types and sizes of nanoparticles.

4.2.2 Safety of Intrauterine Exposure to Nanomaterials

4.2.2.1 Penetration of Blood–Placental Barrier by Nanomaterials

Many nanomaterials such as gold nanoparticles [21–23], carbon nanotubes [24], fullerenes [25, 26], titanium oxide nanoparticles [27, 28], silica nanoparticles [28], polystyrene nanoparticles [29], iron oxide nanoparticles [30], silver nanoparticles [31], and quantum dots [32] have been reported to penetrate the blood–placental barrier (BPB) and to be distributed to fetuses in rodent studies. However, in other studies, gold nanoparticles [33, 34] and quantum dots [35] have been reported to be unable to penetrate the BPB. These conflicting results may be due to differences in detection methods or detection limits. Studies that have demonstrated nanoparticles' penetration of the BPB have used high-sensitivity quantitative methods such as inductively coupled plasma mass spectrometry (ICP-MS), inductively coupled plasma atomic emission spectroscopy (ICP-AES), and radioisotope measurements [21–23, 32]. In contrast, studies that have shown that nanoparticles do not penetrate the BPB have used relatively insensitive methods such as autometallography, spectroscopic examination, and microscopic examination [33, 35]. Although an *ex vivo* human placenta perfusion study that showed that gold nanoparticles do not penetrate the BPB [34] used a quantitative method (ICP-MS), the detection limit of gold in the fetal side of the placenta was only

0.13–0.2 % of the amount detectable in the maternal side. Considering the low transfer rate of gold nanoparticles through the BPB in late pregnancy period by rodent study (about 0.00005–0.07 % of the amount of gold administered to dams) [21–23], the sensitivity of the detection methods might have been insufficient to detect gold in the fetal side. In addition, penetration of the human BPB by polystyrene nanoparticles has been demonstrated by Wick et al. and Grafmüller et al. [36, 37]. Therefore, it is possible that nanomaterials could penetrate the BPB in humans and rodents, although the transfer rate would be low. These reports about transitivity of nanomaterials to fetuses by means of the BPB are summarized in Table 4.1. Some factors that determine the transitivity of nanomaterials through the BPB have been revealed. One of the factors is the size of the nanomaterials: smaller particles were reported to be more easily distributed to the fetus than were larger particles for gold [21, 22], silica [28], and polystyrene [29, 36, 37] nanoparticles as well as quantum dots [32]. The gestational day is also an important factor. Yang et al. showed that 13-nm gold nanoparticles were distributed more readily to fetal tissue before gestational day 9.5 than after gestational day 11.5 [23]. In addition, surface modification or coating with polyethylene glycol (PEG), acids, amino or carboxyl groups, proteins, or SiO_2 can change the nanoparticles' transitivity of the BPB [23, 29, 32]. Therefore, it could be possible to regulate the transitivity of nanomaterials to fetuses by designing appropriate particles or by using nanomaterials during times in the pregnancy term that are determined to be safe.

4.2.2.2 Biological Effects of Nanomaterials on Embryos and Fetuses

Some nanomaterials have been reported to cause hazardous effects on fetuses in rodent studies (Table 4.2). Carbon nanotubes [24, 38–40], fullerenes [25], titanium oxide nanoparticles [28], silica nanoparticles [28], cadmium oxide nanoparticles [41], and quantum dots [32] present hazards leading to miscarriage, fetal death, fetal resorption, fetal growth restriction, or fetal malformation when exposed to dams. In addition, treatment of blastocysts or oocytes by silver nanoparticles [42] or quantum dots [43, 44] has been reported to cause increased resorption of post-implantation embryos and decreased fetal weights. Similar to the case of the transitivity through the BPB, the size and surface modification of the nanomaterials, as well as the pregnancy term, determine the hazard on the fetus. Smaller silica nanoparticles [28] and quantum dots [32] had a greater hazard of causing fetal death, fetal resorption, or fetal growth restriction than did larger particles. Surface modification or coating by PEG, 3-mercaptopropionic acid, amino groups, carboxyl groups, SiO_2, or ZnS could change the nanomaterials' hazard to the fetus [28, 32, 43, 44]. The degree of oxidation of carbon nanotubes was found to contribute to their toxicity [39]. The period of pregnancy during exposure also seems to determine what effects are observed on the fetus. Many studies focused on exposure during the organogenic period have revealed teratogenicity of nanomaterials [25, 38, 39]. On the other hand, exposure to nanomaterials late in pregnancy induced fetal death/resorption or fetal growth restriction [28, 32]. These results

Table 4.1 Distribution of nanomaterials to fetuses

Nanomaterials	Animals	Exposure protocol	Results	References
Gold nanoparticles (5, 30 nm)	Wistar rats	Single intravenous injection on gestational day (GD) 19 at 0.02 mg/rat	Gold nanoparticles were detected in fetus; fetal accumulation was greater for the smaller nanoparticles	[21]
Gold nanoparticles (1.4, 18 nm)	WKY rats	Single intravenous injection in third trimester	Gold nanoparticles were detected in fetus; fetal accumulation was greater for the smaller nanoparticles	[22]
13-nm gold nanoparticles with surface modifications (ferritin, PEG, or citrate)	CD-1 mice	Single intravenous injection at GD 5.5, 7.5, 9.5, 11.5, 13.5, or 15.5 (7.2 μg/g)	Gold nanoparticles were detected in fetal tissue; fetal gold levels declined dramatically post-E11.5; fetal accumulation of ferritin- or PEG-modified nanoparticles was considerably greater than that of citrate-capped nanoparticles	[23]
Oxidized multi-walled carbon nanotubes	Kunming mice	Single intravenous injection on GD 17 at 20 mg/kg	Carbon nanotubes were detected in fetus	[24]
Fullerene (C60)	SLC mice	Single intraperitoneal injection on GD 10 at 25–137 mg/kg	Fullerene was detected in embryos	[25]
Fullerene (C60)	Sprague–Dawley rats	Single intravenous injection on GD 15 at 0.3 mg/kg	Fullerene was detected in fetus	[26]
Titanium dioxide nanoparticles (anatase, 25–70 nm)	ICR mice	Subcutaneous injection on GD 3, 7, 10, and 14 at 0.1 mg/mouse	Titanium dioxide nanoparticles were detected in testes and brain of male offspring	[27]
Titanium dioxide nanoparticles (217 nm), silica nanoparticles (70, 300, 1000 nm), carboxyl-modified silica nanoparticles (70 nm), amine-modified silica nanoparticles (70 nm)	BALB/c mice	Intravenous injection on GD 16 and 17 at 0.8 mg/mouse	Titanium dioxide nanoparticles and silica nanoparticles with diameters of less than 70 nm were detected in fetal liver and brain; larger silica particles (300, 1000 nm) were not detected in fetus	[28]

(continued)

Table 4.1 (continued)

Nanomaterials	Animals	Exposure protocol	Results	References
Carboxyl-modified polystyrene nanoparticles (20, 100, 500 nm), amine-modified polystyrene nanoparticles (200 nm)	Mouse placenta (*ex vivo*)	Injection via extra-embryonic tissue on GD 7.5	20- and 200-nm polystyrene nanoparticles were detected in embryo; 100- and 500-nm polystyrene nanoparticles were not detected	[29]
Iron oxide nanoparticles coated with dimercapto-succinic acid (3–9 nm)	BALB/c mice	Single intraperitoneal injection on GD 8 at 50, 100, 200, and 300 mg/kg	Iron oxide nanoparticles were detected in fetal liver	[30]
Silver nanoparticles (35 nm)	Wistar rats	Single intragastrical administration on GD 20 at 1.69–2.21 mg/kg	Silver nanoparticles were detected in fetus	[31]
CdTe/CdS quantum dots (with various sizes and cappings)	Kunming mice	Single intravenous injection on 20–22 days after female mice were housed with male mice at 20, 50, 86, or 125 μg Cd/mouse	Smaller quantum dots were more easily transferred to fetus than larger ones; capping with an inorganic silica shell or organic polyethylene glycol reduced the transfer of quantum dots to fetus	[32]
Gold nanoparticles (2, 40 nm)	C57BL/6 mice	Single intravenous injection on GD 16 to 18 at 12.13 μg (2-nm gold nanoparticles) or 58.21 μg (40-nm gold nanoparticles)	Gold nanoparticles were not detected in fetal liver	[33]
PEGylated gold nanoparticles (10, 15, 30 nm)	Human placenta (*ex vivo*)	Once-through perfusions (15, 30 nm) or recirculating perfusions (15, 30 nm)	Gold nanoparticles were not detected in fetal outflow	[34]
CdSe/ZnS quantum dots coated with PEG	Wistar rats	Intraperitoneal injection on GD 13, at 0.4 nmol/rat	Quantum dots were not detected in fetus	[35]
Polystyrene nanoparticles (50, 80, 240, 500 nm)	Human placenta (*ex vivo*)	Dual recirculating perfusion	Polystyrene particles with diameter up to 240 nm were able to cross the placental barrier	[36]
Polystyrene nanoparticles (80, 500 nm)	Human placenta (*ex vivo*)	Dual recirculating perfusion	The 80-nm particles were able to cross the placental barrier while the 500-nm particles were not	[37]

Table 4.2 Biological effects of nanomaterials on fetuses

Nanomaterials	Animals	Exposure protocol	Results	References
Oxidized multi-walled carbon nanotubes	Kunming mice	Single intravenous injection on GD 17 at 20 mg/kg	Increased abortion rate	[24]
Single-walled carbon nanotubes functionalized with a hydroxyl group	CD-1 mice	Single oral administration on GD 9 at 10 or 100 mg/kg	Carbon nanotubes administration (10 mg/kg) increased the number of resorptions and resulted in fetal morphological and skeletal abnormalities	[38]
Pristine, oxidized, or ultraoxidized single-walled carbon nanotubes	CD-1 mice	Single intravenous injection on GD 5.5 at 0.01, 0.1, 0.3, 3, or 30 μg/mouse	A high percentage of early miscarriages and fetal malformations were observed in females exposed to single-walled carbon nanotubes, while lower percentages were found in animals exposed to the pristine material; the lowest effective dose was 0.1 μg/mouse	[39]
Multi-walled carbon nanotubes	ICR mice	Single intraperitoneal or intratracheal administration on GD 9 at 2, 3, 4, or 5 mg/kg (intraperitoneal) or 3, 4, or 5 mg/kg (intratracheal)	In the intraperitoneal study, various types of malformation were observed in all carbon nanotube-treated groups. Such malformations were observed in groups given 4 or 5 mg/kg body weight, but not in those treated with 3 mg/kg in the intratracheal study	[40]
Fullerene (C60)	SLC mice	Single intraperitoneal injection on GD 10 at 25–137 mg/kg	Increased fetal death (137 mg/kg) and fetal abnormalities (25, 50, and 137 mg/kg)	[25]

(continued)

Table 4.2 (continued)

Nanomaterials	Animals	Exposure protocol	Results	References
Titanium dioxide nanoparticles (217 nm), silica nanoparticles (70, 300, 1000 nm), carboxyl-modified silica nanoparticles (70 nm), amine-modified silica nanoparticles (70 nm)	BALB/c mice	Intravenous injection on GD 16 and 17 at 0.8 mg/mouse	Titanium dioxide nanoparticles and silica nanoparticles with diameters of less than 70 nm induced reduction of fetal weight and increased resorption rate while other materials did not	[28]
Cadmium oxide nanoparticles (10–15 nm)	CD-1 mice	Inhalation every other day of 100 μg of particles or daily inhalation of 230 μg particles from PND4.5 to 16.5	Daily inhalation of 230 μg particles decreased the incidence of pregnancy, delayed maternal weight gain, altered placental weight, and decreased fetal length	[41]
CdTe/CdS quantum dots (with various sizes and cappings)	Kun Ming mice	Single intravenous injection on 20–22 days after female mice were housed with male mice at 20, 50, 86, or 125 μg Cd/mouse	Smaller quantum dots produced dead pups; PEG or SiO_2 coating could enhance the survival of the pups	[32]

seem reasonable, because teratogenic effects arise mainly following exposure during the organogenic period. It remains to be clarified which period of pregnancy is most susceptible to exposure of nanomaterials. Hazardous effects, such as hepatotoxicity and nephrotoxicity, might be induced in fetuses at doses that do not induce adverse effects on mothers [28]. Since the "no observed adverse effects level" (NOAEL) is lower for fetuses than for mothers, particular attention should be paid to the fetal toxicity of nanomaterials. Unfortunately, the mechanism of these hazardous effects is not well understood and needs to be evaluated further. Our research revealed a partial mechanism of silica nanoparticle–induced fetal growth restriction in mice [28]. In our research, heparin treatment prevented decreased fetal weight caused by silica nanoparticles. Heparin mainly works as anticoagulant. However, heparin is also known to have an anticomplement activation effect [45] and a role as a placental growth factor [46–48]. Therefore, silica nanoparticle–induced fetal growth restriction might involve coagulation, complement activation, or placental dysfunctions. Extensive vascular lesions and increased production of reactive oxygen species (ROS) were also observed in placentas of malformed fetuses by carbon nanotube administration to dams [39]. Oxidative stress in the placenta can cause placental dysfunction and induce pregnancy complications

[49]. Therefore, ROS induction in the placenta and placental dysfunction is a possible mechanism of fetal toxicity by nanomaterials.

4.2.2.3 Postnatal Effects of Intrauterine Exposure to Nanomaterials

In utero exposure to nanomaterials can also induce postnatal effects in rodents (Table 4.3). Hazard information has been collected mainly for titanium oxide nanoparticles and carbon black nanoparticles. After intrauterine exposure, titanium oxide nanoparticles have been observed to distribute to the testes or brain of pups [27]. In addition, they have been shown to induce testicular injury and reduce sperm production [27], as well as brain dysfunctions: altered gene expression [50, 51], altered neurotransmitters [52], increased apoptosis in the olfactory bulb [27], and neurobehavioral alterations [53] of pups. Titanium oxide nanoparticles have also been reported to alter hepatic gene expression of pups [54] and to increase neonatal asthma susceptibility [55]. Carbon black nanoparticles presented hazards similar to those of titanium oxide nanoparticles upon intrauterine exposure, including the risk of causing testicular damage and reduced sperm production [56] (reduced sperm production was even observed in F2 pups [57]), neurobehavioral alterations [58], altered hepatic gene expression [59], hepatic gene damage [60], and renal abnormalities in pups [61]. As for other nanomaterials, decreased growth and abnormal spermatogenesis of pups caused by iron oxide nanoparticles [30] and delayed neonatal growth caused by cadmium oxide nanoparticles [41] have been reported. Taken together, the findings indicate that prenatal exposure to nanomaterials could affect the growth, liver, kidney, brain, and testes of neonates. Although the broad range of tissues and organs affected by the nanomaterials suggests that the toxicity of nanomaterials is not tissue-specific, it is interesting to note that many hazards were observed for the brain and testes of pups. These tissues might have been affected owing to the immaturity of the blood–brain barrier and blood–testis barrier (BTB) during the fetal and juvenile periods [62–65]. Substances that would rarely pass through these barriers in adults, such as nanomaterials or proinflammatory cytokines produced by exposure to nanomaterials, might be more easily distributed to the brain or testes during the fetal and juvenile periods, resulting in increased toxicity for these susceptible tissues. Proinflammatory cytokines, including maternal proinflammatory cytokines, have been shown to affect fetal brain development [66]. In view of these possibilities, more detailed mechanistic analysis of nanomaterials' postnatal effects should be conducted. In addition, for postnatal effects of nanomaterials, information about the relationship between toxicity and physical properties of nanomaterials such as size and surface modification is deficient and should be investigated in future studies.

Table 4.3 Postnatal effects of intrauterine exposure to nanomaterials

Nanomaterials	Animals	Exposure protocol	Results	References
Titanium dioxide nanoparticles (anatase, 25–70 nm)	ICR mice	Subcutaneous injection on GD 3, 7, 10, and 14 at 0.1 mg/mouse	Reduced sperm production and increased apoptosis in olfactory bulb were observed in offspring	[27]
Titanium dioxide nanoparticles (2570 nm)	ICR mice	Subcutaneous injection on GD 6, 9, 12, and 15 at 0.1 mg/mouse	Changes in the expression of genes associated with apoptosis, brain development, response to oxidative stress, neurotransmitters, and psychiatric diseases were found in the brain of pups	[50]
Titanium dioxide nanoparticles (anatase, 25–70 nm)	ICR mice	Subcutaneous injection on GD 6, 9, 12, and 15 at 0.1 mg/mouse	Alteration of gene expression in the cerebral cortex, olfactory bulb, and regions related to dopamine systems of pups	[51]
Titanium dioxide nanoparticles (anatase, 25–70 nm)	ICR mice	Subcutaneous injection on GD 6, 9, 12, 15, and 18 at 0.1 mg/mouse	Dopamine and its metabolites were increased in the prefrontal cortex and the neostriatum of pups	[52]
Titanium dioxide nanoparticles (97 nm)	C57BL/6BomTac mice	Inhalation 1 h/day of 42 mg/m^3 aerosolized powder from GD 8 to 18	Offspring tended to avoid the central zone of the open field and female offspring displayed enhanced prepulse inhibition	[53]
Titanium dioxide nanoparticles (97 nm)	C57BL/6BomTac mice	Inhalation 1 h/day of 42 mg/m^3 aerosolized powder from GD8 to 18	Changes in gene expression related to the retinoic acid signaling pathway in the female pups	[54]
Titanium dioxide nanoparticles	BALB/c mice	Single intranasal administration on GD 14 at 50 μg/mouse	Increased asthma susceptibility in offspring	[55]
Carbon nanoparticles (14 nm)	ICR mice	Intratracheal administration on GD7 and 14 at 0.2 mg/mouse	Histological abnormalities in testes and reduced daily sperm production of pups	[56]

(continued)

Table 4.3 (continued)

Nanomaterials	Animals	Exposure protocol	Results	References
Carbon black nanoparticles (140 nm)	C57BL/6 J mice	Intratracheal administration on GD 7, 10, 15, and 18 at 67 μg/mouse	F2 offspring, whose fathers were prenatally exposed to carbon black nanoparticles, showed lowered sperm production	[57]
Carbon black nanoparticles (140 nm)	C57BL/6BomTac mice	Intratracheal administration on GD 7, 10, 15, and 18 with total doses of 11, 54, and 268 μg/mouse	Female offspring displayed altered habituation pattern during the open-field test	[58]
Carbon black nanoparticles (140 nm)	C57BL/6BomTac mice	Intratracheal administration on GD 7, 10, 15, and 18 with total doses of 11, 54, and 268 μg/mouse	Gene expression changes in pup's liver	[59]
Carbon black nanoparticles (140 nm)	C57BL/6BomTac mice	Inhalation of 42 mg/m^3 carbon black nanoparticles for 1 h/day from GD 8 to 18, or intratracheal administration on GD 7, 10, 15, and 18 with total doses of 11, 54, or 268 μg/mouse	Inhalation exposure induced DNA strand breaks in the liver of offspring, whereas intratracheal administration did not	[60]
Carbon black nanoparticles (14 nm)	ICR mice	Intranasal administration on GD 5 and 9 at 50 μg/mouse	Increased expression of the gene encoding collagen, type VIII, alpha 1 in the tubular cells in the kidney of 12-week-old offspring mice	[61]
Iron oxide nanoparticles coated with dimercaptosuccinic acid (3–9 nm)	BALB/c mice	Single intraperitoneal injection on GD8 at 50, 100, 200, or 300 mg/kg	Decreased growth of pups; decrease in spermatogonia, spermatocytes, spermatids, and mature sperm of pups	[30]
Cadmium oxide nanoparticles (10–15 nm)	CD-1 mice	Inhalation every other day of 100 μg of particles or daily inhalation of 230 μg particles from PND4.5 to 16.5	Daily inhalation of 230 μg particles induced delayed neonatal growth	[41]

4.2.3 Safety Information Regarding Lactational Exposure to Nanomaterials

4.2.3.1 Distribution of Nanomaterials to Breast Milk

The possibility that nanomaterials could be distributed to breast milk has been demonstrated in a few studies. Titanium oxide nanoparticles [67] and silver nanoparticles [31] were detected in neonates after oral administration to lactating dams. However, these results are thought to be insufficient to verify the transitivity of nanomaterials to breast milk, because neonates could be exposed to nanomaterials not only through breast milk but also from contact with the dam's excretion or the dam herself. Among the very few studies that have directly examined nanomaterials' transitivity to breast milk, Sumner et al. showed that fullerenes could be distributed to breast milk after intravenous injection to lactating rats [26] and Hougaard et al. showed that titanium dioxide nanoparticles are not detected in breast milk after inhalation by pregnant mice [53]. Information about the transitivity of other nanoparticles to breast milk is limited. Therefore, the transitivity of nanomaterials to breast milk should be investigated more thoroughly, using various species and sizes of nanoparticles.

4.2.3.2 Biological Effects on Neonates by Lactational Exposure to Nanomaterials

Very little information is available regarding the hazards of neonatal exposure to nanomaterials via lactation, compared to the information available for in utero exposure. Gao X. et al. orally treated lactating rats with 100 mg/kg of titanium oxide nanoparticles from postnatal days 2–21, and they revealed that the offspring's synaptic plasticity, namely, input/output functions, paired pulse reaction, and long-term potentiation in the hippocampal dentate gyrus area, all were attenuated [67]. In addition, they showed that if dams were exposed to titanium oxide nanoparticles during pregnancy, rather than while lactating, only the paired pulse reaction was attenuated in the offspring. These results suggest that the susceptibility of neonates or infants to the nanomaterials varied among pregnancy and lactation periods. Therefore, more investigations focused on lactational exposure to nanomaterials would help to reveal more hazards to neonates, including the identification of target tissues, in addition to the hazards described in Sect. 4.2.2.3.

4.3 Effects of Nanomaterials on Male Reproductive Functions

4.3.1 Penetration of BTB by Nanomaterials

Many nanomaterials such as gold nanoparticles [68–70], carbon nanotubes [71], titanium oxide particles [72, 73], silica nanoparticles [74], iron oxide nanoparticles [75], silver nanoparticles [76–79], ceria nanoparticles [80], magnetic nanoparticles [81, 82], cobalt–chromium nanoparticles [83], and polymethyl methacrylate nanoparticles [84] have been reported to be distributed to the testes (Table 4.4). In addition, smaller nanomaterials were more easily distributed to the testes than were larger nanomaterials [68, 74, 77]. The BTB is the barrier between blood vessels and seminiferous tubules that is formed by tight junctions of Sertoli cells. Distribution to the testes itself does not mean that the BTB has been penetrated, because some interstitial testis cells exist on the external side of the BTB. However, gold nanoparticles [70], titanium oxide particles [72, 73], silica nanoparticles [74], and magnetic nanoparticles [81] have been detected inside seminiferous tubules or Sertoli cells raising the possibility that nanomaterials can penetrate the BTB. Furthermore, gold nanoparticles [70] and silica nanoparticles [74] have been shown to be distributed to male germ cells. Testicular distribution of nanomaterials has some interesting characteristics. Nanomaterials distributed to the testes are retained for a long time compared to those retained in other tissues [78, 79]. Accumulation of gold nanoparticles in testes has been reported to occur from 1 month postinjection [69]. Considering these findings of long retention and late accumulation, further studies on nanomaterials in testes should focus on long-term analysis.

4.3.2 Biological Effects of Nanomaterials on Male Reproductive Functions

Some nanomaterials have been reported to cause hazardous effects on the male reproductive functions of rodents *in vivo* (Table 4.5). Carbon nanotubes [71], carbon black nanoparticles [85], titanium oxide nanoparticles [72, 73, 86], silica nanoparticles [87], silver nanoparticles [88], and cobalt–chromium nanoparticles [83] can cause oxidative stress or tissue damage in the testes. Gold nanoparticles [70], carbon black nanoparticles [85], titanium oxide nanoparticles [20, 72], and nanoparticle-rich diesel exhaust [89, 90] have been shown to disrupt the endocrine activity of the male reproductive system. Carbon black nanoparticles [85], titanium oxide nanoparticles [72, 73, 86, 91], silver nanoparticles (especially smaller silver particles) [88], and cobalt–chromium nanoparticles [83] can affect sperm production or injure sperm (or germ cells). Although such occurrences are thought to be infrequent, male germ cells have been shown to be directly exposed to nanomaterials in some cases [70, 74]. In this regard, hazard information for male

Table 4.4 Distribution of nanomaterials to testes

Nanomaterials	Animals	Exposure protocol	Results	References
Gold nanoparticles (10, 50, 100, 250 nm)	Wistar rats	Single intravenous injection at 77, 96, 89, or 108 μg/rat (for 10-, 50-, 100-, and 250-nm particles, respectively)	Gold nanoparticles were detected in testes; 10-nm nanoparticles were the most easily distributed to testes	[68]
Gold nanoparticles (20 nm)	Wistar rats	Single intravenous injection at 3.02 μg/rat	Gold nanoparticles were detected in testes; significant accumulation of Au in testes took place only after 1–2 months postinjection	[69]
PEG-NH_2-modified or ω-methoxy and ω-aminoethyl poly (ethylene glycol)–modified gold nanoparticles (14 nm)	ICR mice	Single intravenous injection at 45 mg/kg	Gold nanoparticles were detected in testes; PEG-NH_2-modified gold nanoparticles accumulate more easily in testis than do ω-methoxy and ω-aminoethyl poly (ethylene glycol)–modified gold nanoparticles	[70]
Carboxylate-functionalized multi-walled carbon nanotubes	BALB/c mice	Single intravenous injection at 5 mg/kg	Carbon nanotubes were detected in testes	[71]
Titanium dioxide nanoparticles (anatase, 294 nm)	CD-1 mice	Intragastric administration for 90 days at 2.5, 5, or 10 mg/kg	Titanium dioxide nanoparticles were detected inside of the seminiferous tubules	[72]
Titanium dioxide nanoparticles (310 nm)	CD-1 mice	Intragastric administration for 90 days at 2.5, 5, or 10 mg/kg	Titanium dioxide nanoparticles were detected in Sertoli cells	[73]
Silica nanoparticles (70, 300 nm)	BALB/c mice	Intravenous injection on two consecutive days at 0.8 mg/mouse	70-nm silica nanoparticles were detected within Sertoli cells and spermatocytes, while 300-nm silica particles were not	[74]
Iron oxide nanoparticles (144 nm)	Sprague–Dawley rats	Single intratracheal administration at 4 mg/rat	Iron oxide nanoparticles were detected in testes	[75]
Silver nanoparticles (56 nm)	F344 rats	Oral administration for 90 days at 30, 125, or 500 mg/kg	Silver nanoparticles were detected in testes	[76]

(continued)

Table 4.4 (continued)

Nanomaterials	Animals	Exposure protocol	Results	References
Silver nanoparticles (22, 42, 71, 323 nm)	ICR mice	Oral administration for 14 days at 1 mg/kg	Smaller silver nanoparticles (22 nm and 42 nm) were detected in testes, while larger silver nanoparticles (71 and 323 nm) were not	[77]
<20-nm noncoated, or <15-nm polyvinylpyrrolidone-coated silver nanoparticles	Sprague–Dawley rats	Oral administration for 28 days at 90 mg/kg	Silver nanoparticles were detected in testes; silver nanoparticles were not cleared from the testes after 8 weeks post-dosing	[78]
Silver nanoparticles (10, 25 nm)	Sprague–Dawley rats	Oral administration for 28 days at 100 or 500 mg/kg	Silver nanoparticles were detected in testes; silver concentrations in the testes did not clear well after the 4-month recovery period	[79]
Ceria nanoparticles (30 nm)	Sprague–Dawley rats	Single intravenous administration at −100 mg/kg	Ceria nanoparticles were detected in testes	[80]
Silica-overcoated magnetic nanoparticles (50 nm)	ICR mice	Intraperitoneal administration for 4 weeks at 25, 50, or 100 mg/kg	Magnetic nanoparticles were detected inside of the seminiferous tubules	[81]
Magnetic nanoparticles (50 nm)	ICR mice	By nose-only exposure chamber system with a total particle number of 4.89 x 10^5 /cm^3 (low concentration) and 9.34 x 10^5 / cm^3 (high concentration) for 4 weeks (4 h/d, 5 d/wk)	Magnetic nanoparticles were detected in testes	[82]
Cobalt–chromium nanoparticles (55 nm)	Sprague–Dawley rats	Intra-articular administration once a week at 20, 100, or 500 μg/kg for 10 consecutive weeks	Cobalt–chromium nanoparticles were detected in testes	[83]
Polymethyl methacrylate nanoparticles (130 nm)	Wistar rats	Single oral administration	Polymethyl methacrylate nanoparticles were detected in testes	[84]

Table 4.5 Biological effects of nanomaterials on male reproductive functions

Nanomaterials	Animals	Exposure protocol	Results	References
Carboxylate- and amine-functionalized multi-walled carbon nanotubes	BALB/c mice	Intravenous injection every 3 days for 5 times at 5 mg/kg	Nanotubes generated oxidative stress and decreased the thickness of the seminiferous epithelium in the testes at 15 days after the first dose, but the damage was repaired at 60 and 90 days after the first dose	[71]
Carbon black nanoparticles (14, 56, 95 nm)	ICR mice	Intratracheal administration for 10 times every week at 0.1 mg/mouse	Carbon black nanoparticles induced increased serum testosterone, partial vacuolation of the seminiferous tubules, and reduced daily sperm production	[85]
Titanium dioxide nanoparticles (anatase, 294 nm)	CD-1 mice	Intragastric administration for 90 days at 2.5, 5, or 10 mg/kg	Titanium dioxide nanoparticles induced testicular lesions, sperm malformations, alterations in serum sex hormone levels, and altered gene expression in testes	[72]
Titanium dioxide nanoparticles (310 nm)	CD-1 mice	Intragastric administration for 90 days at 2.5, 5, or 10 mg/kg	Titanium dioxide nanoparticles induced testicular oxidative damage and/or apoptosis, altered gene expression in testes, and increased abnormal sperm	[73]
Titanium dioxide nanoparticles (33, 160 nm)	CBAB6F1 mice	Oral administration for 7 days at 40, 200, or 1000 mg/kg	Particles induced increased frequency of spermatids with two and more nuclei (33, 160 nm), apoptosis in testes (only 33 nm)	[86]

(continued)

Table 4.5 (continued)

Nanomaterials	Animals	Exposure protocol	Results	References
Silica nanoparticles (10–15 nm)	Wistar mice	Single oral administration at 333.33 mg/kg	Silica nanoparticles induced testicular lesions	[87]
Silver nanoparticles (20, 200 nm)	Wistar rats	Single intravenous injection at 5 (20 and 200 nm) or 10 (only 20 nm) mg/kg	Silver nanoparticles induced decrease of the epididymal sperm count, DNA damage in germ cells, and change in the testes seminiferous tubule morphometry	[88]
Cobalt–chromium nanoparticles (55 nm)	Sprague–Dawley rats	Intra-articular administration once a week at 20, 100, or 500 μg/kg for 10 consecutive weeks	Cobalt–chromium nanoparticles reduced epididymal sperm motility, viability, and concentration, increased abnormal sperm rate, and induced testicular damage and pathological changes via oxidative stress	[83]
PEG-NH_2-modified or ω-methoxy and ω-aminoethyl poly (ethylene glycol)–modified Gold nanoparticles (14 nm)	ICR mice	Three intravenous injection each other day at 45 or 225 (only for ω-methoxy and ω-aminoethyl poly (ethylene glycol)–modified gold nanoparticles) mg/kg	PEG-NH_2-modified gold nanoparticles increased plasma testosterone levels	[70]
Titanium dioxide nanoparticles	Sprague–Dawley rats	Oral administration for 5 days at 1 or 2 mg/kg	Titanium dioxide nanoparticles increased plasma testosterone levels	[20]
Nanoparticle-rich diesel exhaust	F344 rats	Inhalation for 4, 8, or 12 weeks (5 h/day, 5 days/week) at 15.37, 36.35, or 168.84 μg/m^3	Increased plasma testosterone, plasma inhibin, and testicular testosterone concentration	[89]
Nanoparticle-rich diesel exhaust	F344 rats	Inhalation for 4, 8, or 12 weeks (5 h/day, 5 days/week) at 15.37, 36.35, or 168.84 μg/m^3	Increased plasma testosterone concentration	[90]
Titanium dioxide nanoparticles	ICR mice	Intraperitoneal injection every other day for 5 times at 200 or 500 mg/kg	The high-dose group showed reduced sperm density and motility, increased sperm abnormality, and germ cell apoptosis	[91]

germ cells directly exposed to nanomaterials have been collected by some *in vitro* studies. In these studies, gold nanoparticles [92], magnetic nanoparticles [93], and silver nanoparticles [94] could penetrate into the sperm or the spermatogonial stem cell. Silver nanoparticles were shown to decrease motility and viability of sperm [95], and gold nanoparticles were shown to decrease motility of sperm, increase fragmentation of sperm, and disturb nuclear chromatin decondensation in sperm [92, 96]. In view of these reported hazards, opportunities of nanomaterial exposure to sperm, such as distribution of nanomaterials to seminal vesicle fluid, should be investigated in greater detail. In addition, transgenerational effects through fathers have been reported [97–100]. Therefore, biological effects on neonates from fathers exposed to nanomaterials should also be evaluated.

Some nanomaterials have been reported to have beneficial effects rather than hazardous effects on male reproductive functions *in vivo*. Hydrated fullerenes have been reported to restore decreased weight in reproductive tissues, blood testosterone, sperm motility, and sperm concentration in the epididymis and to mitigate testicular injury in streptozotocin-induced diabetic male rats [101]. In addition, fullerenol can prevent testicular oxidative stress induced by doxorubicin [102]. In humans, rates of male infertility continue to increase and male infertility has been an arduous problem [7]. Therefore, beneficial nanomaterials should be utilized to improve male fertility with consideration of the balance between risk and benefit.

4.4 Conclusion

In this chapter, the biodistribution of nanomaterials to reproductive tissues, fetuses, and infants and the potential effects of nanomaterials on these susceptible tissues and populations have been reviewed. When female rodents are exposed to nanomaterials, the nanomaterials might be distributed to the ovaries and affect sex hormone secretion and fertility. Exposure to nanomaterials during pregnancy results in accumulation of nanomaterials in the fetus and has the potential to cause miscarriage, fetal death, fetal resorption, fetal growth restriction, and fetal malformation. In utero exposure of nanomaterials also presents a risk of causing malfunctions in offspring, including hepatotoxicity, nephrotoxicity, reproductive toxicity, neurotoxicity, and immunotoxicity. Although more detailed studies of lactational exposure effects are needed, nanomaterials might be distributed to breast milk and cause neurotoxicity of breast-fed offspring mice. When male rodents were exposed to nanomaterials, the nanomaterials could be distributed to the testes or male germ cells and could affect sex hormone secretion and sperm production. Smaller nanomaterials are more easily distributed to the fetus or testes through the BPB or BTB. In addition, some hazardous effects are more severe for smaller particles than for larger particles. Therefore, special attention should be paid to nanoparticles, more so than larger particles, when considering reproductive and developmental toxicity. On the other hand, similarly sized particles can induce different biological effects when the surface coating or modification of the particles is varied, which complicates understanding of the safety of nanomaterials. Interactions between biomolecules (such as lipids and proteins) and nanomaterials, to form the so-called corona, are assumed to affect the nanomaterials' biodistribution and biological effects [103]. Thus, it is necessary to reveal the factors that define the reproductive and developmental toxicity of nanomaterials by focusing not only on the physicochemical properties of the nanoparticle but also on the biomolecular corona. The NOAEL is not clear for many of the hazards described in this article. Therefore, determination of the NOAEL for each nanomaterial is also important.

References

1. Faustman EM, Silbernagel SM, Fenske RA, Burbacher TM, Ponce RA. Mechanisms underlying Children's susceptibility to environmental toxicants. Environ Health Perspect. 2000;108 Suppl 1:13–21.
2. Wigle DT, Arbuckle TE, Turner MC, Berube A, Yang Q, Liu S, et al. Epidemiologic evidence of relationships between reproductive and child health outcomes and environmental chemical contaminants. J Toxicol Environ Health B Crit Rev. 2008;11(5–6):373–517. doi:10.1080/10937400801921320.
3. Koopman-Esseboom C, Weisglas-Kuperus N, de Ridder MA, Van der Paauw CG, Tuinstra LG, Sauer PJ. Effects of polychlorinated biphenyl/dioxin exposure and feeding type on infants' mental and psychomotor development. Pediatrics. 1996;97(5):700–6.
4. Santos IS, Matijasevich A, Domingues MR. Maternal caffeine consumption and infant nighttime waking: prospective cohort study. Pediatrics. 2012;129(5):860–8. doi:10.1542/peds.2011-1773.
5. Fujimoto T, Kubo K, Nishikawa Y, Aou S. Postnatal exposure to low-dose bisphenol A influences various emotional conditions. J Toxicol Sci. 2013;38(4):539–46.
6. Healy DL, Trounson AO, Andersen AN. Female infertility: causes and treatment. Lancet. 1994;343(8912):1539–44.
7. Howards SS. Treatment of male infertility. N Engl J Med. 1995;332(5):312–17. doi:10.1056/NEJM199502023320507.
8. Franklin M, Zeka A, Schwartz J. Association between PM2.5 and all-cause and specific-cause mortality in 27 US communities. J Expo Sci Environ Epidemiol. 2007;17(3):279–87. doi:10.1038/sj.jes.7500530.
9. Hammoud A, Carrell DT, Gibson M, Sanderson M, Parker-Jones K, Peterson CM. Decreased sperm motility is associated with air pollution in Salt Lake City. Fertil Steril. 2010;93(6):1875–9. doi:10.1016/j.fertnstert.2008.12.089.
10. Volk HE, Lurmann F, Penfold B, Hertz-Picciotto I, McConnell R. Traffic-related air pollution, particulate matter, and autism. JAMA Psychiatry. 2013;70(1):71–7. doi:10.1001/jamapsychiatry.2013.266.
11. Delfino RJ, Sioutas C, Malik S. Potential role of ultrafine particles in associations between airborne particle mass and cardiovascular health. Environ Health Perspect. 2005;113(8):934–46.
12. McCreanor J, Cullinan P, Nieuwenhuijsen MJ, Stewart-Evans J, Malliarou E, Jarup L, et al. Respiratory effects of exposure to diesel traffic in persons with asthma. N Engl J Med. 2007;357(23):2348–58. doi:10.1056/NEJMoa071535.
13. Bowman DM, van Calster G, Friedrichs S. Nanomaterials and regulation of cosmetics. Nat Nanotechnol. 2010;5(2):92. doi:10.1038/nnano.2010.12.

14. Magnuson BA, Jonaitis TS, Card JW. A brief review of the occurrence, use, and safety of food-related nanomaterials. J Food Sci. 2011;76(6):R126–33. doi:10.1111/j.1750-3841.2011.02170.x.
15. Cheng Z, Al Zaki A, Hui JZ, Muzykantov VR, Tsourkas A. Multifunctional nanoparticles: cost versus benefit of adding targeting and imaging capabilities. Science. 2012;338(6109):903–10. doi:10.1126/science.1226338.
16. Song Y, Li X, Du X. Exposure to nanoparticles is related to pleural effusion, pulmonary fibrosis and granuloma. Eur Respir J. 2009;34(3):559–67. doi:10.1183/09031936.00178308.
17. Liao HY, Chung YT, Lai CH, Lin MH, Liou SH. Sneezing and allergic dermatitis were increased in engineered nanomaterial handling workers. Ind Health. 2014;52(3):199–215.
18. Wu WT, Liao HY, Chung YT, Li WF, Tsou TC, Li LA, et al. Effect of nanoparticles exposure on fractional exhaled nitric oxide (FENO) in workers exposed to nanomaterials. Int J Mol Sci. 2014;15(1):878–94. doi:10.3390/ijms15010878.
19. Gao G, Ze Y, Li B, Zhao X, Zhang T, Sheng L, et al. Ovarian dysfunction and gene-expressed characteristics of female mice caused by long-term exposure to titanium dioxide nanoparticles. J Hazard Mater. 2012;243:19–27. doi:10.1016/j.jhazmat.2012.08.049.
20. Tassinari R, Cubadda F, Moracci G, Aureli F, D'Amato M, Valeri M, et al. Oral, short-term exposure to titanium dioxide nanoparticles in Sprague–Dawley rat: focus on reproductive and endocrine systems and spleen. Nanotoxicology. 2014;8(6):654–62. doi:10.3109/17435390.2013.822114.
21. Takahashi S, Matsuoka O. Cross placental transfer of 198Au-colloid in near term rats. J Radiat Res. 1981;22(2):242–9.
22. Semmler-Behnke M, Fertsch S, Schmid G, Wenk A, Kreyling. Uptake of 1.4 nm versus 18 nm gold nanoparticles in secondary target organs is size dependent in control and pregnant rats after intratracheal or intravenous application. In: EuroNanoForum 2007 – nanotechnology in industrial applications. 2007. Düsseldorf, Germany.
23. Yang H, Sun C, Fan Z, Tian X, Yan L, Du L, et al. Effects of gestational age and surface modification on materno-fetal transfer of nanoparticles in murine pregnancy. Sci Rep. 2012;2:847. doi:10.1038/srep00847.
24. Qi W, Bi J, Zhang X, Wang J, Wang J, Liu P, et al. Damaging effects of multi-walled carbon nanotubes on pregnant mice with different pregnancy times. Sci Rep. 2014;4:4352. doi:10.1038/srep04352.
25. Tsuchiya T, Oguri I, Yamakoshi YN, Miyata N. Novel harmful effects of [60]fullerene on mouse embryos in vitro and in vivo. FEBS Lett. 1996;393(1):139–45.
26. Sumner SC, Fennell TR, Snyder RW, Taylor GF, Lewin AH. Distribution of carbon-14 labeled C60 ([14C]C60) in the pregnant and in the lactating dam and the effect of C60 exposure on the biochemical profile of urine. J Appl Toxicol JAT. 2010;30(4):354–60. doi:10.1002/jat.1503.
27. Takeda K, Suzuki K, Ishihara A, Kubo-Irie M, Fujimoto R, Tabata M, et al. Nanoparticles transferred from pregnant mice to their offspring can damage the genital and cranial nerve systems. J Health Sci. 2009;55:95–102. doi:10.1248/jhs.55.95.
28. Yamashita K, Yoshioka Y, Higashisaka K, Mimura K, Morishita Y, Nozaki M, et al. Silica and titanium dioxide nanoparticles cause pregnancy complications in mice. Nat Nanotechnol. 2011;6(5):321–8. doi:10.1038/nnano.2011.41.
29. Tian F, Razansky D, Estrada GG, Semmler-Behnke M, Beyerle A, Kreyling W, et al. Surface modification and size dependence in particle translocation during early embryonic development. Inhal Toxicol. 2009;21 Suppl 1:92–6. doi:10.1080/08958370902942624.
30. Noori A, Parivar K, Modaresi M, Messripour M, Yousefi MH, Amiri GR, et al. Effect of magnetic iron oxide nanoparticles on pregnancy and testicular development of mice. Afr J Biotechnol. 2011;10(7):1221–7. doi:10.5897/AJB10.1544.
31. Melnik EA, Buzulukov YP, Demin VF, Demin VA, Gmoshinski IV, Tyshko NV, et al. Transfer of Silver Nanoparticles through the Placenta and Breast Milk during in vivo Experiments on Rats. Acta Nat. 2013;5(3):107–15.

32. Chu M, Wu Q, Yang H, Yuan R, Hou S, Yang Y, et al. Transfer of quantum dots from pregnant mice to pups across the placental barrier. Small. 2010;6(5):670–8. doi:10.1002/smll.200902049.
33. Sadauskas E, Wallin H, Stoltenberg M, Vogel U, Doering P, Larsen A, et al. Kupffer cells are central in the removal of nanoparticles from the organism. Part Fibre Toxicol. 2007;4:10. doi:10.1186/1743-8977-4-10.
34. Myllynen PK, Loughran MJ, Howard CV, Sormunen R, Walsh AA, Vahakangas KH. Kinetics of gold nanoparticles in the human placenta. Reprod Toxicol. 2008;26(2):130–7. doi:10.1016/j.reprotox.2008.06.008.
35. Zalgeviciene V, Kulvietis V, Bulotiene D, Didziapetriene J, Rotomskis R. The effect of nanoparticles in rats during critical periods of pregnancy. Medicina. 2012;48(5):256–64.
36. Wick P, Malek A, Manser P, Meili D, Maeder-Althaus X, Diener L, et al. Barrier capacity of human placenta for nanosized materials. Environ Health Perspect. 2010;118(3):432–6. doi:10.1289/ehp.0901200.
37. Grafmuller S, Manser P, Krug HF, Wick P, von Mandach U. Determination of the transport rate of xenobiotics and nanomaterials across the placenta using the ex vivo human placental perfusion model. J Vis Exp JoVE. 2013(76). doi:10.3791/50401.
38. Philbrook NA, Walker VK, Afrooz AR, Saleh NB, Winn LM. Investigating the effects of functionalized carbon nanotubes on reproduction and development in Drosophila melanogaster and CD-1 mice. Reprod Toxicol. 2011;32(4):442–8. doi:10.1016/j.reprotox.2011.09.002.
39. Pietroiusti A, Massimiani M, Fenoglio I, Colonna M, Valentini F, Palleschi G, et al. Low doses of pristine and oxidized single-wall carbon nanotubes affect mammalian embryonic development. ACS Nano. 2011;5(6):4624–33. doi:10.1021/nn200372g.
40. Fujitani T, Ohyama K, Hirose A, Nishimura T, Nakae D, Ogata A. Teratogenicity of multi-wall carbon nanotube (MWCNT) in ICR mice. J Toxicol Sci. 2012;37(1):81–9.
41. Blum JL, Xiong JQ, Hoffman C, Zelikoff JT. Cadmium associated with inhaled cadmium oxide nanoparticles impacts fetal and neonatal development and growth. Toxicol Sci. 2012;126(2):478–86. doi:10.1093/toxsci/kfs008.
42. Li PW, Kuo TH, Chang JH, Yeh JM, Chan WH. Induction of cytotoxicity and apoptosis in mouse blastocysts by silver nanoparticles. Toxicol Lett. 2010;197(2):82–7. doi:10.1016/j.toxlet.2010.05.003.
43. Chan WH, Shiao NH. Cytotoxic effect of CdSe quantum dots on mouse embryonic development. Acta Pharmacol Sin. 2008;29(2):259–66. doi:10.1111/j.1745-7254.2008.00743.x.
44. Hsieh MS, Shiao NH, Chan WH. Cytotoxic effects of CdSe quantum dots on maturation of mouse oocytes, fertilization, and fetal development. Int J Mol Sci. 2009;10(5):2122–35. doi:10.3390/ijms10052122.
45. Girardi G, Redecha P, Salmon JE. Heparin prevents antiphospholipid antibody-induced fetal loss by inhibiting complement activation. Nat Med. 2004;10(11):1222–6. doi:10.1038/nm1121.
46. Li Y, Wang HY, Cho CH. Association of heparin with basic fibroblast growth factor, epidermal growth factor, and constitutive nitric oxide synthase on healing of gastric ulcer in rats. J Pharmacol Exp Ther. 1999;290(2):789–96.
47. Hills FA, Abrahams VM, Gonzalez-Timon B, Francis J, Cloke B, Hinkson L, et al. Heparin prevents programmed cell death in human trophoblast. Mol Hum Reprod. 2006;12(4):237–43. doi:10.1093/molehr/gal026.
48. Hossain N, Schatz F, Paidas MJ. Heparin and maternal fetal interface: why should it work to prevent pregnancy complications? Thromb Res. 2009;124(6):653–5. doi:10.1016/j.thromres.2009.08.001.
49. Myatt L, Cui X. Oxidative stress in the placenta. Histochem Cell Biol. 2004;122(4):369–82. doi:10.1007/s00418-004-0677-x.
50. Shimizu M, Tainaka H, Oba T, Mizuo K, Umezawa M, Takeda K. Maternal exposure to nanoparticulate titanium dioxide during the prenatal period alters gene expression related to

brain development in the mouse. Part Fibre Toxicol. 2009;6:20. doi:10.1186/1743-8977-6-20.

51. Umezawa M, Tainaka H, Kawashima N, Shimizu M, Takeda K. Effect of fetal exposure to titanium dioxide nanoparticle on brain development – brain region information. J Toxicol Sci. 2012;37(6):1247–52.
52. Takahashi Y, Mizuo K, Shinkai Y, Oshio S, Takeda K. Prenatal exposure to titanium dioxide nanoparticles increases dopamine levels in the prefrontal cortex and neostriatum of mice. J Toxicol Sci. 2010;35(5):749–56.
53. Hougaard KS, Jackson P, Jensen KA, Sloth JJ, Loschner K, Larsen EH, et al. Effects of prenatal exposure to surface-coated nanosized titanium dioxide (UV-Titan). A study in mice. Part Fibre Toxicol. 2010;7:16. doi:10.1186/1743-8977-7-16.
54. Jackson P, Halappanavar S, Hougaard KS, Williams A, Madsen AM, Lamson JS, et al. Maternal inhalation of surface-coated nanosized titanium dioxide (UV-Titan) in C57BL/6 mice: effects in prenatally exposed offspring on hepatic DNA damage and gene expression. Nanotoxicology. 2013;7(1):85–96. doi:10.3109/17435390.2011.633715.
55. Fedulov AV, Leme A, Yang Z, Dahl M, Lim R, Mariani TJ, et al. Pulmonary exposure to particles during pregnancy causes increased neonatal asthma susceptibility. Am J Respir Cell Mol Biol. 2008;38(1):57–67. doi:10.1165/rcmb.2007-0124OC.
56. Yoshida S, Hiyoshi K, Oshio S, Takano H, Takeda K, Ichinose T. Effects of fetal exposure to carbon nanoparticles on reproductive function in male offspring. Fertil Steril. 2010;93(5):1695–9. doi:10.1016/j.fertnstert.2009.03.094.
57. Kyjovska ZO, Boisen AM, Jackson P, Wallin H, Vogel U, Hougaard KS. Daily sperm production: application in studies of prenatal exposure to nanoparticles in mice. Reprod Toxicol. 2013;36:88–97. doi:10.1016/j.reprotox.2012.12.005.
58. Jackson P, Vogel U, Wallin H, Hougaard KS. Prenatal exposure to carbon black (printex 90): effects on sexual development and neurofunction. Basic Clin Pharmacol Toxicol. 2011;109(6):434–7. doi:10.1111/j.1742-7843.2011.00745.x.
59. Jackson P, Hougaard KS, Vogel U, Wu D, Casavant L, Williams A, et al. Exposure of pregnant mice to carbon black by intratracheal instillation: toxicogenomic effects in dams and offspring. Mutat Res. 2012;745(1–2):73–83. doi:10.1016/j.mrgentox.2011.09.018.
60. Jackson P, Hougaard KS, Boisen AM, Jacobsen NR, Jensen KA, Moller P, et al. Pulmonary exposure to carbon black by inhalation or instillation in pregnant mice: effects on liver DNA strand breaks in dams and offspring. Nanotoxicology. 2012;6(5):486–500. doi:10.3109/17435390.2011.587902.
61. Umezawa M, Kudo S, Yanagita S, Shinkai Y, Niki R, Oyabu T, et al. Maternal exposure to carbon black nanoparticle increases collagen type VIII expression in the kidney of offspring. J Toxicol Sci. 2011;36(4):461–8.
62. Vitale R, Fawcett DW, Dym M. The normal development of the blood-testis barrier and the effects of clomiphene and estrogen treatment. Anat Rec. 1973;176(3):331–44.
63. Johanson CE. Permeability and vascularity of the developing brain: cerebellum vs cerebral cortex. Brain Res. 1980;190(1):3–16.
64. Chemes HE. Infancy is not a quiescent period of testicular development. Int J Androl. 2001;24(1):2–7.
65. Watson RE, Desesso JM, Hurtt ME, Cappon GD. Postnatal growth and morphological development of the brain: a species comparison. Birth Defects Res A Clin Mol Teratol. 2006;77(5):471–84. doi:10.1002/bdrb.20090.
66. Jonakait GM. The effects of maternal inflammation on neuronal development: possible mechanisms. Int J Dev Neurosci. 2007;25(7):415–25. doi:10.1016/j.ijdevneu.2007.08.017.
67. Gao X, Yin S, Tang M, Chen J, Yang Z, Zhang W, et al. Effects of developmental exposure to TiO2 nanoparticles on synaptic plasticity in hippocampal dentate gyrus area: an in vivo study in anesthetized rats. Biol Trace Elem Res. 2011;143(3):1616–28. doi:10.1007/s12011-011-8990-4.

68. De Jong WH, Hagens WI, Krystek P, Burger MC, Sips AJ, Geertsma RE. Particle size-dependent organ distribution of gold nanoparticles after intravenous administration. Biomaterials. 2008;29(12):1912–19. doi:10.1016/j.biomaterials.2007.12.037.
69. Balasubramanian SK, Jittiwat J, Manikandan J, Ong CN, Yu LE, Ong WY. Biodistribution of gold nanoparticles and gene expression changes in the liver and spleen after intravenous administration in rats. Biomaterials. 2010;31(8):2034–42. doi:10.1016/j.biomaterials.2009.11.079.
70. Li WQ, Wang F, Liu ZM, Wang YC, Wang J, Sun F. Gold nanoparticles elevate plasma testosterone levels in male mice without affecting fertility. Small. 2013;9(9–10):1708–14. doi:10.1002/smll.201201079.
71. Bai Y, Zhang Y, Zhang J, Mu Q, Zhang W, Butch ER, et al. Repeated administrations of carbon nanotubes in male mice cause reversible testis damage without affecting fertility. Nat Nanotechnol. 2010;5(9):683–9. doi:10.1038/nnano.2010.153.
72. Gao G, Ze Y, Zhao X, Sang X, Zheng L, Ze X, et al. Titanium dioxide nanoparticle-induced testicular damage, spermatogenesis suppression, and gene expression alterations in male mice. J Hazard Mater. 2013;258–259:133–43. doi:10.1016/j.jhazmat.2013.04.046.
73. Zhao X, Sheng L, Wang L, Hong J, Yu X, Sang X, et al. Mechanisms of nanosized titanium dioxide-induced testicular oxidative stress and apoptosis in male mice. Part Fibre Toxicol. 2014;11(1):47. doi:10.1186/s12989-014-0047-3.
74. Morishita Y, Yoshioka Y, Satoh H, Nojiri N, Nagano K, Abe Y, et al. Distribution and histologic effects of intravenously administered amorphous nanosilica particles in the testes of mice. Biochem Biophys Res Commun. 2012;420(2):297–301. doi:10.1016/j.bbrc.2012.02.153.
75. Zhu MT, Feng WY, Wang Y, Wang B, Wang M, Ouyang H, et al. Particokinetics and extrapulmonary translocation of intratracheally instilled ferric oxide nanoparticles in rats and the potential health risk assessment. Toxicol Sci. 2009;107(2):342–51. doi:10.1093/toxsci/kfn245.
76. Kim YS, Song MY, Park JD, Song KS, Ryu HR, Chung YH, et al. Subchronic oral toxicity of silver nanoparticles. Parti Fibre Toxicol. 2010;7:20. doi:10.1186/1743-8977-7-20.
77. Park EJ, Bae E, Yi J, Kim Y, Choi K, Lee SH, et al. Repeated-dose toxicity and inflammatory responses in mice by oral administration of silver nanoparticles. Environ Toxicol Pharmacol. 2010;30(2):162–8. doi:10.1016/j.etap.2010.05.004.
78. van der Zande M, Vandebriel RJ, Van Doren E, Kramer E, Herrera Rivera Z, Serrano-Rojero CS, et al. Distribution, elimination, and toxicity of silver nanoparticles and silver ions in rats after 28-day oral exposure. ACS Nano. 2012;6(8):7427–42. doi:10.1021/nn302649p.
79. Lee JH, Kim YS, Song KS, Ryu HR, Sung JH, Park JD, et al. Biopersistence of silver nanoparticles in tissues from Sprague–Dawley rats. Part Fibre Toxicol. 2013;10:36. doi:10.1186/1743-8977-10-36.
80. Yokel RA, Au TC, MacPhail R, Hardas SS, Butterfield DA, Sultana R, et al. Distribution, elimination, and biopersistence to 90 days of a systemically introduced 30 nm ceria-engineered nanomaterial in rats. Toxicol Sci. 2012;127(1):256–68. doi:10.1093/toxsci/kfs067.
81. Kim JS, Yoon TJ, Yu KN, Kim BG, Park SJ, Kim HW, et al. Toxicity and tissue distribution of magnetic nanoparticles in mice. Toxicol Sci. 2006;89(1):338–47. doi:10.1093/toxsci/kfj027.
82. Kwon JT, Hwang SK, Jin H, Kim DS, Minai-Tehrani A, Yoon HJ, et al. Body distribution of inhaled fluorescent magnetic nanoparticles in the mice. J Occup Health. 2008;50(1):1–6.
83. Wang Z, Chen Z, Zuo Q, Song F, Wu D, Cheng W, et al. Reproductive toxicity in adult male rats following intra-articular injection of cobalt-chromium nanoparticles. J Orthop Sci. 2013;18(6):1020–6. doi:10.1007/s00776-013-0458-2.
84. Araujo L, Sheppard M, Löbenberg R, Kreuter J. Uptake of PMMA nanoparticles from the gastrointestinal tract after oral administration to rats: modification of the body distribution

after suspension in surfactant solutions and in oil vehicles. Int J Pharm. 1999;176(2):209–24. doi:10.1016/S0378-5173(98)00314-7.
85. Yoshida S, Hiyoshi K, Ichinose T, Takano H, Oshio S, Sugawara I, et al. Effect of nanoparticles on the male reproductive system of mice. Int J Androl. 2009;32(4):337–42. doi:10.1111/j.1365-2605.2007.00865.x.
86. Sycheva LP, Zhurkov VS, Iurchenko VV, Daugel-Dauge NO, Kovalenko MA, Krivtsova EK, et al. Investigation of genotoxic and cytotoxic effects of micro- and nanosized titanium dioxide in six organs of mice in vivo. Mutat Res. 2011;726(1):8–14. doi:10.1016/j.mrgentox.2011.07.010.
87. Hassankhani R, Esmaeillou M, Tehrani AA, Nasirzadeh K, Khadir F, Maadi H. In vivo toxicity of orally administrated silicon dioxide nanoparticles in healthy adult mice. Environ Sci Pollut Res Int. 2015;22(2):1127–32. doi:10.1007/s11356-014-3413-7.
88. Gromadzka-Ostrowska J, Dziendzikowska K, Lankoff A, Dobrzynska M, Instanes C, Brunborg G, et al. Silver nanoparticles effects on epididymal sperm in rats. Toxicol Lett. 2012;214(3):251–8. doi:10.1016/j.toxlet.2012.08.028.
89. Li C, Taneda S, Taya K, Watanabe G, Li X, Fujitani Y, et al. Effects of inhaled nanoparticle-rich diesel exhaust on regulation of testicular function in adult male rats. Inhal Toxicol. 2009;21(10):803–11. doi:10.1080/08958370802524381.
90. Ramdhan DH, Ito Y, Yanagiba Y, Yamagishi N, Hayashi Y, Li C, et al. Nanoparticle-rich diesel exhaust may disrupt testosterone biosynthesis and metabolism via growth hormone. Toxicol Lett. 2009;191(2–3):103–8. doi:10.1016/j.toxlet.2009.08.013.
91. Guo LL, Liu XH, Qin DX, Gao L, Zhang HM, Liu JY, et al. Effects of nanosized titanium dioxide on the reproductive system of male mice. Zhonghua nan ke xue = Nat J Androl. 2009;15(6):517–22.
92. Wiwanitkit V, Sereemaspun A, Rojanathanes R. Effect of gold nanoparticles on spermatozoa: the first world report. Fertil Steril. 2009;91(1):e7–8. doi:10.1016/j.fertnstert.2007.08.021.
93. Ben-David Makhluf S, Qasem R, Rubinstein S, Gedanken A, Breitbart H. Loading magnetic nanoparticles into sperm cells does not affect their functionality. Langmuir. 2006;22 (23):9480–2. doi:10.1021/la061988z.
94. Braydich-Stolle LK, Lucas B, Schrand A, Murdock RC, Lee T, Schlager JJ, et al. Silver nanoparticles disrupt GDNF/Fyn kinase signaling in spermatogonial stem cells. Toxicol Sci. 2010;116(2):577–89. doi:10.1093/toxsci/kfq148.
95. Terzuoli G, Iacoponi F, Moretti E, Renieri T, Baldi G, Collodel G. In vitro effect of silver engineered nanoparticles on human spermatozoa. J Siena Acad Sci. 2011;3(1):27–9. doi:10.4081/jsas.2011.27.
96. Zakhidow ST, Marshak TL, Malolina EA, Kulibin AY, Zelenina IA, Pavluchenkova SM, et al. Gold nanoparticles disturb nuclear chromatin decondensation in mouse sperm in vitro. Biochem (Moscow) Suppl Ser A Membr Cell Biol. 2010;4(3):293–6. doi:10.1134/S1990747810030074.
97. Carone BR, Fauquier L, Habib N, Shea JM, Hart CE, Li R, et al. Paternally induced transgenerational environmental reprogramming of metabolic gene expression in mammals. Cell. 2010;143(7):1084–96. doi:10.1016/j.cell.2010.12.008.
98. Ng SF, Lin RC, Laybutt DR, Barres R, Owens JA, Morris MJ. Chronic high-fat diet in fathers programs beta-cell dysfunction in female rat offspring. Nature. 2010;467(7318):963–6. doi:10.1038/nature09491.
99. Dias BG, Ressler KJ. Parental olfactory experience influences behavior and neural structure in subsequent generations. Nat Neurosci. 2014;17(1):89–96. doi:10.1038/nn.3594.
100. Gapp K, Jawaid A, Sarkies P, Bohacek J, Pelczar P, Prados J, et al. Implication of sperm RNAs in transgenerational inheritance of the effects of early trauma in mice. Nat Neurosci. 2014;17(5):667–9. doi:10.1038/nn.3695.
101. Bal R, Turk G, Tuzcu M, Yilmaz O, Ozercan I, Kuloglu T, et al. Protective effects of nanostructures of hydrated C(60) fullerene on reproductive function in streptozotocin-diabetic male rats. Toxicology. 2011;282(3):69–81. doi:10.1016/j.tox.2010.12.003.

102. Srdjenovic B, Milic-Torres V, Grujic N, Stankov K, Djordjevic A, Vasovic V. Antioxidant properties of fullerenol C60(OH)24 in rat kidneys, testes, and lungs treated with doxorubicin. Toxicol Mech Methods. 2010;20(6):298–305. doi:10.3109/15376516.2010.485622.
103. Lundqvist M, Stigler J, Elia G, Lynch I, Cedervall T, Dawson KA. Nanoparticle size and surface properties determine the protein corona with possible implications for biological impacts. Proc Natl Acad Sci U S A. 2008;105(38):14265–70. doi:10.1073/pnas.0805135105.

Chapter 5
Fibrogenic and Immunotoxic Responses to Carbon Nanotubes

James C. Bonner

Abstract Carbon nanotubes (CNTs) are a major product of the emerging nanotechnology industry that have numerous applications. Human exposure to CNTs is inevitable as they will be manufactured and incorporated into consumer products. CNTs represent a widely varying class of nanomaterials that vary due to numbers of concentric walls (single versus multiple) and manufacturing process that result in variable rigidity and metal catalyst content. Moreover, post-synthesis functionalization to enhance the properties of CNTs will create a vast array of new nanomaterials that have unknown effects on biological systems. Toxicologists have been proactive in investigating the potential adverse effects of CNTs, and an overwhelming body of evidence shows that fibrosis is a common outcome of pulmonary exposure in rodents. CNTs also have adverse effects on the immune system, including impaired macrophage function and exacerbation of preexisting lung inflammatory diseases. In addition, CNTs may cause systemic immune suppression. A major issue is the potential carcinogenic effects of CNTs, particularly with regards to mesothelioma. The overall goal is to predict and prevent human disease that could occur from CNT exposure.

Keywords Carbon nanotubes • Fibrosis • Immunotoxicity • Lung

5.1 Introduction

The nanotechnology industry emerged only over the past few decades, and yet even in this relatively short period of time, thousands of different types of engineered nanoparticles (ENMs) have been created with a myriad of potential uses in engineering, electronics, and medicine [1, 2]. ENMs produced in the greatest volume include titanium dioxide, cerium oxide, zinc oxide, silver, and carbon nanotubes (CNTs). A concern is that these newly emerging nanoscale particle- and fiber-like

J.C. Bonner (✉)
Department of Biological Sciences, North Carolina State University, Campus Box 7633, Raleigh, NC 27695, USA
e-mail: james_bonner@ncsu.edu

T. Otsuki et al. (eds.), *Biological Effects of Fibrous and Particulate Substances*, Current Topics in Environmental Health and Preventive Medicine,
DOI 10.1007/978-4-431-55732-6_5

structures with widely varying physical dimensions and chemical features will pose a risk for disease through occupational, consumer, or environmental exposure.

Almost all human diseases that have been associated with environmental exposure to particles and fibers involve chronic tissue remodeling that originates from the dysregulation of the immune system. CNTs are no exception and have the potential to cause lung immunotoxic and fibroproliferative responses due their high surface area per unit mass, increased reactivity, greater ability to cross biological barriers, and increased opportunity to directly interact with immune cells [3].

CNTs are graphene sheets rolled into cylinders that are one ("single-walled," SWCNT) or multiple ("multiwalled," MWCNT) layers thick. MWCNTs have unique physical and chemical properties that make them particularly hazardous, including fiber-like shape with increased rigidity reinforced by multiple concentric layers and residual metal catalyst from the manufacturing process [4]. SWCNTs and MWCNTs have numerous useful applications in structural engineering, electronics, and medicine. However, CNTs also represent a risk to human health as they have been shown to cause pulmonary fibrosis and immunotoxicity in rodents following inhalation exposure.

The focus of this chapter is to overview some of the mechanisms of CNT-induced lung fibrogenesis and immunotoxicity. Growing evidence from rodent studies indicate that fibrosis caused by CNT exposure is determined by multiple factors, including rigidity, metal catalyst contamination, dispersion, and post-synthesis functionalization. In addition, the development and utility of *in vitro* cell and tissue culture assays to predict *in vivo* responses in rodents will be discussed as means to more effectively and rapidly test adverse effects on human health in the face of a rapidly growing diversity of ENMs, including CNTs.

5.2 Pulmonary Fibrosis

Fibrosis is a chronic fibroproliferative disease caused by environmental or occupational exposure to a variety of particles, fibers, and metals [5, 6]. Pathological changes can occur within the pulmonary interstitium of the distal lung parenchyma, around the conducting airways or vasculature, or at the subpleura. In severe cases, sustained fibroproliferative responses compromise lung function through progressive accumulation of extracellular matrix that impedes gas exchange. In severe fibrosis cases, including asbestosis, sarcoidosis, and idiopathic pulmonary fibrosis (IPF), fibrosis is the dominant phenotypic outcome and results in respiratory failure. Pulmonary fibrosis is an occupational hazard following exposure to many particles and fibers. CNTs could pose a significant risk for the development of fibrosis because of their increased surface area to mass ratio and ROS-producing potential. CNTs have been compared to asbestos fibers based mainly on rigid fiber-like shape [4]. Asbestos fibers are a known cause of fibrosis and mesothelioma in humans. However, CNTs also have some uniquely different properties from asbestos, including nanoscale width and highly conformal structure. While not yet known, a growing body of evidence from rodent studies suggests that CNTs will cause pulmonary fibrosis in humans [7, 8].

5.2.1 Inhalation Versus Aspiration

Fibrosis has been documented in the lungs of rodents after exposure to CNTs delivered by several methods, including inhalation, instillation, or oropharyngeal aspiration. Inhalation exposure is ideal as it represents a more realistic exposure in terms of deposition patterns in the lung that would occur in occupational settings. The deposition of inhaled CNTs is determined by a number of factors including size, shape, electrostatic charge, and aggregation state. For example, inhalation exposure to well-dispersed MWCNTs results in deposition in the distal regions, i.e., alveolar duct bifurcations and alveolar epithelial surfaces in the lungs of mice or rats [9, 10]. Inhalation of dry MWCNTs or aerosolized MWCNTs in surfactant-containing media causes diffuse interstitial fibrotic lesions within the alveolar and subpleural regions of the lung. Exposure by instillation or oropharyngeal aspiration, which involves a bolus delivery of CNT suspended aqueous media, can also result in deposition at distal sites in the lungs if the nanoparticles are well dispersed. However, a number of studies have reported granulomas in the lungs of rodents that result from agglomerated SWCNTs or MWCNTs that lodge within small airways, which is not observed in most inhalation studies. However, methods for dispersing CNTs in aqueous suspension using surfactant-containing media prior to instillation or aspiration in rats or mice have greatly improved, making this route of exposure generally acceptable [11]. The different types of fibrotic lesions described above are illustrated in Fig. 5.1.

5.2.2 Agglomeration

The relative state of agglomeration is an important determinant of fibrogenic responses to CNTs. Agglomeration refers to nanoparticles that loosely adhere to one another through noncovalent interactions, such as electrostatic charge or van der Waals forces. Agglomerated CNTs can be dispersed by surfactant-containing media. In addition, surface functionalization of CNTs that decrease electrostatic charge reduces agglomeration. Agglomerated CNTs tend to produce granulomatous lesions [12–15]. In contrast, dispersion of MWCNTs with dipalmitoylphosphatidylcholine (DPPC) caused enhanced uptake by macrophages and an increase in diffuse pulmonary fibrosis in mice [16]. Also, in this same study, it was shown that well-dispersed MWCNTs were readily taken up by macrophages and stimulate increased growth factor (PDGF-AA, TGF-β1) and IL-1β production compared with agglomerated MWCNTs. Agglomeration status is also an important determinant for *in vitro* testing cultured cells since agglomerated CNTs tend to remain in the culture

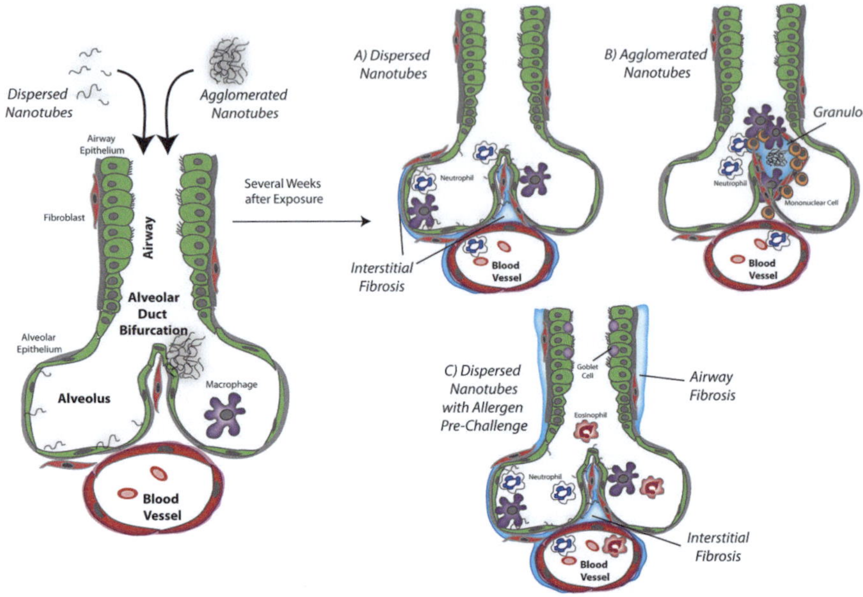

Fig. 5.1 Illustration of different types of fibrotic lesions observed in the lungs of mice after exposure to MWCNTs. (**a**) Interstitial fibrosis associated dispersed MWCNTs in the alveolar region of the lung (**b**). Granuloma formation caused by agglomerated MWCNTs at the alveolar duct bifurcation. (**c**) Airway fibrosis and interstitial fibrosis caused by dispersed MWCNTs in the lungs of mice prechallenged with ovalbumin or house dust mite allergen

medium, whereas dispersed CNTs reach the cell surface more effectively. Therefore, the actual dose at the cell surface can be significantly different when comparing agglomerated versus dispersed CNTs and should be taken into consideration for *in vitro* testing [17].

5.2.3 Rigidity

Long, rigid MWCNTs disrupt macrophage function by causing frustrated phagocytosis, which results in the disruption of cell membranes and cell death [4, 18]. Cell membrane disruption also causes leakage of cellular constituents (e.g., enzymes, cytokines) that can cause injury to surrounding cells and tissues. While CNT length is an important determinant of clearance rate from the lungs, length alone does not necessarily determine CNT persistence. For example, long SWCNTs are flexible and when folded are taken up by macrophages without causing frustrated phagocytosis or impeding macrophage clearance. Rigid MWCNTs disrupt macrophage function if the nanotube length exceeds the width of the engulfing phagocyte. Short, rigid MWCNTs are capable of being taken up by macrophages without causing frustrated phagocytosis. MWCNTs from different manufacturing sources possess different degrees of rigidity even though they may have similar width; some are "curly" whereas others are straight. This comparison is reminiscent of the comparison between asbestos fiber types; chrysotile asbestos is a curly fiber, whereas crocidolite asbestos is a more toxic straight rigid fiber.

5.2.4 Metal Catalysts

A variety of metals are used as catalysts in the manufacture of CNTs by chemical vapor deposition (CVD). For example, cobalt is used as a catalyst in the synthesis of SWCNTs, while nickel or iron is used as a catalyst in the synthesis of MWCNTs. These same metals are known to mediate pulmonary fibrosis in humans in occupational settings [19]. For example, nickel is known to cause occupational asthma and contact dermatitis, whereas iron and cobalt cause interstitial pulmonary fibrosis in occupations related to mining and metallurgy. Metal catalysts used in the CVD manufacturing process become integrated into the carbon structure of nanotubes and mediate some of the pro-inflammatory effects seen after exposure to MWCNTs in rodents. For example, the activation of macrophage inflammasomes and subsequent IL-1β production induced by MWCNT exposure are due at least in part to residual nickel contamination [20]. Acid washing of MWCNTs removes some, but not all, of residual nickel, and intralaboratory comparisons of the pro-inflammatory effects of acid-washed MWCNTs and pristine MWCNTs show that neutrophilic inflammation in the lungs of mice is reduced by partial removal of nickel.

5.2.5 Functionalization

CNTs can be modified post-synthesis by adding molecules to the surface to alter physicochemical characteristics and functionality. Surface functionalization of MWCNTs alters charge and agglomeration status, thereby modifying biological responses *in vitro* and *in vivo*. For example, MWCNTs functionalized with strong cationic polyetherimide (PEI)-MWCNTs induced significant lung fibrosis in mice, while carboxylation of MWCNTs significantly decreased the extent of pulmonary fibrosis compared with pristine MWCNTs [21]. Carboxylated MWCNTs also stimulate less neutrophilic inflammation in mice as compared with pristine MWCNTs [22]. These results demonstrated that surface charge plays an important role in the structure-activity relationships that determine the profibrogenic potential of functionalized CNTs in the lung. Surface functionalization of MWCNTs by atomic layer deposition (ALD) thin film coating, which allows for a highly conformal nanoscale coating, can be achieved with a variety of inorganic and organic substrates. ALD functionalization has been shown to modify the fibrogenic response *in vitro* and *in vivo*. For example, ALD coating of MWCNTs with Al_2O_3 reduces the secretion of profibrogenic cytokines (e.g., osteopontin and tumor necrosis factor-α) in human monocytic THP-1 cells and human peripheral blood monocytes *in vitro*, and this correlates to reduced levels of these cytokines in the lungs of mice *in vivo* [23]. Moreover, Al_2O_3-coated MWCNTs cause less fibrosis in the lungs of mice compared with uncoated MWCNTs. Figure 5.2 shows transmission electron micrographs of MWCNTs before and after ALD functionalization with Al_2O_3 and the resulting lung pathology in mice after exposure to these MWCNTs.

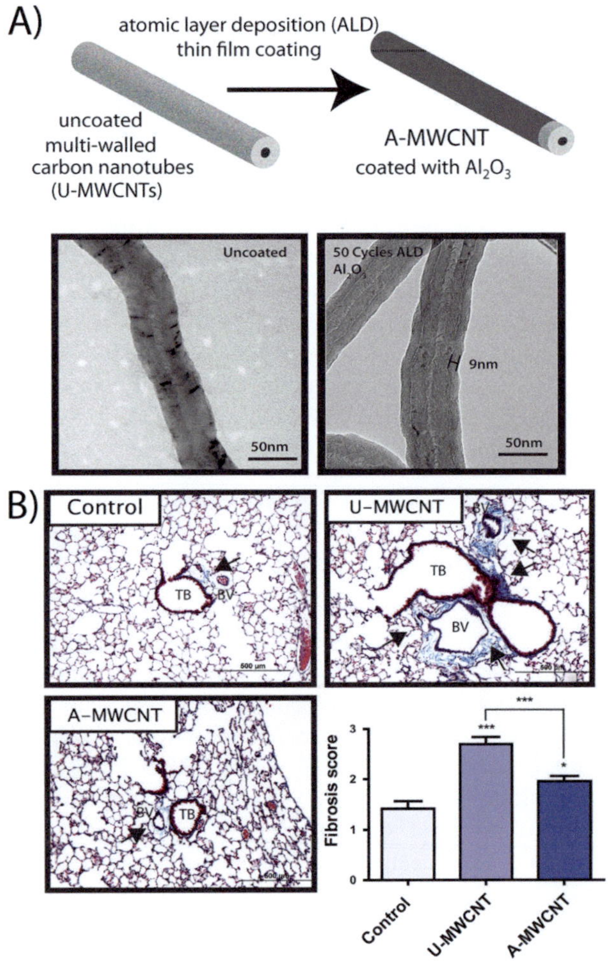

Fig. 5.2 (**a**) Illustration and transmission electron micrographs of pristine uncoated (U)-MWCNT or MWCNT coated with Al_2O_3 (A-MWCNT) by 50 cycles of atomic layer deposition (ALD). (**b**) Representative microscopic images of trichrome-stained slides (20X) and semiquantitative morphometry at 28 days following exposure to 0.1 % pluronic/PBS vehicle (control), U-MWCNT, or A-MWCNT at a dose of 4 mg/kg (Adapted from Ref. [23])

5.2.6 Biocorona Formation

An important concept in nanotoxicology is the formation of a "biocorona" on the surface of the ENMs that alters the interaction of the nanoparticle with other molecules and cell membranes. The biocorona forms in biological systems as nanomaterials adsorb biomolecules [24]. For example, SWCNTs recovered from the bronchoalveolar lavage fluid of mice after delivery by oropharyngeal aspiration adsorbed surfactant phospholipids (phosphatidylcholine, phosphatidylglycerol, and surfactant proteins A, B, and D) as determined by liquid chromatography mass spectrometry (LC-MS) [25]. In this same study, the authors showed that the surfactant biocorona on SWCNTs enhanced uptake of SWCNTs by RAW264.7 mouse macrophages. The consequence of surfactant biocorona formation on CNTs *in vivo* is not clear, but surfactant proteins are critical to lung development, normal lung homeostasis, and protection against nickel-induced lung injury [26]. It is possible that CNTs could disrupt normal lung homeostasis by adsorbing surfactant proteins. Other work has shown that coating CNTs with phospholipids modifies recognition and phagocytosis by macrophages. Coating SWCNTs with phosphatidylserine (PS), a phospholipid on the surface of apoptotic cells that signals macrophage recognition and phagocytosis of dying cells, promoted uptake of SWCNTs *in vitro* by RAW264.7 macrophages and *in vivo* following pharyngeal aspiration in a mouse model [27]. These studies highlight the importance the biocorona in modifying the innate immune response of macrophage to CNTs. SWCNTs and MWCNTs also bind a variety of proteins in cell culture media (FBS-DMEM) which has important implications for studying biological responses *in vitro* [28]. In addition to phospholipids and serum proteins, it is also possible that CNTs could adsorb other biomolecules such as growth factors, cytokines, enzymes, and nucleic acids.

5.2.7 Clearance and Degradation

CNTs taken up by macrophages are removed from the lungs through two primary mechanisms: (1) the mucociliary escalator and (2) the lymphatic drainage system. The mucociliary escalator is driven by ciliary beating of airway epithelial cells that move a layer of mucus up and out of the lungs [29]. Macrophages containing CNTs migrate to the distal portion of small airways where they are transported by the escalator to larger airways and ultimately out of the trachea where they are swallowed or expelled through coughing. A secondary macrophage-mediated clearance passage for CNTs out of the lungs is the lymphatic drainage system, which includes lymphatic vessels that drain into the pleural cavity. Some macrophages containing MWCNTs exit the lung via the pleural lymphatic system and enter the pleural space or can be found in lung-associated lymph nodes [30]. As mentioned above, rigid MWCNTs disrupt macrophage function by causing frustrated phagocytosis, which results in the release of inflammatory mediators (ROS and cytokines) and cell death. The innate immune function of macrophages could also be compromised by the formation of bridges composed of parallel bundles of SWCNTs that link two or more macrophages [31]. As mentioned above, CNTs that are long and rigid impede clearance. Structures longer than 10–15 μm (the approximate width of an alveolar macrophage) are difficult to clear from lung tissues via macrophage-mediated mechanisms. Some MWCNTs are biopersistent and transmission electron microscopy shows that some remain in lung and subpleural tissue for months [32]. However, several studies in recent years have shown that CNTs are susceptible to degradation by naturally occurring enzymes (peroxidases). For example, CNTs can be degraded by neutrophil myeloperoxidase and eosinophil peroxide [33, 34]. Interestingly, myeloperoxidase-deficient mice have impaired clearance of CNTs and enhanced pulmonary inflammation and fibrosis [35].

5.3 Mechanisms of Fibrogenesis

The cellular and molecular mechanisms that mediate pulmonary fibrogenesis in the lung depend on the insulting agent (e.g., metals, fibers, chemotherapeutic drugs, radiation) and genetic susceptibility [5]. A common denominator in the progression of fibrosis is mesenchymal cells (fibroblasts, myofibroblasts, and fibrocytes) that provide the major source of secreted collagen that defines end-stage lung fibrosis. The most notable mesenchymal phenotype that contributes to the majority of secreted matrix during the fibrogenic process is the myofibroblast [6]. Abundant evidence indicates that myofibroblasts provide the major source of collagen that defines the fibrotic lesion and that TGF-β1 is the dominant growth factor that stimulates matrix synthesis by lung mesenchymal cells. Myofibroblast accumulation can result from several possible mechanisms (recruitment of circulating fibrocytes, epithelial-mesenchymal cell transition, or migration and proliferation of resident lung mesenchymal cells). The resolution of fibrosis is determined by degradation of collagen by matrix metalloproteinases and myofibroblast growth arrest/apoptosis. In contrast, progressive fibrosis is the result of sustained matrix deposition or the lack of matrix degradation, coupled with myofibroblast survival.

5.3.1 Oxidative Stress

Like other ENMs, the high surface area per unit mass of CNTs allows for increased potential for ROS production and subsequent cellular damage. Treatment of mice with the antioxidant N-acetyl-L-cysteine has recently been shown to inhibit MWCNT-induced fibrosis, and this is related to NADPH oxidase-dependent inflammasome activation [36]. NADPH-oxidase-deficient mice exhibit increased accumulation of neutrophils and decreased fibrosis [37]. This is further evidence that oxidative stress is linked to fibrogenesis. Studies with a panel of cultured lung cells *in vitro* (BEAS-2B, A549, WI38) show that MWCNTs induced substantial ROS production and mitochondrial damage, which was implicated in the activation of redox-sensitive transcription factor NF-κB and the production of a variety of profibrogenic cytokines and growth factors [38]. Macrophage activation by CNTs involves a complex network of intracellular signaling pathways, some of which are designed as protective responses to oxidative stress and cell injury. For example, long MWCNTs activate nuclear translocation of the antioxidant transcription factor Nrf2 in cultured human THP-1 monocytic cells and cause increased gene expression of Nrf2-regulated genes, heme oxygenase-1(HO-1) and glutathione S-transferase (GST) [39]. Furthermore, this study showed that the long nanotubes increased release of the pro-inflammatory cytokine IL-1β by THP-1 cells, and this effect was inhibited by the antioxidant Trolox, suggesting a role of oxidative stress in the upregulation of this cytokine. MWCNTs also increase levels of the cyclooxygenase-2 (COX-2) enzyme through MAP kinase-dependent activation in mouse RAW264.7 cells *in vitro*, and the initiation of this pathway is oxidant dependent as it is blocked by the antioxidant N-acetyl-L-cysteine [40]. COX-2 is a protective factor against lung disease that is increased to counteract ROS-induced cellular stress, and interestingly, COX-2 knockout mice are susceptible to airway fibrosis caused by exposure to ovalbumin allergen and MWCNTs [41].

5.3.2 Cytokines and Growth Factors

A variety of growth factors, cytokines, and chemokines that stimulate myofibroblast differentiation, growth, migration, and extracellular matrix production are induced in the lungs of rats or mice after exposure to ENMs [5]. SWCNTs or MWCNTs delivered to rats by intratracheal instillation or mice by inhalation or oropharyngeal aspiration increase mRNA and protein levels of platelet-derived growth factor (PDGF) [31, 42, 43]. PDGF stimulates the replication, chemotaxis, and survival of lung mesenchymal cells (fibroblasts, myofibroblasts, and smooth muscle cells) to promote lung fibrogenesis [44]. SWCNTs or MWCNTs delivered to the lungs of mice also increase levels of TGF-β1, a central mediator of collagen production by fibroblasts and myofibroblasts [12, 42]. In addition to TGF-β1, osteopontin (OPN) stimulates collagen deposition and fibroblast migration, and levels of OPN are increased in the lungs of rats exposed to single-walled CNTs [31]. Alveolar macrophages, as well as airway epithelial cells and fibroblasts, produce PDGF, TGF-β1, and OPN. Chemokines for inflammatory cells involved in the innate immune response are also induced by CNT exposure and drive the inflammatory response in the lung. CXCL8 (IL-8), a potent neutrophil chemoattractant, is produced by a human bronchial epithelial cell line *in vitro* after exposure to multiwalled CNTs [45]. CXCL1 (MIP-1) and CXCL2 (KC) are the murine homologues to human CXCL8. Both CXCL1 and CXCL2 are induced in the lungs of mice exposed to MWCNT and correspond to neutrophil influx into the lungs at 1 day postexposure by oropharyngeal aspiration [46]. CCL2, also known as monocyte chemoattractant protein-1 (MCP-1), is produced by macrophages and airway epithelial cells and is increased in the bronchoalveolar lavage fluid of mice after MWCNT inhalation exposure [42]. These are only a few examples of the variety of cytokines, chemokines, and growth factors induced by CNT exposure that contribute to inflammation and the progression of pulmonary fibrosis.

5.4 Immunotoxicity

The immune system has evolved to cope with foreign material entering the body that is "not self" and defend against invading microbes (e.g., viruses, bacteria) and immunogenic particles (e.g., allergens). Most of these foreign structures are at the nanoscale. Therefore, it is not surprising that ENMs will present a challenge to our immune system. Immunotoxicity is defined as any adverse effect on the immune system following toxicant exposure that results in immune stimulation or immune suppression. Immunostimulation increases the incidence of allergic reactions, inflammatory responses, fibrogenesis, or autoimmunity, while immunosuppression suppresses the maturation and proliferation of immune cells, resulting in increased susceptibility to infectious diseases or tumor growth. ENMs, including CNTs, have been reported to have either immunostimulatory or immunosuppressive effects in the lung, and this largely depends on the specific type of ENM in question [47]. However, the effects of ENMs on the immune system can also depend on the context of exposure, for example, repeated ENM exposures versus ENM exposure after the establishment of allergic inflammation.

5.4.1 Impairment of Immune Cell Function

Lung macrophages play a critical role in immune surveillance of pathogens and removal of inhaled particles and fibers. CNTs, like many other inhaled particles and fibers, are avidly taken up by alveolar macrophages. Many of the principles that apply to fiber-like particles, such as frustrated phagocytosis, apply to CNTs. As mentioned above, rigid MWCNTs cause frustrated phagocytosis in macrophages, which results in cell membrane damage and leakage of cellular constituents [4]. Also, as discussed below, the uptake and clearance of bacteria is reduced by exposure to CNTs. Some unusual interactions with macrophages have also been observed with CNTs. For example, SWCNTs and some MWCNTs cause bridge-like structures between two or more macrophages [31]. These CNT structures would almost certainly impede the migration of macrophages.

5.4.2 Inflammasomes

A variety of fiber-like particles, including asbestos, silica, and CNTs, all exert at least part of their pro-inflammatory activity by activating macrophage inflammasomes. Inflammasomes are protein scaffolds that facilitate the action of caspase-1 to cleave pro-IL-1β to a mature, secreted form of IL-1β that has important functions in neutrophil infiltration. Several studies have reported that CNTs stimulate inflammasome activation in macrophages [36, 48, 49]. The dysregulation of inflammasomes has been implicated in a variety of disease states [50]. Inflammasome activation by MWCNTs and other high aspect ratio materials (e.g., nanofibers, TiO_2 nanobelts) is mediated by lysosomal disruption and ROS production [51]. Inflammasome activation leading to the release of mature IL-1β has been proposed as a profibrogenic event [16]. However, macrophage IL-1β release is also an important innate immune response for recruiting neutrophils to the lung to participate in microbial killing and the resolution of inflammation [51]. Inflammasome activation occurs to a greater degree in classically activated macrophages (CAMs), which are important in microbial killing. In allergic asthma or fibrosis, macrophages are polarized to "alternatively activated macrophages" (AAMs) in the presence of Th2 cytokines IL-4 or IL-13. AAMs are thought to play important roles in fibrosis and cancer [52]. A recent study showed that inflammasome activation and IL-1β production are suppressed by the Th2 cytokines IL-4 and IL-13 in human monocytic THP-1 cells *in vitro* and in the lungs of mice sensitized with house dust mite allergen prior to MWCNT exposure by oropharyngeal aspiration [46]. The mechanism of inflammasome suppression by these Th2 cytokines was through an STAT6-dependent decrease in pro-caspase-1, the precursor to caspase-1 which serves as the key inflammasome component that cleaves pro-IL-1β to mature IL-1β. This study also showed that MWCNT exposure exacerbated house dust mite allergen-induced airway fibrosis while reducing numbers of neutrophils in the lung, suggesting that inflammasome activation was not a mechanism of airway fibrosis but may instead serve to resolve tissue injury by recruiting neutrophils. Neutrophilic inflammation in the lung is a classic response to MWCNT exposure. Other work has shown that IL-1 receptor knockout (IL-1R KO) mice do not exhibit neutrophilic inflammation and yet develop pulmonary fibrosis to a greater degree than wild-type mice [53]. Recently, inflammasome activation by MWCNTs in human airway epithelial cells *in vitro* was reported as a possible mechanism of driving profibrogenic responses in fibroblasts [54]. The role of inflammasomes and IL-1β in CNT-induced fibrosis remains controversial, and whether IL-1β is profibrogenic or antifibrogenic may depend on its temporal expression, which in turn could determine the duration of neutrophilic inflammation in the lung.

5.4.3 CNTs and Allergen-Induced Airway Disease

Engineered nanoparticles, including CNTs, could pose the greatest health risk to individuals with preexisting lung disease, including asthma. Asthma is a complex disease characterized by chronic airway remodeling that includes increased levels of Th2 cytokines (e.g., IL-4 and IL-13), eosinophilic inflammation, mucous cell metaplasia, and airway fibrosis. Studies from mouse models of allergen airway inflammation suggest that CNTs exacerbate preexisting asthma. For example, MWCNTs enhance allergic airway inflammation in mice caused by ovalbumin sensitization as evidenced by increased Th2 cytokines and chemokines and serum IgE levels as compared with allergen alone [55]. MWCNTs also exacerbate the development of airway fibrosis in the ovalbumin mouse model [42]. This concept is illustrated in Fig. 5.1. SWCNTs exacerbate allergic airway inflammation in mice by enhancing T-helper cell immunity and increasing oxidative stress [56, 57]. More recent work has shown that rodlike MWCNTs, but not tangled MWCNTs, induce eosinophilia, mucus hypersecretion, and the expression of Th2-type cytokines in the absence of any allergen challenge, suggesting that certain types of CNTs could directly cause asthma-like effects [58]. In addition, this study showed that mast cells partially regulated the inflammation caused by rodlike CNTs. Mast cells play key roles in the allergic immune response and have been shown to participate in the activation of the IL-33/ST2 axis to mediate adverse pulmonary and cardiovascular responses to MWCNTs [59, 60]. Other work suggests that MWCNTs cause IL-33 release from injured airway epithelial cells, which in turn promotes innate lymphoid cell recruitment and the development of an IL-13-dependent inflammatory response [61]. Dendritic cells (DCs) are important immune initiators that serve to capture and present allergens to naïve T cells, thereby driving T cell polarization [62]. The exacerbation of allergen-induced airway disease by CNTs could be due to inappropriate activation of antigen-presenting DCs. Interestingly, CNTs have been reported to inhibit the differentiation of peripheral blood monocytes into DCs [63]. Also, CNTs have direct effects on DCs that result in immune suppression [64]. Genetic susceptibility also plays an important role in the CNT-induced exacerbation of allergic airway disease. For example, deficiencies in the COX-2 enzyme and the STAT1 transcription factor have both been demonstrated to confer susceptibility to MWCNT exacerbation of ovalbumin-induced airway remodeling in mice [41, 65]. Moreover, mice lacking the transcription factor T-bet, which maintains Th1 immunity, develop allergic airway remodeling after exposure to MWCNTs or nickel nanoparticles in the absence of any allergen challenge [66]. While these studies suggest that individuals with allergic asthma are susceptible to lung and airway disease caused by ENMs exposure, it remains unknown whether ENMs will cause or exacerbate asthma in humans.

5.4.4 CNTs, Bacteria, and Viruses

CNT exposure can influence susceptibility to microbial infection (bacteria or viruses) or can modify the inflammation caused by biomolecules derived from microbes. For example, bacterial lipopolysaccharide (LPS) is a potent pro-inflammatory agent and has been implicated in a number of occupational and environmental lung diseases in humans, including bronchitis, chronic obstructive pulmonary disease (COPD), and asthma. Pulmonary inflammation and fibrosis induced by MWCNTs are increased by LPS preexposure in rats [43]. In addition, CNT-induced production of PDGF, a mediator of fibrosis, by rat alveolar macrophages and lung epithelial cells is enhanced by LPS preexposure [43]. These studies provide evidence that LPS-induced lung inflammation is a susceptibility factor that increases the severity of fibroproliferative lung disease caused by CNT exposure. ENMs have also been reported to impair phagocytosis and clearance of live bacteria. For example, mice exposed to SWCNTs have impaired clearance of the bacteria *Listeria monocytogenes* [67]. Decreased bacterial clearance in SWCNT-preexposed mice was associated with decreased phagocytosis of bacteria by macrophages and a decrease in nitric oxide production by these phagocytes. Helical carbon nanotubes delivered in mice infected with *Pseudomonas aeruginosa* inhibited macrophage-mediated phagocytosis of the bacteria [68]. However, clearance of *P. aeruginosa* was not affected because exposure to the helical CNTs primed the immune system for an enhanced inflammatory response to pulmonary infection consisting of an influx of neutrophils and macrophages. CNTs also influence viral infectivity. SWCNTs have been reported to increase pandemic influenza A H1N1 virus infectivity of lung epithelial cells *in vitro* [69]. These *in vitro* observations suggest that CNTs would increase viral infectivity *in vivo*, similar to observations of diesel exhaust particulates, which enhance viral infectivity in mice [70].

5.4.5 Systemic Immunotoxicity

Many types of inhaled ENMs are capable of stimulating or suppressing immune responses systemically, since they can cross lung epithelial and vascular endothelial barriers [71]. While the majority of inhaled CNTs do not enter the circulation, especially in agglomerated form, recent findings have shown that a significant fraction of MWCNTs migrate to lymph nodes and singlet MWCNTs have been detected by enhanced dark-field microscopy in extrapulmonary organs including the brain and kidney [72]. However, CNTs do not necessarily need to translocate to distant organs to have systemic effects since soluble mediators released from the injury site can influence immune status. For example, inhaled MWCNTs cause systemic immunosuppression in mice through a mechanism that involves the release of TGF-β1 from the lungs, which enters the bloodstream to signal

COX-2-mediated increases in PGE_2 and IL-10 in the spleen, to suppress T cell proliferation [73, 74].

5.5 Pleural Disease

Pleural disease is a major concern for CNTs due to their fiber-like similarities to asbestos, which is a known cause of subpleural fibrosis and mesothelioma. As with asbestos, which encompasses a variety different mineral types (e.g., chrysotile, crocidolite, amosite), different types of CNTs may have widely differing effects on pleural injury and subsequent disease.

5.5.1 *Acute Pleural Responses*

CNTs are of particular concern for human health since they have been shown to migrate to the mesothelial lining surrounding the lungs (pleura). CNTs have been shown to interact with the pleural lining directly (i.e., by physically piercing the mesothelial lining driven by forces of lung expansion and contraction during breathing) or macrophages containing CNTs which can interact with the mesothelial lining of the pleura when moving through the stomata from the lung to the pleural cavity. The persistence and durability of CNTs, along with their fiber-like shape and reactivity (i.e., ROS-generating capacity), result in injury to mesothelial cells. MWCNTs delivered to the lungs by inhalation or aspiration migrate to the subpleura, some of which penetrate the mesothelium. An acute response to MWCNTs at the pleura in C57BL6 mice involves focal mononuclear cell accumulation [32]. In this same study, elevated levels of PDGF and CCL2 were observed in bronchoalveolar lavage fluid from MWCNT-exposed mice. Interestingly, PDGF and MWCNTs or Ni nanoparticles synergistically increase CCL2 production by cultured rat mesothelial cells *in vitro* [75]. The accumulation of mononuclear cell foci at the pleural surface after exposure to MWCNTs could be mediated by PDGF secreted by activated macrophages, since in vitro studies with cultured mesothelial cells show that PDGF stimulates the production of CCL2. In turn, CCL2 is a known chemoattractant for monocytes and is a likely candidate for promoting mononuclear cell foci observed at the pleura of mice after inhalation of MWCNTs [32].

5.5.2 *Subpleural Fibrosis*

Subpleural fibrosis, like airway and interstitial pulmonary fibrosis, involves the activation of myofibroblasts to produce collagen and other matrix proteins that define the fibrotic lesion. However, some differences are that communication between mesothelial cells and myofibroblasts is likely an important event in subpleural fibrogenesis, whereas airway epithelial-myofibroblasts interactions or alveolar epithelial-fibroblast interactions (termed epithelial-mesenchymal cell trophic unit) are important in airway or interstitial lung fibrosis, respectively. The concept of a mesothelial-mesenchymal cell trophic unit has not been investigated. Alveolar macrophages that migrate to the subpleural region could also play a role in stimulating subpleural fibrosis by producing growth factors (e.g., PDGF, TGF-β1) for myofibroblasts to stimulate proliferation and collagen deposition, respectively.

5.5.3 Mesothelioma

CNTs, especially MWCNTs, have been proposed to have asbestos-like behavior and long-term immune or inflammatory effects that could lead to pleural cancer (i.e., mesothelioma). Early studies showed that intraperitoneal injection of MWCNTs in mice, a surrogate assay for pleural mesothelial injury, induced inflammation and granuloma formation on the mesothelial surface of the peritoneum [76]. This study showed that long MWCNTs were particularly potent for inducing granulomas as compared with short MWCNTs. Another study showed that mice deficient in the tumor suppressor p53 showed mesothelioma formation in the abdominal cavity after injection of CNTs [77]. However, it has been difficult to translate these studies to definitive answers for CNT-induced mesothelioma formation in the lungs of rodents. Recent work showing MWCNT-induced adenocarcinoma tumors in B6C3F1 mice relied on the use of a tumor initiator, methylcholanthrene (MCA), which alone caused a relatively high background of tumors [78]. This study indicated that MWCNTs could pose a carcinogenic risk but was not conclusive for the issue of mesothelioma. Nevertheless, the fact that some rodlike MWCNT can penetrate the pleura in mice is a cause for concern that they could pose a risk for significant injury to the mesothelial lining and cause mesothelioma [79]. The issue of whether CNTs are capable of causing mesothelioma in humans remains an elusive but important issue for assessing the human health hazards of CNTs.

5.6 Summary

Carbon nanotubes have been extensively studied for toxic effects on cultured cells *in vitro* and in rodents *in vivo*. The overwhelming evidence indicates that CNTs, both SWCNTs and MWCNTs, cause pulmonary fibrosis and should be regarded as a significant occupational health hazard. Growing evidence also indicates that CNTs possess immunotoxicity and can have systemic effects beyond the lungs. The variety of different CNT types, including many of which are functionalized, must be taken into consideration in assessing biological properties and human health effects.

References

1. Nel A, Xia T, Mädler L, Li N. Toxic potential of materials at the nanolevel. Science. 2006;311:622–7.
2. Bonner JC. Nanoparticles as a potential cause of pleural and interstitial lung disease. Proc Am Thorac Soc. 2010;7(2):138–41.
3. Thompson EA, Sayers BC, Glista-Baker EE, Shipkowski KA, Taylor AJ, Bonner JC. Innate immune responses to nanoparticle exposure in the lung. J Environ Immunol Toxicol. 2014;1 (3):150–6.
4. Donaldson K, Murphy FA, Duffin R, et al. Asbestos, carbon nanotubes and the pleural mesothelium: a review of the hypothesis regarding the role of long fibre retention in the parietal pleura, inflammation and mesothelioma. Part Fibre Toxicol. 2010;7:5.
5. Bonner JC. Mesenchymal cell survival in airway and interstitial pulmonary fibrosis. Fibrogenesis Tissue Repair. 2010;3:15.
6. Wilson MS, Wynn TA. Pulmonary fibrosis: pathogenesis, etiology and regulation. Mucosal Immunol. 2009;2(2):103–21.
7. Li JG, Li WX, Xu JY, et al. Comparative study of pathological lesions induced by multiwalled carbon nanotubes in lungs of mice by intratracheal instillation and inhalation. Environ Toxicol. 2007;22:415–21.
8. Porter DW, Hubbs AF, Mercer RR, et al. Mouse pulmonary dose- and time course-responses induced by exposure to multi-walled carbon nanotubes. Toxicology. 2010;269:136–47.
9. Ma-Hock L, Treumann S, Strauss V, et al. Inhalation toxicity of multiwall carbon nanotubes in rats exposed for 3 months. Toxicol Sci. 2009;112(2):468–81.
10. Pauluhn J. Subchronic 13-week inhalation exposure of rats to multiwalled carbon nanotubes: toxic effects are determined by density of agglomerate structures, not fibrillar structures. Toxicol Sci. 2010;113(1):226–42.
11. Mercer RR, Scabilloni J, Wang L, et al. Alteration of deposition pattern and pulmonary response as a result of improved dispersion of aspirated single-walled carbon nanotubes in a mouse model. Am J Physiol. 2008;294:L87–97.
12. Shvedova AA, Kisin ER, Mercer R, Murray AR, Johnson VJ, Potapovich AI, Tyurina YY, Gorelik O, Arepalli S, Schwegler-Berry D, Hubbs AF, Antonini J, Evans DE, Ku BK, Ramsey D, Maynard A, Kagan VE, Castranova V, Baron P. Unusual inflammatory and fibrogenic pulmonary responses to single-walled carbon nanotubes. Am J Physiol. 2005;289 (5):L698–708.
13. Muller J, Huaux F, Moreau N, Misson P, Heilier JF, Delos M, Arras M, Fonseca A, Nagy JB, Lison D. Respiratory toxicity of multi-wall carbon nanotubes. Toxicol Appl Pharmacol. 2005;207:221–31.
14. Murray AR, Kisin ER, Tkach AV, et al. Factoring-in agglomeration of carbon nanotubes and nanofibers for better prediction of their toxicity versus asbestos. Part Fibre Toxicol. 2012;9:10.
15. Warheit DB, Laurence BR, Reed KL, et al. Comparative pulmonary toxicity assessment of single-wall carbon nanotubes in rats. Toxicol Sci. 2004;77:117–25.
16. Wang X, Tian X, Ntim SA, et al. The dispersal state of multi-walled carbon nanotubes influences pro-fibrogenic epithelial and macrophage responses that correlate with the extent of pulmonary fibrosis. ACS Nano. 2011;5(12):9772–87.
17. DeLoid G, Cohen JM, Darrah T, Derk R, Rojanasakul L, Pyrgiotakis G, Wohlleben W, Demokritou P. Estimating the effective density of engineered nanomaterials for in vitro dosimetry. Nat Commun. 2014;5:3514.

18. Murphy FA, Schinwald A, Poland CA, et al. The mechanism of pleural inflammation by long carbon nanotubes: interaction of long fibres with macrophages stimulates them to amplify pro-inflammatory responses in mesothelial cells. Part Fibre Toxicol. 2012;9:8.
19. Kelleher P, Pacheco K, Newman LS. Inorganic dust pneumonias: the metal-related parenchymal disorders. Environ Health Perspect. 2000;108(4):685–96.
20. Hamilton Jr RF, Buford M, Xiang C, et al. NLRP3 inflammasome activation in murine alveolar macrophages and related lung pathology is associated with MWCNT nickel contamination. Inhal Toxicol. 2012;24(14):995–1008.
21. Li R, Wang X, Ji Z, Sun B, Zhang H, Chang CH, Lin S, Meng H, Liao YP, Wang M, Li Z, Hwang AA, Song TB, Xu R, Yang Y, Zink JI, Nel AE, Xia T. Surface charge and cellular processing of covalently functionalized multiwall carbon nanotubes determine pulmonary toxicity. ACS Nano. 2013;7(3):2352–68.
22. Bonner JC, Silva RM, Taylor AJ, Brown JM, Hilderbrand SC, Castranova V, Porter D, Elder A, Oberdörster G, Harkema JR, Bramble LA, Kavanagh TJ, Botta D, Nel A, Pinkerton KE. Interlaboratory evaluation of rodent pulmonary responses to engineered nanomaterials: the NIEHS Nano GO Consortium. Environ Health Perspect. 2013;121(6):676–82.
23. Taylor AJ, McClure CD, Shipkowski KA, Thompson EA, Hussain S, Garantziotis S, Parsons GN, Bonner JC. Atomic layer deposition coating of carbon nanotubes with aluminum oxide alters pro-fibrogenic cytokine expression by human mononuclear phagocytes in vitro and reduces lung fibrosis in mice in vivo. PLoS One. 2014;9(9), e106870.
24. Bhattacharya K, Andón FT, El-Sayed R, Fadeel B. Mechanisms of carbon nanotube-induced toxicity: focus on pulmonary inflammation. Adv Drug Deliv Rev. 2013;65(15):2087–97.
25. Kapralov AA, Feng WH, Amoscato AA, Yanamala N, Balasubramanian K, Winnica DE, Kisin ER, Kotchey GP, Gou P, Sparvero LJ, Ray P, Mallampalli RK, Klein-Seetharaman J, Fadeel B, Star A, Shvedova AA, Kagan VE. Adsorption of surfactant lipids by single-walled carbon nanotubes in mouse lung upon pharyngeal aspiration. ACS Nano. 2012;6(5):4147–56.
26. Bein K, Wesselkamper SC, Liu X, Dietsch M, Majumder N, Concel VJ, Medvedovic M, Sartor MA, Henning LN, Venditto C, Borchers MT, Barchowsky A, Weaver TE, Tichelaar JW, Prows DR, Korfhagen TR, Hardie WD, Bachurski CJ, Leikauf GD. Surfactant-associated protein B is critical to survival in nickel-induced injury in mice. Am J Respir Cell Mol Biol. 2009;41(2):226–36.
27. Konduru NV, Tyurina YY, Feng W, Basova LV, Belikova NA, Bayir H, Clark K, Rubin M, Stolz D, Vallhov H, Scheynius A, Witasp E, Fadeel B, Kichambare PD, Star A, Kisin ER, Murray AR, Shvedova AA, Kagan VE. Phosphatidylserine targets single-walled carbon nanotubes to professional phagocytes in vitro and in vivo. PLoS One. 2009;4(2), e4398.
28. Shannahan JH, Brown JM, Chen R, Ke PC, Lai X, Mitra S, Witzmann FA. Comparison of nanotube-protein corona composition in cell culture media. Small. 2013;9(12):2171–81.
29. Bonner JC. Respiratory toxicology. In: Smart RC, Hodgson E, editors. Molecular and biochemical toxicology. 4th ed. New York: Wiley; 2008. p. 639–70.
30. Mercer RR, Scabilloni JF, Hubbs AF, Wang L, Battelli LA, McKinney W, Castranova V, Porter DW. Extrapulmonary transport of MWCNT following inhalation exposure. Part Fibre Toxicol. 2013;10:38.
31. Mangum JB, Turpin EA, Antao-Menezes A, Cesta MF, Bermudez E, Bonner JC. Single-walled carbon nanotube (SWCNT)-induced interstitial fibrosis in the lungs of rats is associated with increased levels of PDGF mRNA and the formation of unique intercellular carbon structures that bridge alveolar macrophages in situ. Part Fibre Toxicol. 2006;3:15.
32. Ryman-Rasmussen JP, Cesta MF, Brody AR, Shipley-Phillips JK, Everitt JI, Tewksbury EW, Moss OR, Wong BA, Dodd DE, Andersen ME, Bonner JC. Inhaled carbon nanotubes reach the subpleural tissue in mice. Nat Nanotechnol. 2009;4(11):747–51.
33. Kagan VE, Konduru NV, Feng W, Allen BL, Conroy J, Volkov Y, Vlasova II, Belikova NA, Yanamala N, Kapralov A, Tyurina YY, Shi J, Kisin ER, Murray AR, Franks J, Stolz D, Gou P, Klein-Seetharaman J, Fadeel B, Star A, Shvedova AA. Carbon nanotubes degraded by

neutrophil myeloperoxidase induce less pulmonary inflammation. Nat Nanotechnol. 2010;5 (5):354–9.
34. Andón FT, Kapralov AA, Yanamala N, Feng W, Baygan A, Chambers BJ, Hultenby K, Ye F, Toprak MS, Brandner BD, Fornara A, Klein-Seetharaman J, Kotchey GP, Star A, Shvedova AA, Fadeel B, Kagan VE. Biodegradation of single-walled carbon nanotubes by eosinophil peroxidase. Small. 2013;9(16):2721–9.
35. Shvedova AA, Kapralov AA, Feng WH, Kisin ER, Murray AR, Mercer RR, St Croix CM, Lang MA, Watkins SC, Konduru NV, Allen BL, Conroy J, Kotchey GP, Mohamed BM, Meade AD, Volkov Y, Star A, Fadeel B, Kagan VE. Impaired clearance and enhanced pulmonary inflammatory/fibrotic response to carbon nanotubes in myeloperoxidase-deficient mice. PLoS One. 2012;7(3), e30923.
36. Sun B, Wang X, Ji Z, Wang M, Liao YP, Chang CH, Li R, Zhang H, Nel AE, Xia T. NADPH oxidase-dependent NLRP3 inflammasome activation and its important role in lung fibrosis by multiwalled carbon nanotubes. Small. 2015. doi:10.1002/smll.201402859 [Epub ahead of print].
37. Shvedova AA, Kisin ER, Murray AR, Kommineni C, Castranova V, Fadeel B, Kagan VE. Increased accumulation of neutrophils and decreased fibrosis in the lung of NADPH oxidase-deficient c57bl/6 mice exposed to carbon nanotubes. Toxicol Appl Pharmacol. 2008;231:235–40.
38. He X, Young SH, Schwegler-Berry D, Chisholm WP, Fernback JE, Ma Q. Multi-walled carbon nanotubes induced a fibrogenic response by stimulating reactive oxygen species production, activating NF-kB signaling, and promoting fibroblast-to-myofibroblast transformation. Chem Res Toxicol. 2011;24(12):2237–48.
39. Brown DM, Donaldson K, Stone V. Nuclear translocation of Nrf2 and expression of antioxidant defence genes in THP-1 cells exposed to carbon nanotubes. J Biomed Nanotechnol. 2010;6(3):224–33.
40. Lee JK, Sayers BC, Chun KS, Lao HC, Shipley-Phillips JK, Bonner JC, Langenbach R. Multiwalled carbon nanotubes induce COX-2 and iNOS expression via MAP kinase-dependent and -independent mechanisms in mouse RAW264.7 macrophages. Part Fibre Toxicol. 2012;9:14.
41. Sayers BC, Taylor AJ, Glista-Baker EE, Shipley-Phillips JK, Dackor RT, Edin ML, Lih FB, Tomer KB, Zeldin DC, Langenbach R, Bonner JC. Role of cyclooxygenase-2 in exacerbation of allergen-induced airway remodeling by multiwalled carbon nanotubes. Am J Respir Cell Mol Biol. 2013;49(4):525–35.
42. Ryman-Rasmussen JP, Tewksbury EW, Moss OR, Cesta MF, Wong BA, Bonner JC. Inhaled multiwalled carbon nanotubes potentiate airway fibrosis in a murine model of allergic asthma. Am J Respir Cell Mol Biol. 2009;40(3):349–58.
43. Cesta MF, Ryman-Rasmussen JP, Wallace DG, Masinde T, Hurlburt G, Taylor AJ, Bonner JC. Bacterial lipopolysaccharide enhances PDGF signaling and pulmonary fibrosis in rats exposed to carbon nanotubes. Am J Respir Cell Mol Biol. 2010;43(2):142–51.
44. Bonner JC. Regulation of PDGF and its receptors in fibrotic diseases. Cytokine Growth Factor Rev. 2004;15:255–73.
45. Hirano S, Fujitani Y, Furuyama A, et al. Uptake and cytotoxic effects of multi-walled carbon nanotubes in human bronchial epithelial cells. Toxicol Appl Pharmacol. 2010;249(1):8–15.
46. Shipkowski KA, Taylor AJ, Thompson EA, Glista-Baker EE, Sayers BC, Messenger ZJ, Bauer RN, Jaspers I, Bonner JC. An allergic lung microenvironment suppresses carbon nanotube-induced inflammasome activation via STAT6-dependent inhibition of caspase-1. PLoS One. 2015;10(6):e0128888.
47. Hussain S, Vanoirbeek JA, Hoet PH. Interactions of nanomaterials with the immune system. Wiley Interdiscip Rev Nanomed Nanobiotechnol. 2012;4(2):169–83.
48. Palomäki J, Välimäki E, Sund J, et al. Long, needle-like carbon nanotubes and asbestos activate the NLRP3 inflammasome through a similar mechanism. ACS Nano. 2011;5 (9):6861–70.

49. Meunier E, Coste A, Olagnier D, et al. Double-walled carbon nanotubes trigger IL-1β release in human monocytes through Nlrp3 inflammasome activation. Nanomedicine. 2012;8 (6):987–95.
50. Strowig T, Henao-Mejia J, Elinav E, et al. Inflammasomes in health and disease. Nature. 2012;481(7381):278–86.
51. Martinon F, Mayor A, Tschopp J. The inflammasomes: guardians of the body. Annu Rev Immunol. 2009;27:229–65.
52. Gordon S, Martinez FO. Alternative activation of macrophages: mechanism and functions. Immunity. 2010;32(5):593–604.
53. Girtsman TA, Beamer CA, Wu N, Buford M, Holian A. IL-1R signaling is critical for regulation of multi-walled carbon nanotubes-induced acute lung inflammation n C57Bl/6 mice. Nanotoxicology. 2014;8(1):17–27.
54. Hussain S, Sangtian S, Anderson SM, Snyder RJ, Marshburn JD, Rice AB, Bonner JC, Garantziotis S. Inflammasome activation in airway epithelial cells after multi-walled carbon nanotube exposure mediates a profibrotic response in lung fibroblasts. Part Fibre Toxicol. 2014;11:28.
55. Inoue K, Koike E, Yanagisawa R, Hirano S, Nishikawa M, Takano H. Effects of multi-walled carbon nanotubes on a murine allergic airway inflammation model. Toxicol Appl Pharmacol. 2009;237(3):306–16.
56. Inoue K, Yanagisawa R, Koike E, Nishikawa M, Takano H. Repeated pulmonary exposure to single-walled carbon nanotubes exacerbates allergic inflammation of the airway: possible role of oxidative stress. Free Radic Biol Med. 2010;48(7):924–34.
57. Nygaard UC, Hansen JS, Samuelsen M, Alberg T, Marioara CD, Løvik M. Single-walled and multi-walled carbon nanotubes promote allergic immune responses in mice. Toxicol Sci. 2009;109(1):113–23.
58. Rydman EM, Ilves M, Koivisto AJ, Kinaret PA, Fortino V, Savinko TS, Lehto MT, Pulkkinen V, Vippola M, Hämeri KJ, Matikainen S, Wolff H, Savolainen KM, Greco D, Alenius H. Inhalation of rod-like carbon nanotubes causes unconventional allergic airway inflammation. Part Fibre Toxicol. 2014;11:48.
59. Brown JM, Wilson TM, Metcalfe DD. The mast cell and allergic diseases: role in pathogenesis and implications for therapy. Clin Exp Allergy. 2008;38(1):4–18.
60. Katwa P, Wang X, Urankar RN, Podila R, Hilderbrand SC, Fick RB, Rao AM, Ke PC, Wingard CJ, Brown JM. A carbon nanotube toxicity paradigm driven by mast cells and the IL33/ST2 axis. Small. 2012;8(18):2904–12.
61. Beamer CA, Girtsman TA, Seaver BP, Finsaas KJ, Migliaccio CT, Perry VK, Rottman JB, Smith DE, Holian A. IL-33 mediates multi-walled carbon nanotube (MWCNT)-induced airway hyper-reactivity via the mobilization of innate helper cells in the lung. Nanotoxicology. 2013;7(6):1070–81.
62. Gill MA. The role of dendritic cells in asthma. J Allergy Clin Immunol. 2012;129(4):889–901.
63. Laverny G, Casset A, Purohit A, et al. Immunomodulatory properties of multi-walled carbon nanotubes in peripheral blood mononuclear cells from healthy subjects and allergic patients. Toxicol Lett. 2012;217(2):91–101.
64. Tkach AV, Shurin GV, Shurin MR, Kisin ER, Murray AR, Young SH, Star A, Fadeel B, Kagan VE, Shvedova AA. Direct effects of carbon nanotubes on dendritic cells induce immune suppression upon pulmonary exposure. ACS Nano. 2011;5(7):5755–62.
65. Thompson EA, Sayers BC, Glista-Baker EE, Shipkowski KA, Ihrie MD, Duke KS, Taylor AJ, Bonner JC. STAT1 attenuates murine allergen-induced airway remodeling and exacerbation by carbon nanotubes. Am J Respir Cell Mol Biol. 2015; [Epub ahead of print].
66. Glista-Baker EE, Taylor AJ, Sayers BC, Thompson EA, Bonner JC. Nickel nanoparticles cause exaggerated lung and airway remodeling in mice lacking the T-box transcription factor, TBX21 (T-bet). Part Fibre Toxicol. 2014;11:7.
67. Shvedova AA, Fabisiak JP, Kisin ER, Murray AR, Roberts JR, Tyurina YY, Antonini JM, Feng WH, Kommineni C, Reynolds J, Barchowsky A, Castranova V, Kagan VE. Sequential

exposure to carbon nanotubes and bacteria enhances pulmonary inflammation. Am J Respir Cell Mol Biol. 2008;38(5):579–90.
68. Walling BE, Kuang Z, Hao Y, Estrada D, Wood JD, Lian F, Miller LA, Shah AB, Jeffries JL, Haasch RT, Lyding JW, Pop E, Lau GW. Helical carbon nanotubes enhance the early immune response and inhibit macrophage-mediated phagocytosis of Pseudomonas aeruginosa. PLoS One. 2013;8(11), e80283.
69. Sanpui P, Zheng X, Loeb JC, Bisesi Jr JH, Khan IA, Afrooz AR, Liu K, Badireddy A, Wiesner MR, Ferguson P, Saleh NB, Lednicky JA, Sabo-Attwood T. Single-walled carbon nanotubes increase pandemic influenza A H1N1 virus infectivity of lung epithelial cells. Part Fibre Toxicol. 2014;11(1):66.
70. Gowdy KM, Krantz QT, King C, Boykin E, Jaspers I, Linak WP, Gilmour MI. Role of oxidative stress on diesel-enhanced influenza infection in mice. Part Fibre Toxicol. 2010;7:34.
71. Kreyling WG, Hirn S, Schleh C. Nanoparticles in the lung. Nat Biotechnol. 2010;28 (12):1275–6.
72. Mercer RR, Scabilloni JF, Hubbs AF, Wang L, Battelli LA, McKinney W, Castranova V, Porter DW. Extrapulmonary transport of MWCNT following inhalation exposure. Part Fibre Toxicol. 2013;10:38.
73. Mitchell LA, Gao J, Wal RV, et al. Pulmonary and systemic immune response to inhaled multiwalled carbon nanotubes. Toxicol Sci. 2007;100:203–14.
74. Mitchell LA, Lauer FT, Burchiel SW, et al. Mechanisms for how inhaled multiwalled carbon nanotubes suppress systemic immune function in mice. Nature Nanotechnol. 2009;4(7):451–6.
75. Glista-Baker EE, Taylor AJ, Sayers BC, et al. Nickel nanoparticles enhance platelet-derived growth factor-induced chemokine expression by mesothelial cells via prolonged mitogen-activated protein kinase activation. Am J Respir Cell Mol Biol. 2012;47(4):552–61.
76. Poland CA, Duffin R, Kinloch I, et al. Carbon nanotubes introduced into the abdominal cavity of mice show asbestos-like pathogenicity in a pilot study. Nat Nanotechnol. 2008;3(7):423–8.
77. Takagi A, Hirose A, Nishimura T, et al. Induction of mesothelioma in p53 +/− mouse by intraperitoneal application of multi-wall carbon nanotube. J Toxicol Sci. 2008;33:105–16.
78. Mercer RR, Hubbs AF, Scabilloni JF, et al. Distribution and persistence of pleural penetrations by multi-walled carbon nanotubes. Part Fibre Toxicol. 2010;7:28.
79. Sargent LM, Porter DW, Staska LM, Hubbs AF, Lowry DT, Battelli L, Siegrist KJ, Kashon ML, Mercer RR, Bauer AK, Chen BT, Salisbury JL, Frazer D, McKinney W, Andrew M, Tsuruoka S, Endo M, Fluharty KL, Castranova V, Reynolds SH. Promotion of lung adenocarcinoma following inhalation exposure to multi-walled carbon nanotubes. Part Fibre Toxicol. 2014;11:3.

Chapter 6
Potential Hazards of Skin Exposure to Nanoparticles

Toshiro Hirai, Yasuo Yoshioka, Kazuma Higashisaka, and Yasuo Tsutsumi

Abstract Our environment is teeming with nanoparticles—in cosmetics and other consumer products, motor vehicle emissions, and even the soil itself. These nanoparticles bombard us not only through the airways but also skin. However, the health risk of skin exposure to nanoparticles is not yet well established. Qualitative data suggest that nanoparticles penetrate skin only very infrequently. However, the mutagenicity and sensitizing ability of nanoparticles need to be considered, because these adverse effects are sometimes induced even at relatively low-level skin exposure to a chemical substance. Furthermore, although exposure to nanoparticles often occurs simultaneously with exposure to other chemical compounds and environmental allergens, little is known about the hazards of combined skin exposure to nanoparticles and other substances. Here, we summarize current knowledge regarding skin exposure to nanoparticles, especially those in nanomaterials, and discuss its possible health risk. We believe that further study will enable us to coexist safely and beneficially with nanoparticles.

Key words Nanoparticles • Nanomaterials • Skin • Allergy • Atopic dermatitis

---

T. Hirai • K. Higashisaka
Laboratory of Toxicology and Safety Science, Graduate School of Pharmaceutical Sciences, Osaka University, 1-6 Yamadaoka, Suita, Osaka 565-0871, Japan

Y. Yoshioka (✉)
Laboratory of Toxicology and Safety Science, Graduate School of Pharmaceutical Sciences, Osaka University, 1-6 Yamadaoka, Suita, Osaka 565-0871, Japan

Vaccine Creation Project, BIKEN Innovative Vaccine Research Alliance Laboratories, Research Institute for Microbial Diseases, Osaka University, Suita, Japan

BIKEN Center for Innovative Vaccine Research and Development, The Research Foundation for Microbial Diseases of Osaka University, Suita, Osaka, Japan
e-mail: y-yoshioka@biken.osaka-u.ac.jp

Y. Tsutsumi
Laboratory of Toxicology and Safety Science, Graduate School of Pharmaceutical Sciences, Osaka University, 1-6 Yamadaoka, Suita, Osaka 565-0871, Japan

Laboratory of Innovative Antibody Engineering and Design, Center for Drug Innovation and Screening, National Institute of Biomedical Innovation, Saito, Ibaraki, Japan

T. Otsuki et al. (eds.), *Biological Effects of Fibrous and Particulate Substances*, Current Topics in Environmental Health and Preventive Medicine,
DOI 10.1007/978-4-431-55732-6_6

6.1 Introduction

Because of their unique physicochemical properties and functions, manufactured nanoparticles (or nanomaterials) [1, 2] are increasingly used to add value to goods including cosmetics, foods, medicines, and industrial products [3–5]. However, these same features may render nanomaterials hazardous under various conditions [6]. For example, titanium dioxide nanoparticles reportedly increase the leakiness of subcutaneous blood vessels and the number of pulmonary metastases [7]. In addition, silica nanoparticles, but not microparticles, induce pregnancy complications in mice [8]. We must intensively collect more information about the safety of nanomaterials to fully reap their potential benefits.

Emphasizing concerns about health risks associated with nanomaterials, numerous epidemiologic studies indicate that exposure to environmental particulate matters (PMs), such as PM2.5 or Asian dust, induces many adverse effects, including facilitating the onset and severity allergic diseases [9–12]. Furthermore, the adverse effects of PMs might be particularly attributable to nanosized particles [12–14]. Airborne PMs readily enter the body by inhalation and cause adverse responses in the lungs [10, 15]. Because such adverse effects have primarily been attributed to inhaled PMs, safety studies of nanomaterials have largely focused on their effects after inhalational exposure [16]. In contrast, few studies have evaluated the effects of nanoparticles via skin exposure, even though, in the context of environmental exposure, inhalational and skin exposure to airborne PMs occur concurrently. In addition, the small size of nanoparticles increases their likelihood of penetrating skin, one of the most frequent exposure routes for nanomaterials. In this review, we summarize current knowledge regarding skin exposure to nanoparticles, particularly those in nanomaterials, and discuss possible associated health risks.

6.2 Skin Exposure to Nanoparticles

6.2.1 Opportunities for Skin Exposure to Nanoparticles

Nanomaterials have become indispensable in various consumer products. For example, titanium dioxide and zinc oxide nanoparticles are essential in sunscreens because they are colorless and reflect ultraviolet (UV) rays more efficiently than do larger particles [17–19]. Typically used as an anti-setting agent, silica nanoparticles are found in a wide variety of cosmetics [20]. The 60-carbon nanomaterial fullerene is a strong antioxidant and effectively quenches radical oxygen species (ROS), leading to its frequent use as a "radical sponge" in cosmetics and skin-care products [21–23]. Furthermore, opportunities for skin exposure to nanoparticles extend beyond skin-care products. For example, silver nanoparticles are widely applied as antimicrobials to consumer products including apparel, shoes, socks, antibacterial sprays, and household detergents [24, 25]. The workplace is another potential source of skin-acquired nanomaterials [26].

The environment itself can be a source of unintentional skin exposure to nanoparticles. Environmental nanoparticles in urban areas arise primarily from combustion sources such as burning coal, fuel oil, and biomass; and waste and motor vehicle emissions typically account for the greatest proportion of environmental nanoparticles [27, 28]. Comprising only a small proportion of ambient air particles by mass but a large proportion in terms of number [29], airborne nanoparticles are usually present as aggregates (diameter, ~100 nm) of very small (diameter, $\leq$10 nm) primary nanoparticles [28]. Although information regarding the health effects of environmental exposure is limited to effects after inhalation [30], skin exposure to environmental nanoparticles occurs in the same contexts in which they are inhaled.

Recent reports acknowledge that naturally occurring nanoparticles represent a previously unrecognized opportunity for exposure [31]. For example, various metal objects, including earrings and wire, spontaneously generate metal nanoparticles [32], and laundering silver-embedded textiles releases silver nanoparticles [33]. These naturally occurring metal nanoparticles are thought to arise through the nucleation of metal ions released due to chemical or photochemical reduction [32, 34].

Together, these findings suggest that we are exposed to nanoparticles via the skin merely as a consequence of our daily lives—for example, whenever we wear metal accessories or dress in clothes containing or washed with metal-embellished fabric. In addition, nanoparticles abound in nature. Various soils are naturally rich in nanoparticles, and earthquakes generate massive quantities of new soil-derived nanoparticles via mechanical grinding [31]. Although unavoidable, exposure to nanoparticles via the airways and skin is not a new problem but a long-standing facet of everyday life, at least in terms of naturally occurring nanoparticles.

6.2.2 Skin Penetration by Nanoparticles

We know little regarding how naturally occurring nanoparticles or those emitted during industrial processes enter and cross the skin. However, the intense research done to confirm the safety of nanomaterials has taught us about the skin-penetrating characteristics of nanoparticles.

6.2.2.1 Titanium Dioxide and Zinc Oxide

Primary nanoparticles of titanium dioxide and zinc oxide are 10–20 nm in diameter, but they typically exist as 30- to 150-nm aggregates and frequently are used in cosmetics [35]. In a minipig model of human skin, inductively coupled plasma mass spectroscopy failed to detect any significant increase in the titanium concentration in the dermis or at draining lymph nodes after 22 days of sunscreen application [36]; in the same study, transmission electron microscopy (TEM) of the dermis revealed only a few titanium particles, equivalent to 10^{-6} to 10^{-4} % of the total amount applied. In another study, multiphoton microscopy of human skin in vivo 4 h after the application of zinc oxide nanoparticles revealed zinc oxide nanoparticles in the stratum corneum but none in viable epidermis [37]; a similar quantitative analysis was unable to document any noteworthy penetration of the skin by titanium nanoparticles [38]. Therefore, even though aggregates of titanium dioxide nanoparticles and zinc oxide nanoparticles penetrate the skin in some situations, the rate is extremely low or below the limit of detection of most modern methods of quantitation.

6.2.2.2 Silica Nanoparticles

Manufactured synthetic silica nanoparticles are amorphous silica and are divided into two main types: pyrogenic silica and wet-process silica (i.e., precipitated silica and silica gels) [20, 39]. All pyrogenic silica nanoparticles exist as aggregates and agglomerates; some of the wet-process types also are well dispersed. Pyrogenic silica nanoparticles are widely used in cosmetics, but available data regarding the skin penetration of silica nanoparticles largely derive from the wet-process type, which is used for coatings and ink-receptive papers and as a filter aid in food production. In a mouse model involving epicutaneous application ("skin painting") for 3 days or 28 days, TEM analysis revealed well-dispersed silica nanoparticles (diameter, 70 nm) not only in epidermal Langerhans cells but also in the dermis and draining lymph nodes [40, 41], but the images obtained suggested that the penetration rate was minimal, at most. Fluorescence microscopy and flow cytometry showed that fluorescently labeled silica nanoparticles (diameter, 42 nm) enter keratinocytes and Langerhans cells in human tape-stripped epidermis; the authors stated that tape stripping removed part of the stratum corneum and contents of the follicular infundibulum [42]. Although quantitative data regarding skin penetration by silica nanoparticles is currently unavailable, well-dispersed silica nanoparticles likely will enter viable skin at some point during our daily lives.

6.2.2.3 Quantum Dot Nanoparticles

Quantum dot nanoparticles are intrinsically fluorescent, and their dispersion characteristics are easily manipulated by modifying the particle surface; consequently, they are widely used as models to investigate the biodistribution of nanoparticles. In an early study, confocal scanning microscopy suggested that two types of quantum dot nanoparticles with different coatings (PEG [polyethylene glycol]-carboxylic acid and PEG-amine; diameter, 15 to 45 nm) penetrated the epidermis of pigs [43]; however in a follow-up study using TEM and inductively coupled plasma-optical emission spectroscopy, this same group was unable to detect the entry of a similar nanoparticle preparation (40 nm with PEG modification) [44]. In contrast, our TEM analysis revealed that 40-nm quantum dot nanoparticles penetrated slightly into viable skin in mice [40], and confocal microscopy and TEM both demonstrated very low, but qualitatively higher, penetration of quantum dot nanoparticles in UVR-exposed skin compared with intact skin in mice [45]. The findings of another group suggested that, among the preparations and pH conditions they evaluated,

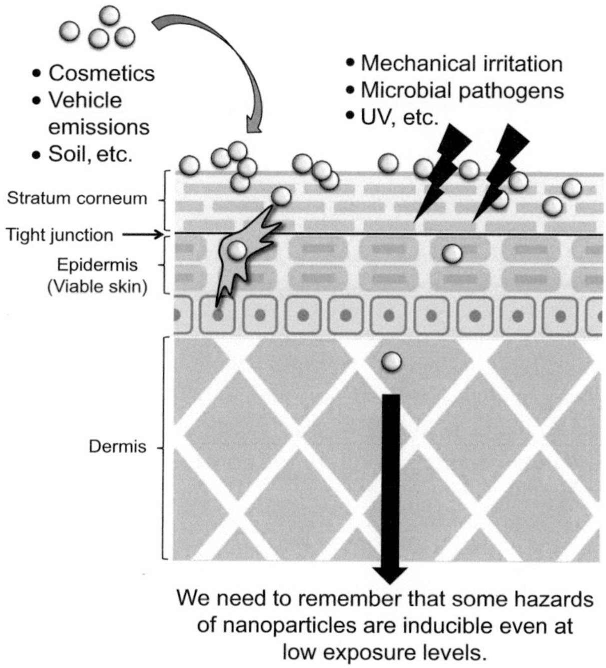

Fig. 6.1 Skin exposure to nanoparticles

only pegylated quantum dot nanoparticles at pH 8.3 penetrated intact human skin [46]. These interesting, but contradictory, observations and quantitative data suggest that, like other nanoparticles, well-dispersed quantum dot nanoparticles can enter our bodies through skin, but the amount that enters is minimal.

The mechanism underlying the penetration of skin by nanoparticles remains unclear. Skin presents two physical barriers: the stratum corneum and tight junctions (TJs). To be absorbed through the skin, a medicine must be less than 500 Da in molecular weight [47]; that is, a compound exceeding 500 Da cannot cross the TJ barrier. Therefore all nanoparticles are thought to be too large to penetrate the TJ barrier, at least when it is fully functional. However, nanoparticles may be able to elude the TJs in hair follicles [48], whose heterogeneously differentiated epithelial cells and their various functions may impart some flexibility in regard to penetration [49]. In addition, Langerhans cells can uptake external antigens despite the presence of an intact TJ barrier [50], thus representing another possible mechanism for the skin penetration of nanoparticles.

The skin is the body's primary defense against the environment and thus is under constant assault from mechanical irritation, microbial pathogens, and chemical insults. Therefore, although the skin barrier is quite strong, it is not always completely protective. For example, tape stripping [51], mechanical flexion [52], and UV exposure [45] all increase nanoparticle penetration in skin. Therefore, in reality, nanoparticles likely gain access into our body through skin that is damaged during the activities of daily living. However, we want to reiterate that the rate of any possible penetration is extremely low, given that state-of-the-art quantitative techniques are unable to detect significant numbers of penetrated particles (Fig. 6.1).

6.3 Potential Hazards of Skin Exposure to Nanoparticles

The potential hazards associated with nanoparticles are divided into two main categories according to the context in which the exposure occurs.

6.3.1 Potential Direct Health Effects of Nanoparticles

Whether nanoparticles are directly inflammatory and cytotoxic currently is the main topic of debate regarding their health risk [53–56]. However, because the rate at which nanoparticles enter through skin is extremely low, we think that they are unlikely to directly cause significant inflammation and cytotoxicity in most situations in skin. Therefore, we now focus on the potential for nanoparticles to lead to mutation and sensitization, adverse effects that are sometimes induced even at relatively low-level skin exposure to a chemical substance.

Many reports suggest that nanoparticles are mutagenic [57–60], but almost all of these studies indicate that the mechanisms underlying the observed mutagenicity were ROS dependent [57–60]. ROS are not "evil" in and of themselves; instead the duration and intensity of exposure determine whether their health effects are harmful or beneficial [61, 62]. For example, high doses of the herbicides, paraquat and juglone, shorten the life span of *Caenorhabditis elegans* by inducing ROS, whereas low doses extend the organism's life span [63, 64]. However, because only very low numbers of nanoparticles enter the body via the skin, the mutagenicity of nanoparticles is unlikely to occur through ROS-dependent mechanisms. Additional research is warranted to address potential mechanisms for the mutagenicity of nanoparticles and the conditions that enhance their entry or accumulation.

Whether nanoparticles act as directly as sensitizing agents has not been determined. A local lymph node assay, which identifies chemical sensitizers by their capacity to induce the proliferation of cells from draining lymph nodes after dermal exposure [65], was unable to detect any sensitizing ability associated with amine-modified polystyrene nanoparticles (diameter, 50 nm) or titanium dioxide primary nanoparticles (diameter, <25 nm) [66]. Another study evaluated the sensitizing ability of two types of wet-process silica nanoparticles, mesoporous silica and colloidal silica, both of which were about 100 nm in diameter [67]. After three consecutive days of skin painting, mesoporous silica but not colloidal silica increased the ear thickness of mice, prompting the authors to conclude that mesoporous silica nanoparticles acted as a chemical sensitizer. However, the changes in ear thickness were slight, and unlike the positive control (2,4-dinitroflourobenzene, a strong chemical sensitizer), the mesoporous silica nanoparticles did not elicit any cell proliferation in the local lymph node assay [67].

To date, the only nanoparticle that is confirmed to be antigenic is fullerene: the immunization of mice with complete Freund's adjuvant and a C_{60} fullerene derivative conjugated to bovine thyroglobulin successfully induced C_{60} fullerene-specific antibodies [68, 69]. However, evaluating the sensitizing ability based on OECD Guideline 406, Ema et al. however could not detect any sensitizability of C_{60} fullerene [69]. These results suggest that C_{60} fullerene must be haptenized to induce specific antibody. However, such haptenization seems unlikely under natural conditions, implying that C_{60} fullerene would be safe in terms of sensitizing ability, according to our current knowledge [70]. Considering all of these findings together, we conclude that the notion that nanoparticles act as chemical sensitizers after skin exposure has not been confirmed.

In contrast, several epidemiologic studies indicate that airborne particulates containing sensitizing metals contribute to the onset of metal allergy [71–73]. Considering metal nanoparticles release metal ions, a supposed cause of metal allergy, metal nanoparticles may act as sensitizers, not because of their own antigenicity, but because of the antigenicity of their released metal ions. Future safety evaluations of nanoparticles need to address this potential function of nanoparticles as indirect sensitizing agents.

6.3.2 Combined Exposure to Nanoparticles and Other Substances

Exposure to nanoparticles often occurs simultaneously with exposure to other chemical compounds and environmental allergens [30]. However, little is known about the hazards of combined skin exposure to nanoparticles and other substances. As mentioned earlier, exposure to environmental nanoparticles facilitates the onset and severity of allergic diseases. Because the most important exposure route for these effects is unknown, the possibility that concurrent skin exposure to nanoparticles and allergen contributes to the onset of allergy needs to be considered.

We first focus on allergic contact dermatitis, which typically is induced by a chemical sensitizer. In one study, injection of titanium dioxide nanoparticles (diameter, 15–25 nm) was done before 2,4-dinitrochlorobenzene-induced expansion of cells from the draining lymph nodes of mice [74]. Furthermore, 3 consecutive days of skin painting with a mixture of mesoporous silica nanoparticles and 2,4-dinitroflourobenzene induced more severe ear swelling in mice than 2,4-dinitroflourobenzene alone did [67]. Furthermore, the fragrances in cosmetics, which frequently contain nanoparticles as well, are a leading cause of allergic contact dermatitis [75]. Additional studies to reveal the mechanisms of these nanoparticle-associated effects and to identify the threshold amount for an adverse response are needed urgently.

Atopic allergies are IgE-related allergic conditions, such as atopic dermatitis. As mentioned earlier, exposure to environmental nanoparticles is one of the most important factors in the induction or aggravation of atopic allergy. Yanagisawa et al. found that intradermal injection of mixture of mite allergen, which is the major cause of atopic dermatitis [76], and titanium dioxide nanoparticles or polystyrene nanoparticles aggravated atopic dermatitis-like skin lesions in the NC/Nga mouse model [77, 78]. We confirmed that intradermal injections of silica nanoparticles caused similar adverse effects, and smaller nanoparticles caused more severe reactions [79]. In contrast, skin painting of zinc oxide nanoparticles with ovalbumin and staphylococcal enterotoxin B did not exacerbate atopic dermatitis-like skin lesions [80]. These findings together suggest that although some nanoparticles might aggravate atopic dermatitis directly, this potential might be weaker under non-laboratory exposure conditions. One potential mechanism for the role of nanoparticles in atopic allergy is that the interaction of nanoparticles and allergen changes the skin penetration kinetics of the allergen and induces IgE-biased immune responses, which are a characteristic feature of human atopic allergies [81, 82]. For this effect, skin penetration by nanoparticles is unnecessary. Therefore studies designed to obviate nanoparticles' possible health risks should focus on not only the direct immunomodulating effects of nanoparticles but also on their potential to interfere with a healthy response to coexisting chemical substances or allergens.

6.4 Conclusion

Existing data are inconclusive regarding the health risk of skin exposure to nanoparticles. Although qualitative data suggest that nanoparticles enter the body via the skin in some situations, almost every quantitative study has concluded that the penetrating amount of nanoparticles is less than the detection limit of present technology, at least in the model used. To continue the discussion regarding the adverse effects of skin-acquired nanoparticles, we propose that further quantitative analyses are needed to determine the rate at which nanoparticles penetrate the skin and any potential for their accumulation. We also believe that additional research should be focused on determining whether nanoparticles cause immunologic sensitization, either directly or by promoting the sensitizing effects of co-exposed substances. These future studies will not only reveal ways through which we can accommodate an environment rich in nanoparticles; they also will provide insight into means to improve the safety and efficacy of nanomedicines for skin care.

References

1. Auffan M, Rose J, Bottero JY, Lowry GV, Jolivet JP, Wiesner MR. Towards a definition of inorganic nanoparticles from an environmental, health and safety perspective. Nat Nanotechnol. 2009;4(10):634–41. doi:10.1038/nnano.2009.242.
2. Cheng Z, Al Zaki A, Hui JZ, Muzykantov VR, Tsourkas A. Multifunctional nanoparticles: cost versus benefit of adding targeting and imaging capabilities. Science. 2012;338(6109):903–10. doi:10.1126/science.1226338.

3. Bowman DM, van Calster G, Friedrichs S. Nanomaterials and regulation of cosmetics. Nat Nanotechnol. 2010;5(2):92. doi:10.1038/nnano.2010.12.
4. Jain RK, Stylianopoulos T. Delivering nanomedicine to solid tumors. Nat Rev Clin Oncol. 2010;7(11):653–64. doi:10.1038/nrclinonc.2010.139.
5. Peters R, Kramer E, Oomen AG, Rivera ZE, Oegema G, Tromp PC, et al. Presence of nano-sized silica during *in vitro* digestion of foods containing silica as a food additive. ACS Nano. 2012;6(3):2441–51. doi:10.1021/nn204728k.
6. Nel A, Xia T, Madler L, Li N. Toxic potential of materials at the nanolevel. Science. 2006;311 (5761):622–7. doi:10.1126/science.1114397.
7. Setyawati MI, Tay CY, Chia SL, Goh SL, Fang W, Neo MJ, et al. Titanium dioxide nanomaterials cause endothelial cell leakiness by disrupting the homophilic interaction of VE-cadherin. Nat Commun. 2013;4:1673. doi:10.1038/ncomms2655.
8. Yamashita K, Yoshioka Y, Higashisaka K, Mimura K, Morishita Y, Nozaki M, et al. Silica and titanium dioxide nanoparticles cause pregnancy complications in mice. Nat Nanotechnol. 2011;6(5):321–8. doi:10.1038/nnano.2011.41.
9. Janssen NA, Brunekreef B, van Vliet P, Aarts F, Meliefste K, Harssema H, et al. The relationship between air pollution from heavy traffic and allergic sensitization, bronchial hyperresponsiveness, and respiratory symptoms in Dutch schoolchildren. Environ Health Perspect. 2003;111(12):1512–18.
10. Kulbok PA, Baldwin JH. From preventive health behavior to health promotion: advancing a positive construct of health. ANS Adv Nurs Sci. 1992;14(4):50–64.
11. Bartra J, Mullol J, del Cuvillo A, Davila I, Ferrer M, Jauregui I, et al. Air pollution and allergens. J Invest Allergol Clin Immunol. 2007;17 Suppl 2:3–8.
12. McCreanor J, Cullinan P, Nieuwenhuijsen MJ, Stewart-Evans J, Malliarou E, Jarup L, et al. Respiratory effects of exposure to diesel traffic in persons with asthma. N Engl J Med. 2007;357(23):2348–58. doi:10.1056/NEJMoa071535.
13. Peters A, Wichmann HE, Tuch T, Heinrich J, Heyder J. Respiratory effects are associated with the number of ultrafine particles. Am J Respir Crit Care Med. 1997;155(4):1376–83. doi:10.1164/ajrccm.155.4.9105082.
14. Delfino RJ, Sioutas C, Malik S. Potential role of ultrafine particles in associations between airborne particle mass and cardiovascular health. Environ Health Perspect. 2005;113 (8):934–46.
15. Maynard AD, Kuempel ED. Airborne nanostructured particles and occupational health. J Nanoparticle Res. 2005;7:587–614.
16. Tsuji JS, Maynard AD, Howard PC, James JT, Lam CW, Warheit DB, et al. Research strategies for safety evaluation of nanomaterials, part IV: risk assessment of nanoparticles. Toxicol Sci. 2006;89(1):42–50. doi:10.1093/toxsci/kfi339.
17. Popov AP, Priezzhev AV, Lademann J, Myllylä R. TiO2 nanoparticles as an effective UV-B radiation skin-protective compound in sunscreens. J Phys D Appl Phys. 2005;38(15):2564–70.
18. Tyner KM, Wokovich AM, Godar DE, Doub WH, Sadrieh N. The state of nano-sized titanium dioxide (TiO_2) may affect sunscreen performance. Int J Cosmet Sci. 2011;33(3):234–44. doi:10.1111/j.1468-2494.2010.00622.x.
19. Weir A, Westerhoff P, Fabricius L, Hristovski K, von Goetz N. Titanium dioxide nanoparticles in food and personal care products. Environ Sci Technol. 2012;46(4):2242–50. doi:10.1021/es204168d.
20. Merget R, Bauer T, Kupper HU, Philippou S, Bauer HD, Breitstadt R, et al. Health hazards due to the inhalation of amorphous silica. Arch Toxicol. 2002;75(11–12):625–34.
21. Yin JJ, Lao F, Fu PP, Wamer WG, Zhao Y, Wang PC, et al. The scavenging of reactive oxygen species and the potential for cell protection by functionalized fullerene materials. Biomaterials. 2009;30(4):611–21. doi:10.1016/j.biomaterials.2008.09.061.
22. Lens M. Use of fullerenes in cosmetics. Recent Patents Biotechnol. 2009;3(2):118–23.
23. Lens M. Recent progresses in application of fullerenes in cosmetics. Recent Patents Biotechnol. 2011;5(2):67–73.

24. Marambio-Jones C, Hoek EMV. A review of the antibacterial effects of silver nanomaterials and potential implications for human health and the environment. J Nanoparticle Res. 2010;12:1531–51.
25. Quadros ME, Marr LC. Silver nanoparticles and total aerosols emitted by nanotechnology-related consumer spray products. Environ Sci Technol. 2011;45(24):10713–19. doi:10.1021/es202770m.
26. Kuhlbusch TA, Asbach C, Fissan H, Gohler D, Stintz M. Nanoparticle exposure at nanotechnology workplaces: a review. Part Fibre Toxicol. 2011;8:22. doi:10.1186/1743-8977-8-22.
27. Lighty JS, Veranth JM, Sarofim AF. Combustion aerosols: factors governing their size and composition and implications to human health. J Air Waste Manage Assoc. 2000;50 (9):1565–618; discussion 619–22.
28. Zhu Y, Hinds WC, Kim S, Sioutas C. Concentration and size distribution of ultrafine particles near a major highway. J Air Waste Manage Assoc. 2002;52(9):1032–42.
29. Donaldson K, Stone V, Seaton A, MacNee W. Ambient particle inhalation and the cardiovascular system: potential mechanisms. Environ Health Perspect. 2001;109 Suppl 4:523–7.
30. Li N, Xia T, Nel AE. The role of oxidative stress in ambient particulate matter-induced lung diseases and its implications in the toxicity of engineered nanoparticles. Free Radic Biol Med. 2008;44(9):1689–99. doi:10.1016/j.freeradbiomed.2008.01.028.
31. Wiesner MR, Lowry GV, Casman E, Bertsch PM, Matson CW, Di Giulio RT, et al. Meditations on the ubiquity and mutability of nano-sized materials in the environment. ACS Nano. 2011;5(11):8466–70. doi:10.1021/nn204118p.
32. Glover RD, Miller JM, Hutchison JE. Generation of metal nanoparticles from silver and copper objects: nanoparticle dynamics on surfaces and potential sources of nanoparticles in the environment. ACS Nano. 2011;5(11):8950–7. doi:10.1021/nn2031319.
33. Mitrano DM, Rimmele E, Wichser A, Erni R, Height M, Nowack B. Presence of nanoparticles in wash water from conventional silver and nano-silver textiles. ACS Nano. 2014;8 (7):7208–19. doi:10.1021/nn502228w.
34. Yin Y, Liu J, Jiang G. Sunlight-induced reduction of ionic Ag and Au to metallic nanoparticles by dissolved organic matter. ACS Nano. 2012;6(9):7910–19. doi:10.1021/nn302293r.
35. Schilling K, Bradford B, Castelli D, Dufour E, Nash JF, Pape W, et al. Human safety review of "nano" titanium dioxide and zinc oxide. Photochem Photobiol Sci. 2010;9(4):495–509. doi:10.1039/b9pp00180h.
36. Sadrieh N, Wokovich AM, Gopee NV, Zheng J, Haines D, Parmiter D, et al. Lack of significant dermal penetration of titanium dioxide from sunscreen formulations containing nano- and submicron-size TiO2 particles. Toxicol Sci. 2010;115(1):156–66. doi:10.1093/toxsci/kfq041.
37. Zvyagin AV, Zhao X, Gierden A, Sanchez W, Ross JA, Roberts MS. Imaging of zinc oxide nanoparticle penetration in human skin *in vitro* and *in vivo*. J Biomed Opt. 2008;13(6):064031. doi:10.1117/1.3041492.
38. Senzui M, Tamura T, Miura K, Ikarashi Y, Watanabe Y, Fujii M. Study on penetration of titanium dioxide (TiO(2)) nanoparticles into intact and damaged skin *in vitro*. J Toxicol Sci. 2010;35(1):107–13.
39. Fruijtier-Polloth C. The toxicological mode of action and the safety of synthetic amorphous silica-a nanostructured material. Toxicology. 2012;294(2–3):61–79. doi:10.1016/j.tox.2012.02.001.
40. Nabeshi H, Yoshikawa T, Matsuyama K, Nakazato Y, Matsuo K, Arimori A, et al. Systemic distribution, nuclear entry and cytotoxicity of amorphous nanosilica following topical application. Biomaterials. 2011;32(11):2713–24. doi:10.1016/j.biomaterials.2010.12.042.
41. Hirai T, Yoshikawa T, Nabeshi H, Yoshida T, Akase T, Yoshioka Y, et al. Dermal absorption of amorphous nanosilica particles after topical exposure for three days. Die Pharmazie. 2012;67(8):742–3.

42. Rancan F, Gao Q, Graf C, Troppens S, Hadam S, Hackbarth S, et al. Skin penetration and cellular uptake of amorphous silica nanoparticles with variable size, surface functionalization, and colloidal stability. ACS Nano. 2012;6(8):6829–42. doi:10.1021/nn301622h.
43. Ryman-Rasmussen JP, Riviere JE, Monteiro-Riviere NA. Penetration of intact skin by quantum dots with diverse physicochemical properties. Toxicol Sci. 2006;91(1):159–65. doi:10.1093/toxsci/kfj122.
44. Zhang LW, Yu WW, Colvin VL, Monteiro-Riviere NA. Biological interactions of quantum dot nanoparticles in skin and in human epidermal keratinocytes. Toxicol Appl Pharmacol. 2008;228(2):200–11. doi:10.1016/j.taap.2007.12.022.
45. Mortensen LJ, Oberdorster G, Pentland AP, Delouise LA. *In vivo* skin penetration of quantum dot nanoparticles in the murine model: the effect of UVR. Nano Lett. 2008;8(9):2779–87. doi:10.1021/nl801323y.
46. Prow TW, Monteiro-Riviere NA, Inman AO, Grice JE, Chen X, Zhao X, et al. Quantum dot penetration into viable human skin. Nanotoxicology. 2012;6(2):173–85. doi:10.3109/17435390.2011.569092.
47. Bos JD, Meinardi MM. The 500 Dalton rule for the skin penetration of chemical compounds and drugs. Exp Dermatol. 2000;9(3):165–9.
48. Hansen S, Lehr CM. Transfollicular delivery takes root: the future for vaccine design? Expert Rev Vaccines. 2014;13(1):5–7. doi:10.1586/14760584.2014.862500.
49. Brandner JM, McIntyre M, Kief S, Wladykowski E, Moll I. Expression and localization of tight junction-associated proteins in human hair follicles. Arch Dermatol Res. 2003;295(5):211–21. doi:10.1007/s00403-003-0418-3.
50. Kubo A, Nagao K, Yokouchi M, Sasaki H, Amagai M. External antigen uptake by Langerhans cells with reorganization of epidermal tight junction barriers. J Exp Med. 2009;206(13):2937–46. doi:10.1084/jem.20091527.
51. Kuchler S, Abdel-Mottaleb M, Lamprecht A, Radowski MR, Haag R, Schafer-Korting M. Influence of nanocarrier type and size on skin delivery of hydrophilic agents. Int J Pharm. 2009;377(1–2):169–72. doi:10.1016/j.ijpharm.2009.04.046.
52. Rouse JG, Yang J, Ryman-Rasmussen JP, Barron AR, Monteiro-Riviere NA. Effects of mechanical flexion on the penetration of fullerene amino acid-derivatized peptide nanoparticles through skin. Nano Lett. 2007;7(1):155–60. doi:10.1021/nl062464m.
53. Winter M, Beer HD, Hornung V, Kramer U, Schins RP, Forster I. Activation of the inflammasome by amorphous silica and TiO_2 nanoparticles in murine dendritic cells. Nanotoxicology. 2011;5(3):326–40. doi:10.3109/17435390.2010.506957.
54. Kumar K, Saini S, Mehta RD, Bumb RA. Contact leucoderma caused by lemon. Indian J Dermatol Venereol Leprol. 1996;62(1):61.
55. Lunov O, Syrovets T, Loos C, Nienhaus GU, Mailander V, Landfester K, et al. Amino-functionalized polystyrene nanoparticles activate the NLRP3 inflammasome in human macrophages. ACS Nano. 2011;5(12):9648–57. doi:10.1021/nn203596e.
56. Stern ST, Adiseshaiah PP, Crist RM. Autophagy and lysosomal dysfunction as emerging mechanisms of nanomaterial toxicity. Part Fibre Toxicol. 2012;9:20. doi:10.1186/1743-8977-9-20.
57. Kang SJ, Kim BM, Lee YJ, Chung HW. Titanium dioxide nanoparticles trigger p53-mediated damage response in peripheral blood lymphocytes. Environ Mol Mutagen. 2008;49(5):399–405. doi:10.1002/em.20399.
58. Trouiller B, Reliene R, Westbrook A, Solaimani P, Schiestl RH. Titanium dioxide nanoparticles induce DNA damage and genetic instability *in vivo* in mice. Cancer Res. 2009;69(22):8784–9. doi:10.1158/0008-5472.CAN-09-2496.
59. Ye Y, Liu J, Xu J, Sun L, Chen M, Lan M. Nano-SiO_2 induces apoptosis via activation of p53 and Bax mediated by oxidative stress in human hepatic cell line. Toxicol In Vitro. 2010;24(3):751–8. doi:10.1016/j.tiv.2010.01.001.

60. Nabeshi H, Yoshikawa T, Matsuyama K, Nakazato Y, Tochigi S, Kondoh S, et al. Amorphous nanosilica induce endocytosis-dependent ROS generation and DNA damage in human keratinocytes. Part Fibre Toxicol. 2011;8:1. doi:10.1186/1743-8977-8-1.
61. Ristow M. Unraveling the truth about antioxidants: mitohormesis explains ROS-induced health benefits. Nat Med. 2014;20(7):709–11. doi:10.1038/nm.3624.
62. Kawagishi H, Finkel T. Unraveling the truth about antioxidants: ROS and disease: finding the right balance. Nat Med. 2014;20(7):711–13. doi:10.1038/nm.3625.
63. Heidler T, Hartwig K, Daniel H, Wenzel U. Caenorhabditis elegans lifespan extension caused by treatment with an orally active ROS-generator is dependent on DAF-16 and SIR-2.1. Biogerontology. 2010;11(2):183–95. doi:10.1007/s10522-009-9239-x.
64. Yang W, Hekimi S. A mitochondrial superoxide signal triggers increased longevity in Caenorhabditis elegans. PLoS Biol. 2010;8(12), e1000556. doi:10.1371/journal.pbio.1000556.
65. Kimber I, Hilton J, Dearman RJ, Gerberick GF, Ryan CA, Basketter DA, et al. An international evaluation of the murine local lymph node assay and comparison of modified procedures. Toxicology. 1995;103(1):63–73.
66. Park YH, Jeong SH, Yi SM, Choi BH, Kim YR, Kim IK, et al. Analysis for the potential of polystyrene and TiO2 nanoparticles to induce skin irritation, phototoxicity, and sensitization. Toxicol In Vitro. 2011;25(8):1863–9. doi:10.1016/j.tiv.2011.05.022.
67. Lee S, Yun HS, Kim SH. The comparative effects of mesoporous silica nanoparticles and colloidal silica on inflammation and apoptosis. Biomaterials. 2011;32(35):9434–43. doi:10.1016/j.biomaterials.2011.08.042.
68. Chen BX, Wilson SR, Das M, Coughlin DJ, Erlanger BF. Antigenicity of fullerenes: antibodies specific for fullerenes and their characteristics. Proc Natl Acad Sci U S A. 1998;95(18):10809–13.
69. Braden BC, Goldbaum FA, Chen BX, Kirschner AN, Wilson SR, Erlanger BF. X-ray crystal structure of an anti-Buckminsterfullerene antibody fab fragment: biomolecular recognition of C(60). Proc Natl Acad Sci U S A. 2000;97(22):12193–7. doi:10.1073/pnas.210396197.
70. Ema M, Matsuda A, Kobayashi N, Naya M, Nakanishi J. Dermal and ocular irritation and skin sensitization studies of fullerene C60 nanoparticles. Cutan Ocul Toxicol. 2013;32(2):128–34. doi:10.3109/15569527.2012.727937.
71. Mann E, Ranft U, Eberwein G, Gladtke D, Sugiri D, Behrendt H, et al. Does airborne nickel exposure induce nickel sensitization? Contact Dermatitis. 2010;62(6):355–62. doi:10.1111/j.1600-0536.2010.01725.x.
72. Otani S, Onishi K, Mu H, Yokoyama Y, Hosoda T, Okamoto M, et al. The relationship between skin symptoms and allergic reactions to Asian dust. Int J Environ Res Pub Health. 2012;9(12):4606–14. doi:10.3390/ijerph9124606.
73. Swinnen I, Goossens A. An update on airborne contact dermatitis: 2007–2011. Contact Dermatitis. 2013;68(4):232–8. doi:10.1111/cod.12022.
74. Hussain S, Smulders S, De Vooght V, Ectors B, Boland S, Marano F, et al. Nano-titanium dioxide modulates the dermal sensitization potency of DNCB. Part Fibre ogy. 2012;9:15. doi:10.1186/1743-8977-9-15.
75. Fonacier LS, Dreskin SC, Leung DY. Allergic skin diseases. J Allergy Clin Immunol. 2010;125(2 Suppl 2):S138–49. doi:10.1016/j.jaci.2009.05.039.
76. Sanda T, Yasue T, Oohashi M, Yasue A. Effectiveness of house dust-mite allergen avoidance through clean room therapy in patients with atopic dermatitis. J Allergy Clin Immunol. 1992;89(3):653–7.
77. Yanagisawa R, Takano H, Inoue K, Koike E, Kamachi T, Sadakane K, et al. Titanium dioxide nanoparticles aggravate atopic dermatitis-like skin lesions in NC/Nga mice. Exp Biol Med. 2009;234(3):314–22. doi:10.3181/0810-RM-304.
78. Yanagisawa R, Takano H, Inoue KI, Koike E, Sadakane K, Ichinose T. Size effects of polystyrene nanoparticles on atopic dermatitislike skin lesions in NC/NGA mice. Int J Immunopathol Pharmacol. 2010;23(1):131–41.

79. Hirai T, Yoshikawa T, Nabeshi H, Yoshida T, Tochigi S, Ichihashi K, et al. Amorphous silica nanoparticles size-dependently aggravate atopic dermatitis-like skin lesions following an intradermal injection. Part Fibre Toxicol. 2012;9:3. doi:10.1186/1743-8977-9-3.
80. Ilves M, Palomaki J, Vippola M, Lehto M, Savolainen K, Savinko T, et al. Topically applied ZnO nanoparticles suppress allergen induced skin inflammation but induce vigorous IgE production in the atopic dermatitis mouse model. Part Fibre Toxicol. 2014;11:38. doi:10.1186/s12989-014-0038-4.
81. Chapman MD, Platts-Mills TA. Measurement of IgG, IgA and IgE antibodies to Dermatophagoides pteronyssinus by antigen-binding assay, using a partially purified fraction of mite extract (F4P1). Clin Exp Immunol. 1978;34(1):126–36.
82. Platts-Mills TA. Local production of IgG, IgA and IgE antibodies in grass pollen hay fever. J Immunol. 1979;122(6):2218–25.

Chapter 7
Health Effects of Silver Nanoparticles and Silver Ions

Takamitsu Miyayama, Yuta Arai, and Seishiro Hirano

Abstract The health effects of silver nanoparticles (AgNPs) have not been well investigated, despite AgNPs now being widely used in consumer products. We introduce living environment, analysis, metabolic behavior, toxicity, and human health effect of AgNPs in comparison to silver nitrate ($AgNO_3$). The American Conference of Governmental Industrial Hygienists (ACGIH) has established separate threshold limit values (TLV) for metallic silver (0.1 mg/m^3) and soluble compounds of silver (0.01 mg/m^3). Argyria and argyrosis are chronic disorders of skin microvessels and eyes in humans, and these disorders reportedly develop following extended oral and inhalational exposure to Ag. In mammals, $AgNO_3$ and AgNPs increased the number of the total cells, neutrophils, and pro-inflammatory cytokine production "IL-1β," and these were distributed in the lung, kidney, and liver. The amount of Ag in the metallothionein (MT)-bound form was related in cellular behavior and toxicity of AgNPs and $AgNO_3$. The cytotoxic effect of AgNPs is a simple function of neither the number nor total surface area. Although the effect may vary among the cell types and the culture conditions, AgNPs were transported to lysosomes and only gradually dissolved in mammals, causing milder inflammatory stimulation.

Keywords Silver nanoparticle • Silver ion • Lysosome • Macrophages • Metallothionein

---

T. Miyayama (✉)
Department of Hygiene and Public Health I, School of Medicine, Tokyo Women's Medical University, Shinjyuku-ku, Tokyo, Japan

Environmental Nanotoxicology Project, RCER, National Institute for Environmental Studies, Tsukuba, Ibaraki, Japan
e-mail: t-miyayama@research.twmu.ac.jp

Y. Arai
Graduate School of Pharmaceutical Sciences, Chiba University, Chiba, Japan

S. Hirano
Environmental Nanotoxicology Project, RCER, National Institute for Environmental Studies, Tsukuba, Ibaraki, Japan

Graduate School of Pharmaceutical Sciences, Chiba University, Chiba, Japan

T. Otsuki et al. (eds.), *Biological Effects of Fibrous and Particulate Substances*, Current Topics in Environmental Health and Preventive Medicine, DOI 10.1007/978-4-431-55732-6_7

7.1 AgNPs in Environment

7.1.1 Chemistry and Commercial Use of AgNPs

Ag is a chemical element with atomic number 47. It is composed of two stable isotopes, ^{107}Ag and ^{109}Ag. The natural abundances between ^{107}Ag and ^{109}Ag are 51.839 % and 48.161 %, respectively. Ag atomic weight is 107.8682 g/mol. A soft, white, lustrous transition metal, it possesses the highest electrical conductivity of any element and the highest thermal conductivity and reflectivity of any metal. Ag occurs naturally in its pure, free form, as an alloy with gold and other metals. Almost all Ag is produced as a by-product of copper, gold, lead, and zinc refining. AgCl argentometry is based on a famous reaction in Ag chemistry, where colorless aqueous $AgNO_3$ and colorless solution of NaCl produce white precipitates of AgCl. This reaction is important to investigate the metabolic behavior of Ag both in vitro and in vivo, because body fluids and culture medium contain chloride ions at a concentration about 4000 ppm and the reaction may take place on the surface of AgNPs. AgNPs are suspended in either citrate or polyvinylpyrrolidone (PVP), which increases dispersion and stability in solution [1]. Citrate and PVP serve as capping agents and stabilize the formed nanoparticles against agglomeration but also play a role in the formation of specific nanoparticles [2]. PVP suspended particles (20 and 110 nm) were taken up by mammalian cells to a greater degree when compared to citrate suspended particles of the same size and shape [3]. On the other hand, the other researchers reported that 10 nm citrate- and PVP-coated AgNPs were not difference in uptake [4].

AgNPs are currently used in consumer products such as cosmetics, food storage containers, medical supplies, and pharmaceuticals [5]. Among over 1800 commercially available products, identified as containing nanomaterials according to manufacturers' reports, about 25 % contain AgNPs [6]. Recently, there are increasing concerns about potential risks of AgNPs to humans and to the environment because of Ag behavior in mammals. Ag has antibacterial properties, and it was used for surgical prosthesis, splints, and fungicides. Soluble Ag compounds, such as silver salts, have been used in treating mental illness, epilepsy, nicotine addiction, gastroenteritis, and infectious diseases. It has been shown that Ag is deposited in the skin, eyes, and other organs in workers processing Ag-containing materials [7, 8]. Argyria and argyrosis are chronic disorders of skin microvessels and eyes in humans, and these disorders reportedly develop following extended oral and inhalational exposure to Ag in occupational exposures. Despite the knowledge about increasing discharge of AgNPs into environment as wastewater and its potential toxicity to microorganisms [9], the interaction of AgNPs with heavy metals in the biological removal process remains poorly understood.

7.1.2 Characterization of AgNPs

The assessment of the physicochemical and biological properties of AgNPs is complicated because these properties depend on a number of parameters such as size, shape, charge, dispersion state, and surface functionality. Therefore, the comparison of the results from different groups is typically difficult because either different particles were used or different chemical or biological methods were applied [2]. Most researchers evaluate primary size, hydrodynamic diameter, and zeta-potential of metal nanoparticles by transmission electron microscope (TEM) and dynamic light scattering (DLS). As the results of TEM and DLS analysis, the addition of fetal bovine serum (FBS) enhanced the stability of the particle suspension by steric hindrance [10, 11]. The presence of proteins reduces the surface energy of a nanoparticle and decreases adhesion of the nanoparticles to the cellular membranes [12, 13]. Because FBS used for the cell culture contains bovine serum albumin, the use of albumin is reasonable to disperse particulate substances and diminish the propensity of nanoparticles to agglomerate in in vivo and in vitro studies [14].

7.1.3 Exposure Limits

Ag can be absorbed into the systemic circulation from the drinking water and also through parenteral routes such as inhalation and dermal exposure [15]. ACGIH has established separate TLV for metallic silver (0.1 mg/m^3) and soluble compounds of silver (0.01 mg/m^3). Occupational Safety and Health Administration (OSHA) and Mine Safety and Health Administration (MSHA) proposed that a permissible exposure limit (PEL) for both metallic and most soluble Ag compounds should be 0.01 mg/m^3 [16]. Argentina, Bulgaria, Columbia, Jordan, Korea, New Zealand, Singapore, and Vietnam recognize the American Conference of Governmental Industrial Hygienists (ACGIH) threshold limit values (TLV) of 0.1 mg/m^3 for metallic Ag, while Austria, Denmark, Germany, the Netherlands, Norway, Switzerland, and Japan recognize 0.01 mg/m^3 as the occupational exposure limit for all forms [17]. There is thus a high probability of exposure to AgNPs through ingestion, skin contact, and inhalation, which raises a potential health risk of Ag in humans.

7.1.4 Measurement and Analysis of AgNPs

Metal analysis provides important information on cellular uptake and tissue distribution of administered metals and also identification and quantification of metal- or metalloid-containing biomolecules. Atomic absorption spectrometry (AAS) and inductively coupled plasma-atomic emission spectrometry (ICP-AES) have been used for metal analysis of biological samples because of their sensitivity and accuracy. Inductively coupled plasma-mass spectrometry (ICP-MS) has higher sensitivity and accuracy for the detection of multielements than AAS and ICP-AES. Particularly, ICP-MS is able to analyze isotopes, which enables the use of enriched stable isotopes as tracers in biological studies. The use of stable isotopes rather than radioisotopes is recommended for biological research [18].

7.1.5 Speciation of Ag in Biological Samples

Speciation is the analytical methods of identifying and/or measuring the quantities of one or more individual chemical species in biological samples as blood plasma, tissue extract, urine, digested spots from electrophoresis, and cell extract [19]. High-performance liquid chromatography (HPLC) coupled with ICP-MS has a multi-separation of biological samples and a high sensitivity and specificity of metal detections. It is suitable for the screening of Ag distribution in tissue and culture cells. In mammals following exposure to AgNPs and $AgNO_3$, it has been reported that Ag-bound metallothioneins (Ag-MT) were determined by HPLC-ICP-MS [20–22]. MT-I, MT-II, MT-III, and MT-IV are low-molecular-weight proteins (MW ~7 kDa). MT-I and MT-II can bind to a variety of essential and toxic metals, such as copper, zinc, cadmium, mercury, and Ag [23–26]. The induction of MTs protects cells against heavy metal toxicity by chelating those metals with cysteine residues and by reducing reactive oxygen species (ROS) generation [27]. It has been reported that $AgNO_3$ and AgNPs were incorporated into cells, where the Ag ion induced de novo synthesis of MT-I and MT-II [28]. These reports suggested that the amount of Ag in the MT-bound form was related to cellular behavior of AgNPs and $AgNO_3$. The analytical collaborations between HPLC-ICP-MS and molecular biological techniques may reveal Ag behavior in mammals.

7.2 Metabolic Behavior of AgNPs

7.2.1 Inhalated AgNPs

There is a high probability of exposure to AgNPs through inhalation, which raises a potential health risk of silver in humans. Inhaled AgNPs are typically cleared from the respiratory tract by coughing, mucociliary transport, and phagocytosis of alveolar macrophages. The major deposition mechanism for particles smaller than 0.5 μm is diffusion. In the lung, squamous alveolar (type I) cells form the structure of the alveolar wall, whereas cuboidal alveolar (type II) cells continuously release pulmonary surfactant by exocytosis. Once AgNPs reach the alveoli, further barriers to diffusion into the blood circulation are limited. This is because the epithelium that separates the inhaled air from the blood capillaries is very thin (<0.5 μm), consisting of a monolayer of type I and type II epithelial cells [6]. Therefore AgNPs can penetrate deeply into the alveolar region, where clearance may be insufficient. Any cellular or protein damage in this region could not only have an impact on pulmonary homeostasis but would also determine possible translocations of AgNPs to other organs and allow them to elicit toxic effects at extrapulmonary sites. Hence, the first interactions of AgNPs with the lung epithelium urgently need to be addressed, in order to predict their adverse effects, provide guidelines for their safe use, and direct the regulation of AgNPs.

7.2.2 AgNPs Exposed via Other Routes

Adult-male C57BL/6 N mice received intraperitoneal administration (i.p.) of 25 nm AgNPs at doses of 100, 500, or 1000 mg/kg, and effects of AgNPs on gene expression in various regions of the mouse brain were investigated. It was suggested that AgNPs may produce neurotoxicity by generating free radical-induced oxidative stress and by altering gene expression, producing apoptosis and neurotoxicity [29]. The study showed the transdermal uptake of Ag by AgNP-containing wound dressings in male rats leading to elevated Ag levels in blood, feces, brain, testis, lung, heart, and muscle tissue after a burn trauma. The Ag blood levels showed a significant increase after 3 weeks of external application of two commercially available Ag wound care products (AgNPs and Ag sulfate). After 6 weeks of application, a significant accumulation of Ag was detected in all analyzed organs and tissue specimens (spleen, kidney, liver, brain, testis, lung, heart, and muscle tissue). AgNPs resulted in higher Ag levels in the organs than the Ag sulfate-containing product [30].

7.3 Toxicity of AgNPs

7.3.1 Toxic Mechanism of AgNPs

AgNPs may enter the cell via phagocytosis, macropinocytosis, or endocytosis and, then, be distributed to cytoplasmic compartments such as endosome, lysosomes, mitochondria, and nucleus. Cellular effects of AgNPs occur as a result of intracellular release of Ag^+, leading to oxidative damage to the cell [31]. It was reported that dissolution of metal nanoparticles to ions in the acid environment of the lysosomes causes lysosomal destabilization and cell death [32]. However, cytotoxicity of AgNPs in human hepatoma cell (HepG2) appeared to be mediated by oxidative stress independent of Ag^+ release [33]. The cytotoxicity mechanisms of

AgNPs depend on not only their concentration, size, shape, and surface modification but also on the target cell type.

7.3.2 Toxicity of AgNPs In Vivo

In mice, $AgNO_3$ and AgNPs increased the number of the total cells, neutrophils, pro-inflammatory and cytokine production "IL-1β" and were distributed in the lung, kidney, and liver after 24 h instillation. Other researchers reported that a single intratracheal instillation of AgNPs (average diameter, 243.8 ± 176.7 nm) caused helper type 2-dominant inflammatory responses, pro-inflammatory cytokine production, and lung tissue damage [34]. Subchronic inhalation exposure of Sprague-Dawley rats to different concentrations of AgNPs (average diameter 18–19 nm) showed that AgNPs were mainly distributed to the lungs and liver and caused lung inflammation and bile-duct hyperplasia [35]. These researchers suggested that the no-observable-adverse-effect level (NOAEL) was calculated to be 100 $\mu g/m^3$. An in vivo study based on oral administration of 15 nm AgNPs to rats indicates the accumulation of Ag in the kidney and liver [21]. The Ag is relatively labile, being eliminated after 30 days. Ag is homogeneously distributed in the liver, whereas in the kidney, it is preferentially located in the cortex. Ag speciation determined Ag-MT in the kidney and liver. The presence of intact AgNPs in rat feces was detected and excreted about 50 % of administrated AgNPs.

7.3.3 Toxicity of AgNPs In Vitro

In mammalian cells, one of the major toxicological interests regarding Ag used in commercial products is the difference in cellular uptake, tissue distribution, and toxicity between ionic (Ag^+) and nanoparticulate forms. Exposure to $AgNO_3$ in vitro decreased the cell viability dose dependently in various types of cells such as rat hepatocytes [36], human dermal fibroblasts [37], Jurkat cells [38], human leukocytes [39], and neuronal PC12 rat pheochromocytoma cells [40]. Silver ion interacts with a variety of biomolecules, such as nucleic acids, cell wall components, and sulfhydryl groups of metabolic enzymes, MTs, and glutathione (GSH), which leads to cellular dysfunction [41, 42]. The toxicity of $AgNO_3$ and AgNPs arises in part from their inhibitory effect on mitochondrial function and cellular energy metabolism [15, 43]. The cytotoxic effects of $AgNO_3$ and AgNPs seem to be associated with oxidative stress [15, 44] and apoptosis signaling [31, 45]. It was reported that the viability of macrophages decreased dose and size dependently following 24-h exposure to 15, 30, and 55 nm AgNPs at concentrations ranging from 10 to 75 μg/mL [43]. The similar effects were reported using titanium oxide and silica nanoparticles [46, 47]. We reported the cytotoxicity, induction of MTs, and intracellular distribution of Ag in $AgNO_3$- or AgNP-exposed

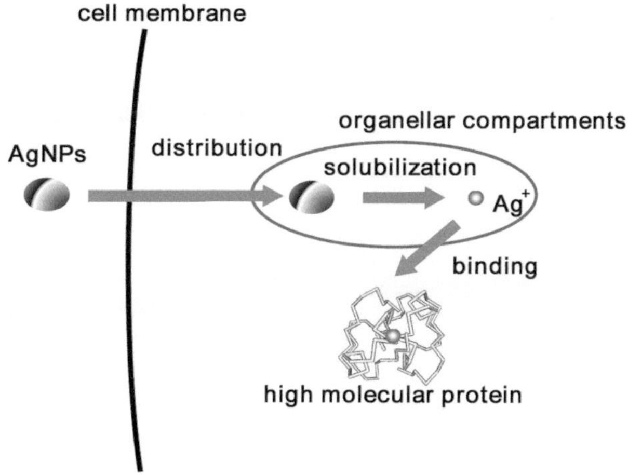

Fig. 7.1 Distribution and behavior of AgNPs in J774.1 murine macrophage cells. AgNPs were accumulated in the lysosomes. It is plausible that AgNPs gradually dissolved and liberated Ag ions bound to intracellular proteins without inducing MTs in J774.1 cells

J774.1 murine macrophage cells [20]. The cytotoxic EC_{50} values of the 20, 60, and 100 nm AgNPs were 38.4, 27.9, and 51.8 μg Ag/mL, respectively, in J774.1 murine macrophage cells, suggesting that smaller Ag particles were slightly more cytotoxic and the cytotoxic effect of AgNPs was not a simple function of either the number or total surface area [20]. In this study chemical speciation analyses of silver in the supernatant of cell lysate were performed. The amount of Ag in the soluble fraction of the cell lysate was higher than that in the insoluble fraction in $AgNO_3$-exposed cells, while the amount of Ag in the insoluble fraction was higher than that in the soluble fraction in AgNP-treated cells. In the HPLC-ICP-MS elution profile of Ag, the intensity of the Ag peak in the MT fraction increased in the $AgNO_3$-treated J774.1 cells, whereas no Ag-bound MT was observed in the AgNP-exposed cells; instead, Ag eluted in a high-molecular protein fraction. It is also indicated that intracellular glutathione level did not play a role in the cytotoxic effect of $AgNO_3$. The phase-contrast images of AgNPs colocalized with fluorescent images of lysosomes in AgNP-exposed cells. AgNPs may be transported to lysosomes and only gradually dissolved in the macrophages (Fig. 7.1), causing milder inflammatory stimulation in the mouse lung compared to $AgNO_3$.

7.4 Effects of AgNPs on Humans

The most common health effects associated with prolonged exposure to Ag are the development of a characteristic, irreversible pigmentation of the skin (argyria), and the eyes (argyrosis). The affected area becomes bluish gray or ash gray and is most prominent in areas of the body exposed to sunlight [48, 49]. Argyria and argyrosis are chronic disorders of skin microvessels and eyes in humans, and these disorders reportedly develop following extended oral and inhalational exposure to $AgNO_3$

[50], silver oxide [51, 52], and particulate and colloidal Ag [7]. Excessive nasal exposure to a Ag-protein complex resulted in a blue-grey pigmentation in the skin due to intradermal silver deposition [53, 54]. Generalized argyria was most often reported that $AgNO_3$ makers were in occupational exposures [51]. The lung and liver were the main target tissues for prolonged AgNP exposure, and NOAEL of AgNPs was determined as 100 $\mu g/m^3$ [35]. Actually, bronchitis, emphysema, and a reduction in pulmonary volume were observed when silver polishers were exposed to Ag [17, 51]. Mayr M et al. reported the patient of argyria in 2009 [55]. The patient, a former laboratory technician, produced a silver colloid solution. The diagnosis was argyrosis of the kidney and discrete signs of benign nephroangiosclerosis. The history of severe hypertension led to the assumption that the cause of the decreased kidney function was benign nephroangiosclerosis. Pala G et al. reported the patient of argyrosis in 2008 [56]. The patient was a 71-year-old man, working from the age of 17 as a craftsman producing a variety of Ag items, including vases, plates, trays, and frames. The working bench was situated approximately 30–40 cm from patient's face, who never wore any ocular or respiratory protective devices. No aspiration systems were present in the workplace. Ocular examination revealed a bilateral, marked blue-gray discoloration of the tarsal and bulbar conjunctive and of the cornea. These case reports highlight the hazard of Ag workers without adequate protection and indicate that occupational ocular argyria and argyrosis may still be observed in clinical practice today.

7.5 Conclusion

AgNPs have been gaining attention in both research and industry. Cytotoxicity of AgNPs not only depends on concentration, size, shape, and surface modification but also on the target cell type. Multidimensional approaches were used to reveal the toxicological mechanisms for AgNPs and also Ag ions in cells. These approaches include analysis for chemical species of Ag in cells and tissues by HPLC-ICP-MS, molecular imaging, transcriptional induction, gene product expression, and localization of target proteins in AgNP- or Ag ion-exposed mammalian cells.

References

1. Shannahan JH, Podila R, Aldossari AA, Emerson H, Powell BA, Ke PC, et al. Formation of a protein corona on silver nanoparticles mediates cellular toxicity via scavenger receptors. Toxicol Sci. 2015;143(1):136–46. doi:10.1093/toxsci/kfu217.
2. Ahlberg S, Antonopulos A, Diendorf J, Dringen R, Epple M, Flock R, et al. PVP-coated, negatively charged silver nanoparticles: a multi-center study of their physicochemical characteristics, cell culture and *in vivo* experiments. Beilstein J Nanotechnol. 2014;5:1944–65. doi:10.3762/bjnano.5.205.

3. Aldossari AA, Shannahan JH, Podila R, Brown JM. Influence of physicochemical properties of silver nanoparticles on mast cell activation and degranulation. Toxicol In Vitro. 2015;29 (1):195–203. doi:10.1016/j.tiv.2014.10.008.
4. Gliga AR, Skoglund S, Wallinder IO, Fadeel B, Karlsson HL. Size-dependent cytotoxicity of silver nanoparticles in human lung cells: the role of cellular uptake, agglomeration and Ag release. Part Fibre Toxicol. 2014;11:11. doi:10.1186/1743-8977-11-11.
5. Ahamed M, Karns M, Goodson M, Rowe J, Hussain SM, Schlager JJ, et al. DNA damage response to different surface chemistry of silver nanoparticles in mammalian cells. Toxicol Appl Pharmacol. 2008;233(3):404–10. 10.1016/j.taap.2008.09.015 S0041-008X(08)00388-8 [pii].
6. Theodorou IG, Ryan MP, Tetley TD, Porter AE. Inhalation of silver nanomaterials-seeing the risks. Int J Mol Sci. 2014;15(12):23936–74. doi:10.3390/ijms151223936.
7. Atiyeh BS, Costagliola M, Hayek SN, Dibo SA. Effect of silver on burn wound infection control and healing: review of the literature. Burns. 2007;33(2):139–48. doi:10.1016/j.burns.2006.06.010.
8. Lansdown AB. Silver in health care: antimicrobial effects and safety in use. Curr Probl Dermatol. 2006;33:17–34. 93928 [pii] 10.1159/000093928.
9. Zuo Y, Chen G, Zeng G, Li Z, Yan M, Chen A, et al. Transport, fate, and stimulating impact of silver nanoparticles on the removal of Cd(II) by Phanerochaete chrysosporium in aqueous solutions. J Hazard Mater. 2015;285:236–44. doi:10.1016/j.jhazmat.2014.12.003.
10. Murdock RC, Braydich-Stolle L, Schrand AM, Schlager JJ, Hussain SM. Characterization of nanomaterial dispersion in solution prior to in vitro exposure using dynamic light scattering technique. Toxicol Sci. 2008;101(2):239–53. kfm240 [pii] 10.1093/toxsci/kfm240.
11. Foldbjerg R, Olesen P, Hougaard M, Dang DA, Hoffmann HJ, Autrup H. PVP-coated silver nanoparticles and silver ions induce reactive oxygen species, apoptosis and necrosis in THP-1 monocytes. Toxicol Lett. 2009;190(2):156–62. doi:10.1016/j.toxlet.2009.07.009.
12. Lesniak A, Salvati A, Santos-Martinez MJ, Radomski MW, Dawson KA, Aberg C. Nanoparticle adhesion to the cell membrane and its effect on nanoparticle uptake efficiency. J Am Chem Soc. 2013;135(4):1438–44. doi:10.1021/ja309812z.
13. Hayashi Y, Miclaus T, Scavenius C, Kwiatkowska K, Sobota A, Engelmann P, et al. Species differences take shape at nanoparticles: protein corona made of the native repertoire assists cellular interaction. Environ Sci Technol. 2013;47(24):14367–75. doi:10.1021/es404132w.
14. Kvitek L, Panacek A, Soukupova J, Kolar M, Vecerova R, Prucek R, et al. Effect of surfactants and polymers on stability and antibacterial activity of silver nanoparticles (NPs). J Phys Chem C. 2008;112(15):5825–34. doi:10.1021/Jp711616v.
15. Miyayama T, Arai Y, Suzuki N, Hirano S. Mitochondrial electron transport is inhibited by disappearance of metallothionein in human bronchial epithelial cells following exposure to silver nitrate. Toxicology. 2013;305:20–9. 10.1016/j.tox.2013.01.004 S0300-483X(13)00009-7 [pii].
16. Miyayama T, Arai Y, Hirano S. Environmental exposure to silver and its health effects. Nihon Eiseigaku Zasshi. 2012;67(3):383–9. doi:DN/JST.JSTAGE/jjh/67.383 [pii].
17. Drake PL, Hazelwood KJ. Exposure-related health effects of silver and silver compounds: a review. Ann Occup Hyg. 2005;49(7):575–85. mei019 [pii] 10.1093/annhyg/mei019.
18. Suzuki KT. Simultaneous speciation of endogenous and exogenous elements by HPLC/ICP-MS with enriched stable isotopes. Tohoku J Exp Med. 1996;178(1):27–35.
19. Miyayama T, Ogra Y, Suzuki KT. Separation of metallothionein isoforms extracted from isoform-specific knockdown cells on two-dimensional micro high-performance liquid chromatography hyphenated with inductively coupled plasma-mass spectrometry. J Anal At Spectrom. 2007;22(2):179–82. doi:10.1039/B613662c.
20. Arai Y, Miyayama T, Hirano S. Difference in the toxicity mechanism between ion and nanoparticle forms of silver in the mouse lung and in macrophages. Toxicology. 2014;328C:84–92. doi:10.1016/j.tox.2014.12.014.

21. Jimenez-Lamana J, Laborda F, Bolea E, Abad-Alvaro I, Castillo JR, Bianga J, et al. An insight into silver nanoparticles bioavailability in rats. Metallomics. 2014;6(12):2242–9. doi:10.1039/c4mt00200h.
22. Miyayama T, Arai Y, Suzuki N, Hirano S. Cellular distribution and behavior of metallothionein in mammalian cells following exposure to silver nanoparticles and silver ions. Yakugaku Zasshi J Pharm Soc Jpn. 2014;134(6):723–9.
23. Haq F, Mahoney M, Koropatnick J. Signaling events for metallothionein induction. Mutat Res. 2003;533(1–2):211–26. doi:S0027510703002185.
24. Nordberg M, Nordberg GF. Toxicological aspects of metallothionein. Cell Mol Biol (Noisy-le-Grand). 2000;46(2):451–63.
25. Maret W. The function of zinc metallothionein: a link between cellular zinc and redox state. J Nutr. 2000;130(5S Suppl):1455S–8.
26. Kagi JH, Schaffer A. Biochemistry of metallothionein. Biochemistry. 1988;27(23):8509–15.
27. Fu Z, Guo J, Jing L, Li R, Zhang T, Peng S. Enhanced toxicity and ROS generation by doxorubicin in primary cultures of cardiomyocytes from neonatal metallothionein-I/II null mice. Toxicol In Vitro. 2010;24(6):1584–91. 10.1016/j.tiv.2010.06.009 S0887-2333(10)00151-7 [pii].
28. Lansdown AB. Metallothioneins: potential therapeutic aids for wound healing in the skin. Wound Repair Regen. 2002;10(3):130–2.
29. Rahman MF, Wang J, Patterson TA, Saini UT, Robinson BL, Newport GD, et al. Expression of genes related to oxidative stress in the mouse brain after exposure to silver-25 nanoparticles. Toxicol Lett. 2009;187(1):15–21. doi:10.1016/j.toxlet.2009.01.020.
30. Pfurtscheller K, Petnehazy T, Goessler W, Bubalo V, Kamolz LP, Trop M. Transdermal uptake and organ distribution of silver from two different wound dressings in rats after a burn trauma. Wound Repair Regen. 2014;22(5):654–9. doi:10.1111/wrr.12209.
31. Wilkinson LJ, White RJ, Chipman JK. Silver and nanoparticles of silver in wound dressings: a review of efficacy and safety. J Wound Care. 2011;20(11):543–9.
32. Cho WS, Duffin R, Howie SE, Scotton CJ, Wallace WA, Macnee W, et al. Progressive severe lung injury by zinc oxide nanoparticles; the role of Zn2+ dissolution inside lysosomes. Part Fibre Toxicol. 2011;8:27. doi:10.1186/1743-8977-8-27.
33. Kim S, Choi JE, Choi J, Chung KH, Park K, Yi J, et al. Oxidative stress-dependent toxicity of silver nanoparticles in human hepatoma cells. Toxicol In Vitro. 2009;23(6):1076–84. S0887-2333(09)00129-5 [pii] 10.1016/j.tiv.2009.06.001.
34. Park EJ, Choi K, Park K. Induction of inflammatory responses and gene expression by intratracheal instillation of silver nanoparticles in mice. Arch Pharm Res. 2011;34(2):299–307. doi:10.1007/s12272-011-0216-y.
35. Sung JH, Ji JH, Park JD, Yoon JU, Kim DS, Jeon KS, et al. Subchronic inhalation toxicity of silver nanoparticles. Toxicol Sci. 2009;108(2):452–61. kfn246 [pii] 10.1093/toxsci/kfn246.
36. Baldi C, Minoia C, Di Nucci A, Capodaglio E, Manzo L. Effects of silver in isolated rat hepatocytes. Toxicol Lett. 1988;41(3):261–8.
37. Hidalgo E, Domínguez C. Study of cytotoxicity mechanisms of silver nitrate in human dermal fibroblasts. Toxicol Lett. 1998;98(3):169–79.
38. Eom HJ, Choi J. p38 MAPK activation, DNA damage, cell cycle arrest and apoptosis as mechanisms of toxicity of silver nanoparticles in Jurkat T cells. Environ Sci Technol. 2010;44(21):8337–42. doi:10.1021/es1020668.
39. Jansson G, Harms-Ringdahl M. Stimulating effects of mercuric- and silver ions on the superoxide anion production in human polymorphonuclear leukocytes. Free Radic Res Commun. 1993;18(2):87–98.
40. Powers CM, Wrench N, Ryde IT, Smith AM, Seidler FJ, Slotkin TA. Silver impairs neurodevelopment: studies in PC12 cells. Environ Health Perspect. 2010;118(1):73–9. doi:10.1289/ehp.0901149.

41. Greulich C, Diendorf J, Simon T, Eggeler G, Epple M, Köller M. Uptake and intracellular distribution of silver nanoparticles in human mesenchymal stem cells. Acta Biomater. 2011;7 (1):347–54. doi:10.1016/j.actbio.2010.08.003.
42. Arora S, Jain J, Rajwade JM, Paknikar KM. Interactions of silver nanoparticles with primary mouse fibroblasts and liver cells. Toxicol Appl Pharmacol. 2009;236(3):310–8. 10.1016/j.taap. 2009.02.020 S0041-008X(09)00087-8 [pii].
43. Carlson C, Hussain SM, Schrand AM, Braydich-Stolle LK, Hess KL, Jones RL, et al. Unique cellular interaction of silver nanoparticles: size-dependent generation of reactive oxygen species. J Phys Chem B. 2008;112(43):13608–19. doi:10.1021/jp712087m.
44. Hussain SM, Hess KL, Gearhart JM, Geiss KT, Schlager JJ. In vitro toxicity of nanoparticles in BRL 3A rat liver cells. Toxicol In Vitro. 2005;19(7):975–83. S0887-2333(05)00126-8 [pii] 10. 1016/j.tiv.2005.06.034.
45. Almofti MR, Ichikawa T, Yamashita K, Terada H, Shinohara Y. Silver ion induces a cyclosporine a-insensitive permeability transition in rat liver mitochondria and release of apoptogenic cytochrome C. J Biochem. 2003;134(1):43–9.
46. Oberdorster G, Ferin J, Finkelstein J, Soderholm S. Thermal degradation events as health hazards: particle vs gas phase effects, mechanistic studies with particles. Acta Astronaut. 1992;27:251–6.
47. Sandberg WJ, Lag M, Holme JA, Friede B, Gualtieri M, Kruszewski M, et al. Comparison of non-crystalline silica nanoparticles in IL-1beta release from macrophages. Part Fibre Toxicol. 2012;9:32. doi:10.1186/1743-8977-9-32-1743-8977-9-32.
48. Shelley WB, Shelley ED, Burmeister V. Argyria: the intradermal "photograph," a manifestation of passive photosensitivity. J Am Acad Dermatol. 1987;16(1 Pt 2):211–7.
49. Gulbranson SH, Hud JA, Hansen RC. Argyria following the use of dietary supplements containing colloidal silver protein. Cutis. 2000;66(5):373–4.
50. Stafeeva K, Erlanger M, Velez-Montoya R, Olson JL. Ocular argyrosis secondary to long-term ingestion of silver nitrate salts. Clin Ophthalmol. 2012;6:2033–6. doi:10.2147/OPTH.S37898 opth-6-2033.
51. Rosenman KD, Moss A, Kon S. Argyria: clinical implications of exposure to silver nitrate and silver oxide. J Occup Med. 1979;21(6):430–5.
52. Moss AP, Sugar A, Hargett NA, Atkin A, Wolkstein M, Rosenman KD. The ocular manifestations and functional effects of occupational argyrosis. Arch Ophthalmol. 1979;97(5):906–8.
53. Lansdown AB. A pharmacological and toxicological profile of silver as an antimicrobial agent in medical devices. Adv Pharm Sci. 2010;2010:910686. doi:10.1155/2010/910686.
54. Tomi NS, Kranke B, Aberer W. A silver man. Lancet. 2004;363(9408):532.
55. Mayr M, Kim MJ, Wanner D, Helmut H, Schroeder J, Mihatsch MJ. Argyria and decreased kidney function: are silver compounds toxic to the kidney? Am J Kidney Dis. 2009;53(5):890–4. doi:10.1053/j.ajkd.2008.08.028.
56. Pala G, Fronterre A, Scafa F, Scelsi M, Ceccuzzi R, Gentile E, et al. Ocular argyrosis in a silver craftsman. J Occup Health. 2008;50(6):521–4. doi:JST.JSTAGE/joh/N8001 [pii].

Chapter 8
Multiwalled Carbon Nanotube-Induced Pulmonary Fibrogenesis

Jonathan H. Shannahan and Jared M. Brown

Abstract Engineered nanomaterials are increasingly being incorporated into a variety of technologies and applications due to their unique properties. In particular, multiwalled carbon nanotubes (MWCNT) hold great promise for many different industries. MWCNTs are made of carbon and have a cylindrical structure which can be synthesized with diameters in the nanometer-sized range and variable lengths into the micron range. MWCNTs have unique properties allowing for high electrical and thermal conductance, high tensile strength, low weight, and the ability to be manufactured with a variety of physicochemical properties and to undergo numerous surface modifications. Along with their vast potential, there is growing concern regarding human exposure and the possibility for adverse health effects. The primary route of human exposure to MWCNT is through inhalation in both occupational and environmental settings. Based on a commonality of properties including high aspect ratio and biopersistence within the lung, there is concern of asbestos-like toxicity following inhalation of MWCNTs. To date there has been sufficient toxicological evaluation in cell culture and animal models establishing the fibrogenic potential of MWCNTs. This chapter summarizes our current understanding regarding MWCNT-induced pulmonary fibrosis specifically examining current occupational human exposure levels, pulmonary deposition, susceptibility, and mechanisms of MWCNT-induced fibrogenesis. Further gaps in our current knowledge and likely areas of future study are highlighted throughout.

Keywords Multiwalled carbon nanotube • Pulmonary fibrosis • Inflammasome • Nanotoxicology • Mast cell

---

J.H. Shannahan, Ph.D. • J.M. Brown, Ph.D. (✉)
Department of Pharmaceutical Sciences, Skaggs School of Pharmacy and Pharmaceutical Sciences, The University of Colorado, Anschutz Medical Campus, Aurora, CO 80045, USA
e-mail: jared.brown@ucdenver.edu

T. Otsuki et al. (eds.), *Biological Effects of Fibrous and Particulate Substances*, Current Topics in Environmental Health and Preventive Medicine,
DOI 10.1007/978-4-431-55732-6_8

8.1 Introduction

Engineered nanomaterials are increasingly being incorporated into numerous fields of study and applications thereby influencing almost all aspects of society. Engineered nanomaterials are defined as synthesized materials existing with at least one dimension of 100 nm or less. The inclusion of engineered nanomaterials has revolutionized a variety of technologies including construction, consumer products, renewable energy, and the biomedical field [1]. These nanomaterials have broad-reaching potential due to their diverse physicochemical properties such as size, shape, chemical composition, and surface functionalization. Based on this recent rapid development and utilization of engineered nanomaterials, it is likely that human exposures will increase and necessitate toxicological evaluation.

Exposure to engineered nanomaterials is likely to occur in a variety of scenarios incorporating both environmental and occupational settings. Due to their vast applicability, there is potential for all routes of human exposure to engineered nanomaterials including oral, dermal, parenteral, and inhalation. Inhalation exposure to engineered nanomaterials represents an occupational and consumer exposure concern due to their small size and potential to deposit deep within the lung allowing for them to circumvent mechanisms that the pulmonary system uses to clear larger particles [2]. Further, it has been postulated that inhalation of engineered nanomaterials is increasingly toxic compared to larger particles due to their increased surface area, particle number based on mass, surface reactivity, and deposition potential [3]. Specifically, exposure of animals to metal- and carbon-based engineered nanomaterials by inhalation has demonstrated multiple mechanisms of pulmonary toxicity including cytotoxicity, inflammation, apoptosis, oxidative stress, and damage to the epithelial air interface [4–9]. Based on the emerging evaluation of engineered nanomaterial exposure, one of the primary health and safety concerns following exposure is the development of pulmonary fibrosis resulting in impaired pulmonary function.

Pulmonary fibrosis typically occurs following lung inflammation and tissue injury resulting in fibroblast activation and the deposition of excess collagen forming scar tissue. The development of excess fibrotic connective tissue or scar tissue within the lung reduces the functionally active tissue of the lung and causes impaired pulmonary function. One of the most well-recognized inhalable exposures to cause pulmonary fibrogenesis is asbestos [10, 11]. Asbestos is known to cause fibrosis through a sustained pulmonary inflammatory response due to its biopersistence within the lung. This biopersistence is related to the asbestos fibers' high aspect ratio, rigidity, and chemical composition. Multiwalled carbon nanotubes (MWCNTs) are a class of engineered nanomaterials that represent a similar concern in regard to the development of pulmonary fibrosis. This concern is related to their similar characteristics to asbestos fibers such as high aspect ratio, rigidity, and vast surface area for interaction with lung cells and tissue.

Human exposures to MWCNTs will likely increase based on their inclusion in current products and technologies as well as their future potential for widespread use. Of specific concern are pulmonary responses to MWCNTs due to their inhalation in occupational and environmental settings. This concern has resulted in an increase in research studies on the health and safety of MWCNTs focusing on the development of pulmonary fibrosis following exposure.

8.1.1 Multiwalled Carbon Nanotubes

Carbon nanotubes are composed of sp^2-hybridized carbon with a cylindrical structure. Single-walled carbon nanotubes exist as a single roll of graphene, whereas MWCNTs have layers of rolled graphene. Typically, these materials can be synthesized with diameters in the nano range, while the length is often measured in microns. These high aspect ratios, similar to asbestos fibers, are of concern regarding possible toxicity. Carbon nanotubes have unique properties including high electrical and thermal conductance, high tensile strength, low weight, and the ability to be synthesized with a variety of physicochemical properties (length, diameter, surface coatings, etc.). Further, carbon nanotubes can undergo various surface modifications through the addition of amino acids, peptides, and other molecules. These surface modifications modify the function of carbon nanotubes by allowing for their use in a variety of nanomedicine applications, for example. Modifications to the surface however also can have toxicological implications by influencing cytotoxicity, cellular uptake, oxidative stress, and biodistribution. To date, MWCNT appears to be the most utilized carbon nanotube for industrial and biomedical applications based on its wide range of applications. MWCNTs can be synthesized through a variety of processes including chemical vapor deposition, arc discharge, and laser ablation. These processes are able to precisely produce MWCNTs of reproducible dimensions. Currently, chemical vapor deposition is the most common method for the production of carbon nanotubes. These methods of production however often utilize a metal catalyst, which could impact the purity of the MWCNTs and influence toxicity through increasing surface reactivity. This diversity of MWCNT features along with their increased usage makes evaluation of their toxicity necessary in order to prevent adverse human health effects and specifically the development of pulmonary fibrosis.

8.1.2 Occupational Human Exposure Levels

To date, there is limited research on the direct effects of MWCNT exposure on humans; however, a growing number of animal and cellular studies have demonstrated that exposure could result in pulmonary health effects. One significant hurdle in the assessment of MWCNT-induced health effects is determining human exposure levels especially in occupational settings where MWCNTs are being synthesized and utilized in manufacturing processes. Without appropriate exposure assessments in occupational settings, it is impossible to perform relevant toxicological studies in animal and cell models. Exposure to elemental carbon occurring at eight US-based manufacturers of MWCNTs was analyzed using personal breathing zone sample [12]. The mean concentration for these occupational settings was determined to be 10.6 $\mu g/m^3$, which equated to an average deposited dose of 4.07 μg/day in a human and is equivalent to 2 ng/day for a mouse. The highest concentration observed at one MWCNT manufacturing facility was 79.6 $\mu g/m^3$. This study assumed that 25 % of this concentration would be respirable resulting in an average respirable fraction of 2.65 $\mu g/m^3$. Based on studies such as this and other exposure assessments, the US National Institute of Occupational Safety and Health (NIOSH) has adjusted their relative exposure limit for carbon nanotubes from 7 to 1 $\mu g/m^3$ for an 8 h time-weighted average of elemental carbon [13]. This exposure limit is based on the respirable fraction of carbon and not the total. This study begins to provide context to relate occupational exposure assessment with human relevant dosimetry for in vivo toxicology evaluation of MWCNT. Further evaluations regarding the concentrations to which individuals are exposed to MWCNTs in occupational and environmental settings are needed for impactful human relevant in vivo animal studies. Additional research is also needed to compare characteristics of airborne MWCNTs in an occupational setting compared to MWCNT being utilized for animal- and cell-based studies.

Based on the potential for increased occupational exposure as well as the possibility for the resulting disease progression of pulmonary fibrosis, the NIOSH has made recommendations for employers regarding worker exposures [13]. In summary, some of these recommendations include establishing engineering controls, routine evaluation of airborne exposure levels, development of procedures for spills, implementation of medical screening, and worker education. Most importantly, employers need to provide access to proper personal protective equipment such as respirators, lab coats, and gloves and provide facilities for routine handwashing as well as showering and clothes-changing areas to mitigate cross-contamination of nonwork areas. These recommendations are necessary as information regarding the possible health effects of MWCNTs are being continually studied and confirmed.

8.1.3 MWCNT Deposition

Sites of deposition following inhalation typically correspond to the location of pathogenesis within the lung. Due to their size, MWCNTs may have a unique deposition profile. Many studies have utilized various exposure techniques including aspiration, instillation, and inhalation, of which the latter is the most relevant for human exposures. These various exposure techniques influence deposition and sites of fibrosis within the lung. Fifty-six days following aspiration of MWCNTs, the majority of MWCNTs are found within or penetrating alveolar macrophages (68 %)

[14]. The other sites of deposition included granulomatous lesions within the alveolar airspace (20 %), the interstitium of the alveolar tissue (8 %), and the subpleural region (1.6 %). The granulomas that formed were located near the terminal bronchioles of the lung likely due to this being a primary site of deposition following oropharyngeal aspiration. There are inherent issues with delivering MWCNTs as well as any other toxicant via oropharyngeal aspiration and/or instillation. Of primary concern regarding these methods is a difference in deposition of the material compared to inhalation as well as the effect of delivering a bolus dose. Most studies that deliver MWCNTs through instillation or aspiration show agglomeration of MWCNTs at the terminal bronchioles, which will likely influence responses. A comparison of deposition of MWCNTs following instillation and inhalation demonstrates differences in deposition profile due to the mechanism of delivery. Following an inhalation exposure to 10 mg/m^3 of MWCNTs for 4 days and collection of lungs 1-day postexposure, the total lung burden was 13 ug [15]. This lung burden of MWCNTs was distributed to the airways (24 %) and the alveolar region (76 %). Specifically, these MWCNTs were found in macrophages and interacting with the lung tissue, while a few were identified at the pleural wall. In general, delivery by aspiration and instillation results in deposition of MWCNT agglomerates near or at the terminal bronchioles, while inhalation allows for single nanotube delivery into the deeper regions of the lung. These differences in deposition patterns likely are responsible for variations in sites of fibrosis development within the lung. Comparisons are difficult between inhalation studies evaluating deposition as MWCNT properties such as length, diameter, and flexibility are likely crucial to the deposition profile. These deposition studies however have been used to inform mechanistic in vitro studies allowing them to focus on specific cell types within the lung including macrophages and airway epithelial cells.

8.1.4 MWCNT-Induced Pulmonary Inflammation

The toxicological response to MWCNT exposure within the lung includes a robust acute inflammatory response and progressive fibrosis. The acute inflammatory response has been shown to peak at 7 days and taper off slowly through 56 days [16]. Studies have demonstrated various outcomes investigating inflammatory responses following MWCNT exposure. For example, a comparison of intratracheal instillation and inhalation in the Sprague-Dawley rat model demonstrated similar localization of MWCNTs within alveolar macrophages by both routes [17]. However, administration of MWCNTs by intratracheal instillation resulted in significant neutrophilia that was unseen in inhalation-exposed animals [17]. Inflammation in this study as measured by increased bronchoalveolar lavage neutrophil counts returned to baseline by 21 days postexposure. These variations in inflammatory response are likely related to differences in the physicochemical properties of the MWCNT, differences in animal models, and route of exposure.

Collectively, these studies have raised enough concern to limit human exposures to MWCNTs due to the likely development of fibrotic lung diseases following exposure.

8.2 Fibrosis Studies

Inhalation is the major route of exposure for MWCNT thereby making the lung a critical site for the investigation of toxicity. Based on their size, MWCNTs are able to gain access into the deep alveolar regions of the lung. Due to their asbestos-like qualities such as their biopersistence, surface reactivity, and high-aspect ratio, there is significant concern regarding possible lung toxicity and a need to mitigate human exposures. A growing body of evidence from animal studies has indicated a number of pulmonary pathologic responses that occur following exposure including inflammation, oxidative stress, genotoxicity, formation of granulomas, fibrosis, and decrements in pulmonary function.

8.2.1 MWCNT Physicochemical Properties and Fibrosis

MWCNTs can be synthesized to have a wide range of physicochemical properties including adjustments to diameter and length. These modifiable properties likely are responsible for variations in fibrotic response. Variations in lengths of MWCNTs (0.8 vs 4 um) have been shown to result in differential pulmonary fibrotic responses [18]. Although both lengths of MWCNT were determined to induce fibrosis, the longer MWCNT type (4 um) was found to induce more severe fibrosis as compared to the shorter (0.8 um). This enhanced fibrotic response to the long MWCNT type corresponded to a unique fibrotic gene expression profile compared to the short MWCNT type. Specifically, the long MWCNT type was found to induce greater expression of genes related to TGF-β1 signaling as compared to the short MWCNT type. These results demonstrate the influence of MWCNT characteristics on fibrotic response. However, due to the limitless modifications and combinations of MWCNT characteristics, this raises concerns regarding the evaluation and diversity of MWCNT fibrogenic potential.

Modifications in surface functionalization can influence the pulmonary inflammatory response following exposure. Pulmonary instillation of original, purified (acid washed), and carboxylic acid functionalized MWCNTs has demonstrated differences in inflammatory response, which may alter the development of fibrosis [17]. Following exposure to all three MWCNT types, a concentration-dependent inflammatory response was observed that included increases in neutrophilic influx at 1-day postexposure. Specifically, original MWCNTs induced a more robust acute inflammatory response at 1-day postexposure compared to purified and carboxylic acid functionalized MWCNTs as measured by neutrophilia and histopathological scoring of inflammation. This inflammatory response was resolved by 21 days following exposure, although MWCNTs persisted within the lung, primarily internalized in alveolar macrophages. Macrophages more readily internalized carboxylic acid functionalized MWCNTs as compared to the other MWCNT types at 21 days postexposure. These findings demonstrate differences in the acute inflammatory response as well as macrophage retention based on surface functionalization. These differences in inflammatory response may equate to variations in fibrogenic potential following repeated exposures.

The dispersion of MWCNTs in instillation studies is important as agglomerates within the sample administered may drive many of the effects observed in these studies. These agglomerates may not form during real-world exposures where inhalation is occurring in environmental and/or occupational settings. Examination of different dispersion solutions has demonstrated that addition of a surfactant and protein combination (dipalmitoylphosphatidylcholine (DPPC) and bovine serum albumin (BSA)) results in a more stable suspension of MWCNTs. These well-dispersed MWCNTs induce greater fibrosis compared to non-dispersed MWCNTs in a C57BL/6 mouse model 21 days following a single oropharyngeal instillation [19]. Specifically, compared to a non-dispersed sample, a well-dispersed MWCNT sample induced higher levels of TGF-β1 and platelet-derived growth factor-AA (PDGF-AA) in the bronchoalveolar lavage fluid while also causing increased fibrosis as measured by collagen deposition. This study also demonstrated concentration-dependent responses (0.5, 1, 2, or 4 mg/kg) in these endpoints of bronchoalveolar lavage fluid TGF-β1 and PDGF-AA protein levels and collagen deposition. Ultimately, this demonstrates the importance of MWCNT dispersion for administration of MWCNTs through instillation. Further, these findings suggest that agglomeration of MWCNTs may reduce their potency for the generation of fibrotic responses and may result in an underestimation of the biological response.

8.2.2 Interlaboratory Evaluation of MMWCNT-Induced Fibrosis

Reproducibility of findings between laboratories is necessary for the assessment of MWCNT-induced fibrosis as well as the development of exposure guidelines. A National Institutes of Health interlaboratory evaluation of three different MWCNTs was performed in the C57BL/6 mouse model and two rat models including Sprague-Dawley and Fisher 344 rats [20]. The C57BL/6 mouse model was evaluated for responses to MWCNTs in four independent laboratories, while the rat models were assessed for MWCNT responses in three independent laboratories. These three MWCNTs included original, purified (acid washed), and carboxylic acid functionalized. All MWCNTs were found to induce neutrophilia 1 day following exposure in three out of the four labs using mice and in all labs utilizing rat models. These findings also confirmed the ability of MWCNTs to induce an acute inflammatory response, which may establish a pulmonary environment conducive to the development of fibrotic lung disease. Through the use of standardized methods and materials, many inconsistencies between laboratories can be minimized. These interlaboratory assessments can be highly informative and can produce data necessary for risk assessment of nanomaterials.

8.2.3 Susceptibility to MWCNT-Induced Fibrosis

MWCNTs also have the potential to promote or exacerbate fibrotic response when an underlying disease state may exist. Allergic asthma is a respiratory condition with pathogenesis that includes chronic remodeling of airways, eosinophilia, mucus secretion, thickening of airway smooth muscle, and airway fibrosis. The population of individuals affected by this disease is large and growing and may be particularly susceptible to the effects of MWCNTs. To understand this population's likely susceptibility to MWCNT exposure, an asthmatic mouse model was utilized [21]. Following induction of an asthmatic condition by ovalbumin sensitization, mice were exposed via inhalation to MWCNTs and assessed for markers of fibrosis. The combination of asthmatic disease and MWCNT exposure resulted in increased collagen deposition as well as increased mRNA expression of IL-5. These findings demonstrate how an underlying respiratory condition may enhance pulmonary fibrotic responses to MWCNTs.

Individuals in occupation settings likely will not be exposed to only MWCNTs, rather it is highly likely that co-exposures may occur. One co-exposure that could occur is inhalation of bacteria, which may exacerbate MWCNT-induced fibrosis. To assess this, MWCNT-induced fibrosis has been examined following a co-exposure to LPS. In this scenario, exposure to MWCNTs+LPS increased pulmonary fibrosis compared to MWCNTs alone [4]. Further, the mediator PDGF-AA was synergistically enhanced in animals receiving LPS and MWCNTs compared to MWCNT alone. In vitro studies determined these responses were related to PDGF-AA produced by macrophages and epithelial cells and increased fibroblast expression of the PDGF-Rα within the lung. Overall, this model demonstrates that individuals with conditions that have a pulmonary inflammatory component may be at increased risk for fibrogenesis following subsequent MWCNT exposure.

It is likely that there are gender differences in the development of fibrosis following MWCNT inhalation based on gender-related variations in deposition following inhalation. In a 13-week inhalation exposure study utilizing male and female rats, focal fibrosis of the alveolar walls was observed in both sexes [22]. This study also demonstrated similar concentration-dependent inflammatory responses in both sexes. Interestingly, males were shown to have a greater lung burden following exposure than females. This difference in lung burden is likely due to gender-related differences in minute volume. Overall, this study demonstrates that a long-term inhalation exposure to MWCNT can induce fibrosis, which was not gender specific even though males were found to accumulate more MWCNTs within their lungs. It is likely that due to differences in deposition that males may be more susceptible to fibrosis over long-term exposures. Furthermore, it may be that females are more sensitive to MWCNT-induced fibrogenesis as they demonstrated similar fibrotic lesions with less lung burden. Future studies however are needed to evaluate gender differences in MWCNT-induced pulmonary fibrosis and to elucidate possible variations in mechanism.

8.2.4 Mechanisms of MWCNT-Induced Fibrogenesis

It has been hypothesized that MWCNTs induce fibrosis through the activation of multiple cell types within the lung leading to the release of proinflammatory and profibrotic mediators. A study utilizing a variety of cell lines assessing this mechanism demonstrated that in vitro exposure of alveolar epithelial and fibroblast cell lines to MWCNTs induced concentration-dependent cytotoxicity, reactive oxygen species production, and mitochondrial damage [23]. This generation of oxidative stress within these cells can promote cell death and activation of specific profibrotic signaling pathways leading to the development of pulmonary fibrosis. Further, exposure to MWCNTs was found to activate NF-kB signaling leading to secretion of inflammatory mediators including TNF-α, IL-1β, IL-6, IL-10, and MCP-1 as well as profibrotic factors TGF-β1 and PDGF. Incubation of lung fibroblasts with the supernatants from macrophages exposed to MWCNTs containing the inflammatory and profibrotic mediators resulted in transformation of these cells into myofibroblasts. This transformation is a key step in the development of fibrosis resulting in the synthesis, deposition, and remodeling of the collagen matrix of the lung.

Recently, the contribution of the NLRP3 inflammasome to the development of pulmonary fibrosis following exposure to silica, asbestos, and bleomycin has been postulated [24]. Following formation of the NLRP3 inflammasome complex, activation of caspase-3 occurs resulting in the cleavage of IL-1β and IL-18. Inhibition of the inflammasome pathway as well as inhibition of inflammasome-associated cytokines has been shown to reduce the fibrotic response in cell and animal models of fibrosis. Activation of the NLRP3 inflammasome by MWCNT-induced NADPH oxidase generation of reactive oxygen species has been hypothesized to be a mechanism by which fibrosis occurs [25]. Specifically, knockout of phox47, a cystolic component of the NADPH oxidase complex, has been shown to inhibit MWCNT-induced increases in IL-1β and fibrosis. Treatment with *n*-acetyl cysteine was determined to attenuate MWCNT-induced IL-1β and fibrosis further supporting the role of reactive oxygen species generation in MWCNT-induced fibrosis.

Another source of reactive oxygen species are the metal catalysts used to synthesize MWCNTs by chemical vapor deposition. This provides a source of contaminants that likely contributes to induction of cytotoxicity, oxidative stress, and inflammation. These contaminants are often removed through acid washing, which modifies the surface of the MWCNT. Further, MWCNTs can be functionalized via the addition of carboxyl groups to their surface. Alterations in the surface of MWCNTs also influence toxicity and cellular response. Specifically, unmodified MWCNTs have been shown to induce greater IL-1β production and cytotoxicity compared to purified MWCNTs in alveolar macrophages [26]. Interestingly, carboxylation of raw and purified MWCNTs was found to almost completely inhibit IL-1β production and cytotoxicity. Further IL-1β production was reduced through various inhibitors of the inflammasome supporting its role in MWCNT-induced responses. Taken together these studies demonstrate a likely mechanism by which MWCNT induce fibrosis through activation of the inflammasome. Also these studies demonstrate how activation of the inflammasome can be modified through alterations in the surfaces of MWCNTs.

Deposition studies have demonstrated that following introduction into the lung, MWCNTs can reach the alveolar space and interact with epithelial cells within this region. Small airway epithelial cells in vitro demonstrate oxidative stress and alterations in gene and protein expression following MWCNT exposure [27]. Specifically, quantitative PCR determined 24 genes to be significantly downregulated and 29 genes to be significantly upregulated following exposure to MWCNTs. Following a functional analysis of these MWCNT-altered genes, biological functions including cellular development, cellular growth and proliferation, cell signaling, small molecule biochemistry, and cellular movement were established as modified pathways. Analysis of upstream regulators of these MWCNT-induced genes identified active involvement of two potential regulators NF-kB and IL-1β. This study provided specific gene responses, which may lead to the development of pulmonary fibrosis. These genes possibly represent specific gene profiles involved in MWCNT-induced fibrosis.

8.2.5 IL-33/ST2 Receptor and Mast Cell-Mediated Fibrosis

Recent research examined the role of mast cells in the pulmonary fibrotic response to MWCNTs and signaling through the IL-33/ST2 axis [28, 29, 9]. Specifically, a study investigated the ability of exposure to increasing concentrations of MWCNTs (1, 2, or 4 mg/kg) to produce pulmonary fibrosis and decrements in pulmonary function 30 days following exposure in C57BL/6 mice [9]. Although concentration-dependent increases were seen in bronchoalveolar inflammatory cell populations (macrophages, neutrophils, and eosinophils), significant collagen deposition and fibrosis were only observed at the highest concentration (4 mg/kg). These fibrotic changes equated to decrements in pulmonary function consistent with obstructive pulmonary pathology such as fibrosis. Decrements in pulmonary function consisted of increased Newtonian resistance and total lung resistance with decreased lung compliance. One cytokine of interest that was induced following exposure to MWCNTs was IL-33. IL-33 is a member of the IL-1 cytokine family and is the only known ligand for the ST2 receptor. Due to its role in activating an immune response, IL-33 has been termed an "alarmin." Investigation utilizing an IL-33$^{-/-}$ mouse model has shown an inhibition of MWCNT-induced fibrosis and an alleviation of the decrements seen in pulmonary function in the wild-type C57BL/6 model [29]. In addition, pretreatment with the steroid methylprednisolone was determined to inhibit the robust inflammatory response following MWCNT exposure and thereby inhibited the development of fibrosis and decrements in pulmonary function. Treatment with albuterol however did not alleviate alterations in pulmonary function suggesting that these decrements in function are due to the MWCNT-induced fibrotic lesions at the terminal bronchioles and not smooth muscle contraction or hypertrophy.

One understudied cell type in regard to its role in immunotoxicological responses is the mast cell. Mast cells express the ST2 receptor on their surface, and IL-33 can activate this receptor leading to release of inflammatory cytokines and fibrotic growth factors. In contrast to C57BL/6 mice, exposure to MWCNT was found not to induce fibrosis or a decrement in pulmonary function in mice lacking either mast cells or the ST2 receptor [28]. These findings suggest that release of IL-33 following MWCNT exposure can cause mast cell activation through the ST2 receptor. This mast cell response then initiates and contributes to the acute inflammation that occurs in the lung following MWCNT exposure and is involved in the development of pulmonary fibrosis.

8.3 Areas of Future Study and Conclusions

Currently, our understanding of MWCNT-induced pulmonary fibrosis is lacking in several key areas. To appropriately assess human disease potential, it is necessary to first understand environmental and occupational human exposure levels. For impactful in vivo and in vitro studies to be performed this information is needed to determine appropriate experimental exposure concentrations. There are also discrepancies in response to MWCNTs due to route of exposure (e.g., instillation vs inhalation). This issue can be remediated by an understanding of differences in deposition patterns and human exposure assessment data. By having accurate human exposure assessment data, studies can more appropriately translate concentrations of instillation studies to accurately depict inhalation studies. Further, an understanding of airborne MWCNT characteristics is required to more accurately evaluate real-world exposures. To date, it is difficult to translate laboratory research findings to human exposure risk, as there is a vast amount of physicochemical diversity in the MWCNTs that have been evaluated. This diversity has resulted in not all studies demonstrating fibrosis following MWCNT exposure. These negative studies are likely due to differences in physicochemical properties, which do not elicit fibrogenic effects. Therefore, a thorough systematic evaluation is needed in assessing variations in MWCNT physicochemical properties and fibrotic lung disease. There is also a lack of studies evaluating models of underlying disease states, as these may represent susceptible populations of individuals to the fibrotic effects of MWCNT exposure. Furthermore, of the studies performed, genetic diversity in animal models was not taken into consideration. For example, studies utilizing animal models, which elicit a minor inflammatory response, may under represent possible human inflammation and progression to fibrosis. Lastly, studies need to be expanded in evaluating mechanisms of MWCNT-induced toxicity, which lead to the development of pulmonary fibrosis.

Although studies investigating MWCNT-induced pulmonary disease development are ongoing, significant research has confirmed possible adverse health effects following inhalation. Therefore, mitigation techniques should be put into place, especially within occupational settings, to protect individuals. These protections include knowledge of exposure levels within the workplace and environments as well as the use of personal protective equipment such as fume hoods and respirators. Through the use of these controls, the potential risks from MWCNT exposure for the individual can be mitigated.

In conclusion, due to their rapidly expanding applications and their increased usage, there is concern regarding increased human exposures to MWCNTs. To date, a sufficient amount of research in both animal models and cell culture has been performed demonstrating that exposure to MWCNTs can promote pulmonary fibrosis. In order to mitigate possible adverse human health concerns, controls should be in place to limit inhalation of MWCNTs especially in occupational settings where exposure may be elevated.

References

1. Martin CR, Kohli P. The emerging field of nanotube biotechnology. Nat Rev Drug Discov. 2003;2(1):29–37. doi:10.1038/nrd988.
2. Sanchez-Crespo A, Klepczynska-Nystrom A, Lundin A, Larsson BM, Svartengren M. (1)(1)(1)Indium-labeled ultrafine carbon particles; a novel aerosol for pulmonary deposition and retention studies. Inhal Toxicol. 2011;23(3):121–8. doi:10.3109/08958378.2010.549856.
3. Frampton MW. Systemic and cardiovascular effects of airway injury and inflammation: ultrafine particle exposure in humans. Environ Health Perspect. 2001;109 Suppl 4:529–32.
4. Cesta MF, Ryman-Rasmussen JP, Wallace DG, Masinde T, Hurlburt G, Taylor AJ, et al. Bacterial lipopolysaccharide enhances PDGF signaling and pulmonary fibrosis in rats exposed to carbon nanotubes. Am J Respir Cell Mol Biol. 2010;43(2):142–51. doi:10.1165/rcmb.2009-0113OC.
5. Park EJ, Choi K, Park K. Induction of inflammatory responses and gene expression by intratracheal instillation of silver nanoparticles in mice. Arch Pharm Res. 2011;34(2):299–307. doi:10.1007/s12272-011-0216-y.
6. Sayers BC, Taylor AJ, Glista-Baker EE, Shipley-Phillips JK, Dackor RT, Edin ML, et al. Role of cyclooxygenase-2 in exacerbation of allergen-induced airway remodeling by multiwalled carbon nanotubes. Am J Respir Cell Mol Biol. 2013;49(4):525–35. doi:10.1165/rcmb.2013-0019OC.
7. Shannahan JH, Kodavanti UP, Brown JM. Manufactured and airborne nanoparticle cardiopulmonary interactions: a review of mechanisms and the possible contribution of mast cells. Inhal Toxicol. 2012;24(5):320–39. doi:10.3109/08958378.2012.668229.

8. Wang L, Ding W, Zhang F. Acute toxicity of ferric oxide and zinc oxide nanoparticles in rats. J Nanosci Nanotechnol. 2010;10(12):8617–24.
9. Wang X, Katwa P, Podila R, Chen P, Ke PC, Rao AM, et al. Multi-walled carbon nanotube instillation impairs pulmonary function in C57BL/6 mice. Part Fibre Toxicol. 2011;8:24. doi:10.1186/1743-8977-8-24.
10. Padilla-Carlin DJ, Schladweiler MC, Shannahan JH, Kodavanti UP, Nyska A, Burgoon LD, et al. Pulmonary inflammatory and fibrotic responses in Fischer 344 rats after intratracheal instillation exposure to Libby amphibole. J Toxicol Environ Health A. 2011;74(17):1111–32. doi:10.1080/15287394.2011.586940.
11. Shannahan JH, Nyska A, Cesta M, Schladweiler MC, Vallant BD, Ward WO, et al. Subchronic pulmonary pathology, iron overload, and transcriptional activity after Libby amphibole exposure in rat models of cardiovascular disease. Environ Health Perspect. 2012;120(1):85–91. doi:10.1289/ehp.1103990.
12. Erdely A, Dahm M, Chen BT, Zeidler-Erdely PC, Fernback JE, Birch ME, et al. Carbon nanotube dosimetry: from workplace exposure assessment to inhalation toxicology. Part Fibre Toxicol. 2013;10(1):53. doi:10.1186/1743-8977-10-53.
13. NIOSH DoHaHSC. Current Intelligence Bulletin 65 – occupational exposure to carbon nanotubes and nanofibers. NIOSH Publications and Products 2013. Available from: http://www.cdc.gov/niosh/docs/2013-145/b4.
14. Mercer RR, Hubbs AF, Scabilloni JF, Wang L, Battelli LA, Friend S, et al. Pulmonary fibrotic response to aspiration of multi-walled carbon nanotubes. Part Fibre Toxicol. 2011;8:21. doi:10.1186/1743-8977-8-21.
15. Porter DW, Hubbs AF, Chen BT, McKinney W, Mercer RR, Wolfarth MG, et al. Acute pulmonary dose-responses to inhaled multi-walled carbon nanotubes. Nanotoxicology. 2013;7(7):1179–94. doi:10.3109/17435390.2012.719649.
16. Porter DW, Hubbs AF, Mercer RR, Wu N, Wolfarth MG, Sriram K, et al. Mouse pulmonary dose- and time course-responses induced by exposure to multi-walled carbon nanotubes. Toxicology. 2010;269(2–3):136–47. doi:10.1016/j.tox.2009.10.017.
17. Silva RM, Doudrick K, Franzi LM, TeeSy C, Anderson DS, Wu Z, et al. Instillation versus inhalation of multiwalled carbon nanotubes: exposure-related health effects, clearance, and the role of particle characteristics. ACS Nano. 2014;8(9):8911–31. doi:10.1021/nn503887r.
18. Poulsen SS, Saber AT, Williams A, Andersen O, Kobler C, Atluri R, et al. MWCNTs of different physicochemical properties cause similar inflammatory responses, but differences in transcriptional and histological markers of fibrosis in mouse lungs. Toxicol Appl Pharmacol. 2015;284(1):16–32. doi:10.1016/j.taap.2014.12.011.
19. Wang X, Xia T, Ntim SA, Ji Z, Lin S, Meng H, et al. Dispersal state of multiwalled carbon nanotubes elicits profibrogenic cellular responses that correlate with fibrogenesis biomarkers and fibrosis in the murine lung. ACS Nano. 2011;5(12):9772–87. doi:10.1021/nn2033055.
20. Bonner JC, Silva RM, Taylor AJ, Brown JM, Hilderbrand SC, Castranova V, et al. Interlaboratory evaluation of rodent pulmonary responses to engineered nanomaterials: the NIEHS Nano GO Consortium. Environ Health Perspect. 2013;121(6):676–82. doi:10.1289/ehp.1205693.
21. Ryman-Rasmussen JP, Tewksbury EW, Moss OR, Cesta MF, Wong BA, Bonner JC. Inhaled multiwalled carbon nanotubes potentiate airway fibrosis in murine allergic asthma. Am J Respir Cell Mol Biol. 2009;40(3):349–58. doi:10.1165/rcmb.2008-0276OC.
22. Kasai T, Umeda Y, Ohnishi M, Kondo H, Takeuchi T, Aiso S, et al. Thirteen-week study of toxicity of fiber-like multi-walled carbon nanotubes with whole-body inhalation exposure in rats. Nanotoxicology. 2014;9(4):413–22. doi:10.3109/17435390.2014.933903.
23. He X, Young SH, Schwegler-Berry D, Chisholm WP, Fernback JE, Ma Q. Multiwalled carbon nanotubes induce a fibrogenic response by stimulating reactive oxygen species production, activating NF-kappaB signaling, and promoting fibroblast-to-myofibroblast transformation. Chem Res Toxicol. 2011;24(12):2237–48. doi:10.1021/tx200351d.

24. Rastrick J, Birrell M. The role of the inflammasome in fibrotic respiratory diseases. Minerva Med. 2014;105(1):9–23.
25. Sun B, Wang X, Ji Z, Wang M, Liao YP, Chang CH, et al. NADPH oxidase-dependent NLRP3 inflammasome activation and its important role in lung fibrosis by multiwalled carbon nanotubes. Small. 2015. doi:10.1002/smll.201402859.
26. Hamilton Jr RF, Xiang C, Li M, Ka I, Yang F, Ma D, et al. Purification and sidewall functionalization of multiwalled carbon nanotubes and resulting bioactivity in two macrophage models. Inhal Toxicol. 2013;25(4):199–210. doi:10.3109/08958378.2013.775197.
27. Snyder-Talkington BN, Pacurari M, Dong C, Leonard SS, Schwegler-Berry D, Castranova V, et al. Systematic analysis of multiwalled carbon nanotube-induced cellular signaling and gene expression in human small airway epithelial cells. Toxicol Sci. 2013;133(1):79–89. doi:10.1093/toxsci/kft019.
28. Katwa P, Wang X, Urankar RN, Podila R, Hilderbrand SC, Fick RB, et al. A carbon nanotube toxicity paradigm driven by mast cells and the IL-(3)(3)/ST(2) axis. Small. 2012;8(18):2904–12. doi:10.1002/smll.201200873.
29. Wang X, Shannahan JH, Brown JM. IL-33 modulates chronic airway resistance changes induced by multi-walled carbon nanotubes. Inhal Toxicol. 2014;26(4):240–9. doi:10.3109/08958378.2014.880202.

Chapter 9
Silicates and Autoimmunity

Jessica M. Mayeux, Rahul D. Pawar, and K. Michael Pollard

Abstract Inhalation of particulate matter is associated with a number of acute and chronic disorders including autoimmune rheumatic diseases. The strongest evidence for a link with autoimmune disease comes from epidemiological studies describing the association of occupational exposure to crystalline silica dust with the systemic autoimmune diseases SLE and RA. Very little is known regarding the mechanism by which silica exposure leads to systemic autoimmune disease. However, in the case of silicosis, there is an extensive research literature that can help identify disease processes that may precede development of autoimmunity. The pathophysiology of silicosis consists of deposition of particles into the alveoli of the lung where they cannot be cleared. Ingestion of deposited particles by alveolar macrophages initiates an inflammatory response which then stimulates fibroblasts to proliferate and produce collagen. Silica particles are enveloped by collagen leading to fibrosis and nodular lesions. These findings are consistent with an autoimmune pathogenesis that begins with activation of the innate immune system leading to proinflammatory cytokine production, inflammation of the lung leading to activation of adaptive immunity, breaking of tolerance, autoantibodies, and tissue damage. The variable frequency of these features following silica exposure suggests significant genetic involvement and gene/environment interaction in silica-induced autoimmunity.

Keywords Silica • Asbestos • Silicosis • Autoimmunity • Animal model

9.1 Introduction

Particulate matter (PM) is a complex mixture of extremely small particles and liquid droplets. It is made up of a number of components, including acids, organic chemicals, metals, and soil or dust particles. Particulate matter is categorized according to size, which defines its facility to be retained in the lungs. PM10 (particles up to 10 μm in diameter) deposit in the nasal passages or larger airways,

J.M. Mayeux • R.D. Pawar • K.M. Pollard (✉)
Department of Molecular and Experimental Medicine, The Scripps Research Institute, 10550 North Torrey Pines Road, La Jolla, CA, USA
e-mail: mpollard@scripps.edu

T. Otsuki et al. (eds.), *Biological Effects of Fibrous and Particulate Substances*, Current Topics in Environmental Health and Preventive Medicine,
DOI 10.1007/978-4-431-55732-6_9

while PM2.5 (particles smaller than 2.5 μm in diameter) can reach the alveoli [1]. Inhalation of particulate matter is associated with a number of acute and chronic disorders [1, 2] including autoimmune rheumatic diseases [3, 4]. The strongest evidence for a link with autoimmune disease comes from studies describing the association of exposure to crystalline silica with the systemic autoimmune diseases systemic lupus erythematosus (SLE), rheumatoid arthritis (RA), systemic sclerosis (SSc), and anti-neutrophil cytoplasmic antibodies (ANCA)-related vasculitis [5]. Another silicate, asbestos, has been linked with RA and the presence of autoimmune features in the absence of diagnosed disease [5, 6]. In this chapter, the relationship between exposure to silicates and autoimmunity is examined with particular reference to silica and asbestos; the controversial relationship between silicone-containing breast implants and autoimmunity [7] is not reviewed here because, although silicone contains silicon, they have very different physical and chemical properties. The role of animal models in replicating observations of silicate-induced human autoimmunity is discussed. The limited information on possible mechanisms of silicate-induced autoimmunity, deduced from both human and animal studies, are compared and contrasted, and themes for future research suggested.

9.2 Silica and Autoimmunity in Humans

Silica (SiO_2) is an oxide of silicon and can exist in mineral form as well as being produced synthetically. Crystalline silica exists in seven types or polymorphs. Quartz is the most common form in nature and exists in two forms, α- and β-quartz, with α-quartz being the only stable form under normal conditions [8]. Occupational exposure to respirable crystalline silica (<10 μm) occurs in many situations where materials containing crystalline silica, such as rocks, are reduced to dust or when fine particles containing silica are disturbed. Occupations include drilling, mining, sand blasting, grinding, and cutting and are often referred to as the dusty trades [9, 10]. While oral ingestion of silica is essentially nontoxic, inhalation of crystalline silica dust can lead to silicosis, airway disease, cancer, and autoimmune diseases [9]. Silicosis is characterized by chronic inflammation and scaring in the upper lobes of the lung and can be classified based on the amount inhaled, time course, and duration of exposure as chronic simple silicosis, accelerated silicosis, and acute silicosis (silicoproteinosis) [8, 9, 11]. Chronic simple silicosis is the most common form and occurs after 10–15 years of exposure to low to moderate levels of respirable crystalline silica. A hallmark of the disease is the presence of silicotic nodules. A complicated form occurs when smaller lesions amalgamate to form nodules of greater than 2 cm. Accelerated silicosis occurs in a shorter time span, 5–10 years after first exposure to higher exposure levels. Acute silicosis can develop within weeks to several years following exposure to extremely high levels of respirable crystalline silica. It has a rapid onset of symptoms and is the most severe form of silicosis. The pathophysiology of silicosis, especially the chronic form, consists of deposition of particles into the alveoli of the lung where they cannot be cleared. Ingestion of deposited particles by alveolar macrophages initiates an inflammatory response which then stimulates fibroblasts to proliferate and produce collagen. Silica particles are enveloped by collagen leading to fibrosis and nodular lesions [9].

A number of epidemiological studies support the association of silica exposure with autoimmune diseases in humans [5, 12–16]. It is unclear if silicosis is required for the expression of silica-induced autoimmune diseases, although high exposure levels were associated with SLE [10]. Other studies identified an association between the intensity of exposure and the production of autoantibodies but found no relationship between autoantibodies and silicosis [17, 18]. Importantly, autoantibodies specific to connective tissue diseases (SLE, SSc) were found in exposed individuals including anti-DNA, anti-SS-A/Ro, anti-SS-B/La, anti-centromere, and anti-topoisomerase I [17, 18]. A study of silicotics found no association between histocompatibility antigens and ANA, RF, or serum IgG and IgM; however, there was increased prevalence of B44 and A29 which supported previous observations of a link between HLA and silicosis [19] although the nature of the requirement requires further study. In some individuals the presence of disease-specific autoantibodies preceded the appearance of autoimmune disease [18]. Several studies found increased occurrence of different diseases in individual study populations [10]. Because clinical features and autoantibodies can overlap between diseases, this suggests that silica exposure may trigger a common mechanism among systemic autoimmune diseases.

Although the relative risk of a specific connective tissue disease (CTD) following silica exposure can increase manyfold [16], with the exception of rheumatoid arthritis (RA), most occur at 1 % or less in silica-exposed populations [5, 10, 16, 17]. However, the prevalence of non-disease-specific immunological features associated with autoimmunity occurs in far greater numbers. Antinuclear autoantibodies (ANAs) can be found in up to 30 % of silica-exposed individuals without CTD symptoms, with higher frequencies and titers associated with the development of CTDs [17, 20]. In patients with silicosis, hypergammaglobulinemia can occur in over 65 % of patients [21], and ANA prevalence can be 34 % or higher [22, 23]. ANA often occurs in association with increased cytokines [24]. Even in ANA-negative individuals [25, 26], silica exposure can be associated with changes in cell surface markers and cytokines [26, 27]. Proinflammatory cytokines and inflammation in the lung are thought to be precursors to silicosis [28] which can occur in 47–77 % of individuals with adequate follow-up after silica exposure [29]. End-stage renal disease due to silica exposure occurs in about 5 % of exposed individuals [29]. The mechanism of silica nephropathy is unclear but appears to have two components: a direct nephrotoxicity and induction of autoimmune disease [30]. These findings are consistent with a disease progression that begins with activation of the innate immune system leading to proinflammatory cytokine production, inflammation of the lung leading to activation of adaptive immunity, breaking of tolerance, autoantibodies, and renal damage [9, 28, 31, 32].

9.3 Asbestos and Autoimmunity in Humans

Asbestos consists of six naturally occurring silicate minerals with a characteristic external shape (crystal habit) consisting of long, thin fibrous crystals, with each visible fiber consisting of microscopic fibrils that can be released by abrasion [8]. There are two classes: serpentine and amphibole. Chrysotile is one of the three different polymorphs of the serpentine class; the other two are antigorite and lizardite. Amphibole fibers are needle-like and include the following members: amosite, crocidolite, tremolite, anthophyllite, and actinolite. Chrysotile, unlike amphibole, is sensitive to acidic environments and disassociates from its crystalline state [33]. This may help explain differences in chronic inflammation and pathology, including cancer, induced by exposure to these two forms of asbestos [6, 8, 33]. Prolonged exposure to asbestos results in asbestosis, a chronic lung disease caused by scarring of the lung tissue, which has a pathophysiology similar to that described above for silicosis [34].

In contrast to silica, there is insufficient evidence that asbestos exposure is linked to autoimmune diseases [5, 6]. A case-control study of current and former residents of Libby, Montana, who were exposed to vermiculite contaminated with asbestos found an association with development of RA [35], but no medical records were evaluated to confirm the self-reported diagnoses. Another small case-control study in Sweden found an association with asbestos exposure in men with newly diagnosed RA [36]. A number of studies have suggested an association of asbestos exposure with immune activation or features of autoimmunity (e.g., elevated immunoglobulins, RF, ANA, or ANCA) [5, 6]. For the most part, these studies produced variable results making a definitive assessment of the potential of asbestos exposure to elicit autoimmunity difficult. This may stem in part from the difficulty in defining the contribution of asbestos and silica in concurrent exposures, identifying the important features of asbestos fibers in inflammation and disease, and identifying appropriate study cohorts and diagnostic criteria [5, 6, 34, 37].

9.4 Animal Models of Silica-Induced Autoimmunity

Although there is great confidence that silica exposure is a significant risk factor for human autoimmunity [38], there are few studies of silica-induced autoimmunity in nonhuman species [9, 34, 35]. The paucity of animal studies led a recent National Institutes of Environmental Health Sciences (NIEHS) workshop to note that the lack of a suitable animal model of silica-induced autoimmunity is a critical barrier to progress in understanding how silica exposure leads to autoimmunity [39]. Induction of autoimmunity following silica exposure has been examined in the SLE-prone NZM2410 mouse [40] and in the brown Norway rat [41, 42]. Intranasal instillation of 1 mg of crystalline silica (Min-U-Sil 5, with an average crystal length of 1.5–2.0 μM) twice over a two-week period resulted in exacerbation of autoimmunity in NZM2410 mice compared to controls over the 22-week observation period. Silica-exposed mice had reduced survival, increased proteinuria, circulating immune complexes, renal deposits of IgG and C3, autoantibodies, and pulmonary inflammation and fibrotic lesions. Unlike their human counterparts, the mice had reduced levels of serum IgG. A follow-up study confirmed the reduced IgG and IgG1 as well as showing increased proinflammatory cytokines in bronchoalveolar lavage fluid (BALF), increased B1a B cells and $CD4^+$ T cells in lymph nodes, and an alteration in the ratio of $CD4^+$ T-to-$CD4^+CD25^+$ T cells [43]. Brown Norway rats exposed to 3 mg of sodium silicate ($NaSiO_4$) by oral or subcutaneous administration once a week for 5 weeks developed differing autoantibody responses. After 7 and 14 weeks, it was found that subcutaneous administration resulted in a greater number of ANA-positive animals, but specific autoantibodies (i.e., anti-double-stranded DNA, anti-Sm, anti-SS-A, anti-SS-B) were infrequently detected [42]. A subsequent study revealed that most of the ANA-positive samples also had anti-RNP reactivity [41]. The only other studies to examine the effect of silica on autoimmunity employed its toxic effects to deplete macrophages in a chicken model of autoimmune thyroiditis [44] and in rat [45, 46] and mouse [47] models of diabetes.

9.5 Animal Models of Asbestos-Induced Autoimmunity

Ironically, even though less is known of the relationship between asbestos and human autoimmunity compared with silica, there have been more studies using animal models and asbestos or asbestos-like material. Exposure of female C57BL/6 mice to two doses of 60 μg of Korean tremolite one week apart resulted in an increased frequency of ANA, anti-DNA, anti-SS-A/Ro, and IgG renal deposits [48]. Exposed mice also had decreased percentage of $CD4^+CD25^+$ T cells as well as decreased serum IgG. To explore possible differences in response to amphibole and chrysotile, female C57BL/6 mice were exposed to Libby 6-Mix or intermediate chrysotile by intratracheal instillation twice over 3–4 weeks (60 μg in total). While both materials induced inflammatory responses, only amphibole asbestos increased the frequency of ANA and levels of IL-17 [49]. In a companion study female C57BL/6 mice were exposed to erionite, an asbestos-like fibrous material, and compared to responses to amphibole (Libby 6-Mix, Korean tremolite) and chrysotile asbestos [50]. Erionite-treated mice had increases in serum ANA, IL-17, and TNF-α as well as renal deposits of IgG. Libby 6-Mix amphibole also elicited increased ANA but chrysotile did not. These studies highlight the importance of the properties of asbestos fibers in determining inflammation and autoimmunity.

The Libby 6-Mix amphibole has also been used in animal studies to determine if asbestos exposure can exacerbate RA [51] based on the observation that amphibole exposure in Libby, Montana, was associated with increased risk of RA in humans [35]. Prior to induction of arthritis by either collagen or peptidoglycan-polysaccharide (PG-PS) injection, female Lewis rats received either Libby amphibole or amosite by intratracheal instillation over a 13-week period. Asbestos exposure consisted of a range of doses from 0 to 5 mg in total. Neither exposure affected development of collagen-induced arthritis or production of RF or anti-cyclic citrullinated peptide antibodies. Prior exposure to Libby amphibole reduced features of disease in the PG-PS model. However, both exposures elicited ANA in PG-PS and non-arthritis controls but not rats receiving collagen injections. A follow-up publication attempted to identify the ANA specificity following Libby amphibole exposure and to determine if other features of systemic autoimmunity were present [52]. Although elevated ANA was detected as early as 8 weeks after exposure to the highest dose of Libby amphibole, this could not be explained by reactivity to an extract of soluble nuclear antigens (ENA) or selected nuclear antigens (e.g., Sm, RNP, SS-A/Ro, SS-B/La, Scl-70, DNA). Asbestos exposure was not associated with changes in kidney histology or renal deposition of immunoglobulin or complement, although evidence of proteinuria was found. Intriguingly, almost all of the sera reactive with the soluble nuclear extract were found to react with the Jo-1 antigen, a cytoplasmic protein. Antibodies to Jo-1 are specific for histidyl-tRNA synthetase which is one of a group of autoantibodies against aminoacyl-tRNA synthetases (ARS) which are the key features of the anti-synthetase syndrome (aSS), characterized in part by interstitial lung disease [53]. This raises the interesting possibility that an anti-Jo-1 response may indicate interstitial lung disease following asbestos exposure. However, it remains to be determined if this autoantibody response is common among different forms of asbestos, if it occurs following exposure to other silicates and whether it plays a role in disease pathogenesis.

9.6 Mechanisms of Silicate-Induced Autoimmunity

9.6.1 Human Studies

Very little is known regarding the mechanism by which silica exposure leads to systemic autoimmune disease particularly in relevant patient populations [5]. However, a number of observations, made in a cohort of Japanese brickyard workers diagnosed with silicosis, have been argued as providing insight into immune abnormalities that arise following silica exposure and that might precede development of autoimmune disease [54]. These studies come with two caveats. First, none of the patients studied had evidence of symptoms of autoimmune diseases [54], specifically sclerotic skin, Raynaud's phenomenon, facial erythema, or arthralgia [31]. Thus, the absence of disease makes it difficult to determine if any of the observations gathered are relevant to the development of systemic autoimmune disease. Moreover, as the patient population appears to number less than 100 [55–57], the chance of any individual patient developing a specific systemic autoimmune disease is relatively remote given the low prevalence of systemic autoimmune diseases like RA [58] and SLE [59] in the Japanese population. Second, there is conflicting data concerning the relationship between development of silicosis and autoimmune disease following silica exposure [10]. Therefore, it is unclear if a population of silicotics is the most relevant group in which to study immune abnormalities that may herald impending development of systemic autoimmune disease following silica exposure.

This group of patients was described as having higher titers of ANA than a control group [54], including antibodies to DNA topoisomerase I (also known as anti-Scl-70) [60], an autoantibody response useful in predicting scleroderma patients at higher risk for interstitial fibrosis/restrictive lung disease [61]. Other studies identified the presence of autoantibodies against CD95/Fas [62], caspase-8 [63], and desmoglein [64]. These findings support other observations of a range of autoantibody specificities in silica-exposed individuals [17, 18, 20] together with evidence of a disease-related specificity. The observation that apoptosis-related molecules (CD95/Fas, caspase-8) were targets of autoantibodies led to an examination of Fas expression which identified increased levels of soluble Fas, presence of alternatively spliced versions of Fas lacking the transmembrane domain, and increased expression of decoy receptor 3 (DcR3) which functions to inhibit Fas [54]. These findings suggested inefficient Fas-mediated cell death in silicosis which may allow prolonged survival of self-reactive lymphocytes. Analysis of cell surface markers, coupled with in vitro responses to silica particles, of peripheral blood cells from silicosis patients suggested the presence of two T cell populations. The first being chronically activated T cells resistant to Fas-mediated apoptosis, and the second chronically activated T regulatory cells sensitive to Fas-mediated apoptosis [31, 54]. These findings have received some support from animal model studies where alterations in the ratio of $CD4^+$-to-$CD4^+CD25^+$ T cells have been found following silica exposure of NZM2410 mice [40], and reduced $CD4^+CD25^+$ T cell numbers have been found in C57BL/6 mice exposed to asbestos [48]. However, it is clear that much more probing of mechanism needs to be done especially with larger study populations if there is to be insight into how silicates induce and/or exacerbate autoimmunity and autoimmune disease in humans.

9.6.2 Animal Studies

The scarcity of studies on silica-induced autoimmunity in animal models significantly restricts discussion of mechanisms that might explain development of disease [65]. However, clues to the sequence of events that may eventually lead to autoimmunity may be found in the inflammation and pathology that follows crystalline silica exposure. Strain-specific responses have been found for exposure to silica and induction of silicosis [66–68]. Six different strains exposed to 5 mg of α-quartz by intratracheal instillation showed three different levels of response after 4 weeks [67]. The most responsive strains included the DBA/2, C57BL/10, and BALB/c, while the C57BL/6 and C3H/He had intermediate responses and the

CBA/J the least response. However, all strains had extensive disease compared to saline controls. Comparison of the fibrotic response to intratracheally administered silica also showed strain-dependent responses in eight strains with the C57BL/6 showing the greatest hydroxyproline content and CBA/J the least [68]. Breeding studies and genome-wide linkage analysis identified quantitative trait loci (QTL) on chromosome 4 and suggestive QTL on chromosomes 3 and 18 [68]. Inflammation and fibrosis can be uncoupled in NMRI mice by administration of anti-inflammatory molecules which reduced inflammation and proinflammatory cytokines (IL-1β and TNF-α) but had no significant effect on fibrosis or expression of the fibrogenic cytokines TGF-β and IL-10 [69]. Intense silicosis does not develop with inhalation of amorphous quartz silica, but the more biologically active polymorph crystalline silica produces more extensive disease in an orderly dose-time relationship with little disease activity observed before 3–4 months after exposure [66]. C3H/HeN mice demonstrated histopathological silicotic lesions and enlarged bronchus-associated lymphoid tissue (BALT) and increased lung wet weight; bronchoalveolar lavage (BAL) recovery of macrophages, lymphocytes, and neutrophils; and total lung collagen (hydroxyproline). BALB/c mice developed slight pulmonary lesions, while autoimmune-prone MRL/MpJ mice demonstrated prominent pulmonary infiltrates with lymphocytes, and NZB mice developed extensive alveolar proteinaceous deposits, inflammation, and fibrosis [66]. BALT was particularly numerous in the MRL/MpJ. These regions are of particular interest as recent studies argue that inducible BALT provides a niche for T cell priming and B cell education [70]. The differences in response among strains were attributed to genetic differences, involving histocompatibility loci and other unrelated genetic differences among the strains [66]. These findings show that strain differences exist in response to silica exposure and that a genetic predisposition to autoimmunity is associated with more aggressive pulmonary inflammation arguing that gene-environment interaction may be important in development of frank autoimmune disease.

9.6.2.1 Silica-Induced Autoimmune Phenotypes in Mice

Another critical barrier to progress in understanding the link between particulate exposure and autoimmunity is the lack of criteria for identifying human autoimmune disease phenotypes associated with environmental-induced autoimmunity [71]. However, in the case of silica, there is a rich literature of human and animal research because of the well-documented association with occupational disease [9, 10, 16, 28, 29, 31]. The silica-induced immunological responses in mice and rats include lung inflammation [66, 67, 69], proinflammatory cytokines [72–75], activated adaptive immunity [76–79], autoantibodies [40, 42, 48, 51, 52], and renal disease [40, 48].

The immunological responses to silica which lead to autoimmunity are believed to begin with an inflammatory response in the lung associated with production of proinflammatory cytokines which leads to recruitment of the adaptive immune system characterized by helper CD4^{+} T cell activation and reduced T regulatory cell function [28, 31, 80]. This milieu allows breaking of tolerance and autoantibody production and tissue pathology [10, 20, 25]. The first pathological indices following silica exposure are pulmonary inflammation followed by fibrosis which, although nonspecific in terms of autoimmune disease, are common in inbred mice, and both high and low responders show similar patterns of inflammation and fibrosis which are specific to silica exposure [67]; autoimmune-prone mice appear to have more pronounced responses [66]. Whether silicosis is a precursor of autoimmunity [10] is less clear as inflammation requires only cells of the innate immune system [81], and pulmonary inflammation can be dispensable for the development of fibrosis [69].

9.6.2.2 Involvement of Innate Immunity in Silica-Induced Autoimmunity

The findings that the innate immune response is sufficient for the development of silicosis [81] beg the question as to which innate immune cells and pathways play predominant roles. Silica deposition in the lungs leads to participation of alveolar macrophages in an attempt to clear the particles. This involves scavenger receptors such as macrophage receptor with collagenous structure (MARCO) and can result in cell death [82]. It has been recently appreciated that such cell death allows release of endogenous stores of IL-1α which precedes expression of IL-1β and inflammation consisting predominantly of neutrophils [83]. IL-1β expression requires activation of the inflammasome and caspase-1 in both silica and asbestos exposures [84, 85]. This appears to involve lysosomal destabilization particularly by particles less than 3 μm in length [86] and generation of reactive oxygen species (ROS) [87] leading to cathepsin B activation [84]. However, it is possible that lysosomal destabilization may not be essential for IL-1β production if silica binding to the cell membrane results in potassium ion efflux [88]. In vitro studies suggest that chrysotile asbestos and amphibole (Libby 6-Mix) induce different inflammatory events with chrysotile better at inflammasome activation, while amphibole generated more ROS [89].

Proinflammatory cytokine expression has not been directly compared among different mouse strains, but several strains, including C57BL/6 and A/J, show increases in TNF-α, IL-1β, IFN-γ, and IL-6, particularly in BAL fluid [75, 77, 90–92]. Neutralization of IL-1β attenuates silica-induced lung inflammation and fibrosis in C57BL/6 mice [57] and inflammation, and macrophage apoptosis following silica exposure was found to be induced by IL-1β and nitric oxide [76]. This is not unexpected given the importance of these cytokines to pulmonary inflammation and silicosis [28, 93]. Silica-activated macrophages expressed high levels of IL-10 in the lung of silica-sensitive but not silica-resistant strains of mice, indicating that besides chronic lung inflammation, a pronounced anti-inflammatory reaction may also contribute to the extension of silica-induced lung fibrosis and represent an alternative pathway leading to lung fibrosis [95]. Cytokine expression can be transient lasting hours up to several days following exposure [75, 91]. However, cytokine expression is found in the blood of silica-exposed individuals [26, 27] suggesting that repeated exposure leads to systemic expression. Given that individual genes, such as TNF-α [94] and IFN-γ [93], are required for silicosis, it is possible that genetic heterogeneity in cytokine expression may significantly impact immune responses to silica.

9.6.2.3 Involvement of Adaptive Immunity in Silica-Induced Autoimmunity

Although innate immunity is sufficient for silicosis in mice [81], pulmonary inflammation is also characterized by the presence of T and B cells [93, 95–98], and anti-CD4 treatment reduces fibrosis [97]. Lupus-prone NZM mice have increased numbers of $CD4^+$ but not $CD4^+CD25^+$ T cells following silica exposure [43]. This is reminiscent of the reduced expression of CD25 (IL-2Rα) in human silicosis [24, 26, 99] and supports the suggestion that silica exposure results in the loss of T regulatory cell function [99, 100]. This may be associated with increased presence of soluble CD25 in silicosis [101] which has the ability to promote autoimmune disease and enhance Th17 responses through its ability to sequester IL-2 [102]. In experimental silicosis, production of IL-17A by $\Upsilon\delta$ T and Th17 cells induces acute alveolitis, but is not necessary for the development of the late inflammatory and fibrotic lung responses to silica [97].

Elevation in immunoglobulin levels in both serum and BAL has been observed in response to silica in rodents [79, 103, 104]; however, in autoimmune NZM2410 mice, serum IgG was reduced even though autoimmunity, including autoantibodies, was exacerbated [40, 43]. Asbestos exposure also reduced serum IgG while inducing autoantibodies in C57BL/6 mice [48]. Effects on immunoglobulin levels can also vary in human populations with studies showing increases [21, 105–107] or no change [26]. Other factors may also impact immunoglobulin levels including cytokines [79]. ANAs are quite common in both mice and rats following exposure to silica, asbestos, or sodium silicate with 50–100 % of animals being positive [40, 42, 48, 52] although this was influenced by the site of exposure [42] and the presence of ANA in control animals [48]. Although ANAs can exhibit disease specificity [108], they have been found to occur before clinical onset of disease with some specificities (e.g., anti-SS-B/La, anti-SS-A/Ro) more prevalent than disease-specific autoantibodies (e.g., anti-dsDNA, anti-Sm) [109]. Anti-dsDNA, anti-SS-B/La, and anti-SS-A/Ro have been found to occur in up to 50 % of rodents exposed to silica or asbestos [42, 48].

9.6.2.4 Silica-Induced Nephropathy

Kidney disease is a complication of silicosis and may have an autoimmune component. Apart from evidence of immune deposits in autoimmune-prone NZM2410 mice given silica [40] and C57BL/6 mice exposed to asbestos [48], there has been little done to define the requirements for silica-induced nephropathy in experimental animals. The mechanism of silica nephropathy is unclear but appears to have two components: a direct nephrotoxicity and induction of autoimmune disease [30]. These findings are consistent with a disease progression that begins with activation of the innate immune system leading to proinflammatory cytokine production, inflammation of the lung leading to activation of adaptive immunity, breaking of tolerance, autoantibodies, and renal damage [9, 28, 31, 32]. The variable frequency of these disease features suggests significant genetic involvement and gene-environment interaction.

9.7 Genetic Requirements of Silica-Induced Autoimmunity

There is very little known about the genetic requirements of silica-induced autoimmunity; however, as noted above studies of silicosis in mice have identified significant genetic involvement. Silica-induced pulmonary inflammation is dependent on IFN-γ [93], but not Th2 cytokines such as IL-4 and IL-13 [79] or IL-12 [110]. Innate immunity mediates this process as SiO_2-induced inflammation and fibrosis can occur in the absence of T, B, NK T, or NK cells [81]. Notably, although acute lung inflammation requires IL-17 [78], chronic inflammation is dependent on type 1 IFN and IRF7 [72]. The NLRP3 inflammasome and caspase-1 and IL-1β are also required for silicosis [85, 111–113], as is IL-1α [83]. MyD88 which links TLR signaling to proinflammatory cytokine production is required for silica-induced inflammation but not fibrosis [114]. Deficiency of either scavenger receptors MARCO or CD204, expressed mainly on macrophages, impairs silica clearance and exacerbates silica-induced lung inflammation [115, 116]. Significantly, both MARCO and CD204 have been argued to promote tolerance to apoptotic cell material [117]. Thus, the immunological response to silica requires genes involved in both innate and adaptive immunity. There have been no studies identifying the genetic loci required for silica-induced autoimmunity. A quantitative trait locus (QTL) study of murine silicosis identified a major QTL on chromosome 4 and suggestive loci on chromosomes 3 and 18 [68] suggesting that responses to silica involve multiple genes.

9.8 Conclusions and Future Research

Epidemiological data has established a solid link between silica dust exposure and several systemic autoimmune diseases. However, limited research has been done to unravel the mechanism of this effect. This stems in part from a lack of suitable human cohorts to study but also limited studies toward development of a suitable animal model. The variable frequency of features of silica-induced inflammation and subsequent autoimmune features in human subjects suggests significant genetic involvement as well as gene/environment interaction. This is reflected in the differences in response to silica by inbred mouse strains. Development of a model expressing this heterogeneity of response is unlikely to come from studies of inbred mice. This obstacle may be overcome by the use of outbred strains such as the Diversity Outbred [118] where genetic diversity may lead to a more appropriate representation of the heterogeneity of human responses. On the other hand, the extensive literature on silica-induced responses in the mouse including genetic requirements for both inflammation and fibrosis provides a foundation from which to explore the requirements for silicate-induced autoimmunity. A deeper understanding of the contribution of inflammation to fibrosis is required, as is an understanding of how both inflammation and fibrosis contribute to the induction and development of autoimmunity. The contribution of BALT also needs examination as this feature may be essential in the adaptive (auto)immune response following silica exposure, and the development of these discrete foci in the lung may be a site of either the genesis and/or expansion of autoreactive lymphocytes. These are just some of the unresolved issues that plague our understanding of particulate matter and particularly silica-induced autoimmunity. However, given the active research in this area, it is very likely that the next few years will see a significant increase in our understanding of the relevant mechanisms.

References

1. Grunig G, Marsh LM, Esmaeil N, Jackson K, Gordon T, Reibman J, et al. Perspective: ambient air pollution: inflammatory response and effects on the lung's vasculature. Pulm Circ. 2014;4(1):25–35.
2. van Berlo D, Hullmann M, Schins RP. Toxicology of ambient particulate matter. EXS. 2012;101:165–217.
3. Farhat SC, Silva CA, Orione MA, Campos LM, Sallum AM, Braga AL. Air pollution in autoimmune rheumatic diseases: a review. Autoimmun Rev. 2011;11(1):14–21.
4. Bernatsky S, Fournier M, Pineau CA, Clarke AE, Vinet E, Smargiassi A. Associations between ambient fine particulate levels and disease activity in patients with systemic lupus erythematosus (SLE). Environ Health Perspect. 2011;119(1):45–9.
5. Miller FW, Alfredsson L, Costenbader KH, Kamen DL, Nelson LM, Norris JM, et al. Epidemiology of environmental exposures and human autoimmune diseases: findings from a National Institute of Environmental Health Sciences Expert Panel Workshop. J Autoimmun. 2012;39(4):259–71.
6. Pfau JC, Serve KM, Noonan CW. Autoimmunity and asbestos exposure. Autoimmune Dis. 2014;2014:782045.
7. Al Aranji G, White D, Solanki K. Scleroderma renal crisis following silicone breast implant rupture: a case report and review of the literature. Clin Exp Rheumatol. 2014;32(2):262–6.
8. Mossman BT, Glenn RE. Bioreactivity of the crystalline silica polymorphs, quartz and cristobalite, and implications for occupational exposure limits (OELs). Crit Rev Toxicol. 2013;43(8):632–60.
9. Leung CC, Yu IT, Chen W. Silicosis Lancet. 2012;379(9830):2008–18.
10. Parks CG, Conrad K, Cooper GS. Occupational exposure to crystalline silica and autoimmune disease. Environ Health Perspect. 1999;107 Suppl 5:793–802.

11. Castranova V, Vallyathan V. Silicosis and coal workers' pneumoconiosis. Environ Health Perspect. 2000;108 Suppl 4:675–84.
12. Pollard KM. Gender differences in autoimmunity associated with exposure to environmental factors. J Autoimmun. 2012;38(2-3):J177–86.
13. Parks CG, Cooper GS, Nylander-French LA, Sanderson WT, Dement JM, Cohen PL, et al. Occupational exposure to crystalline silica and risk of systemic lupus erythematosus: a population-based, case-control study in the southeastern United States. Arthritis Rheum. 2002;46(7):1840–50.
14. Cooper GS, Wither J, Bernatsky S, Claudio JO, Clarke A, Rioux JD, et al. Occupational and environmental exposures and risk of systemic lupus erythematosus: silica, sunlight, solvents. Rheumatology (Oxford). 2010;49(11):2172–80.
15. Khuder SA, Peshimam AZ, Agraharam S. Environmental risk factors for rheumatoid arthritis. Rev Environ Health. 2002;17(4):307–15.
16. Makol A, Reilly MJ, Rosenman KD. Prevalence of connective tissue disease in silicosis (1985–2006)-a report from the state of Michigan surveillance system for silicosis. Am J Ind Med. 2011;54(4):255–62.
17. Conrad K, Mehlhorn J, Luthke K, Dorner T, Frank KH. Systemic lupus erythematosus after heavy exposure to quartz dust in uranium mines: clinical and serological characteristics. Lupus. 1996;5(1):62–9.
18. Conrad K, Stahnke G, Liedvogel B, Mehlhorn J, Barth J, Blasum C, et al. Anti-CENP-B response in sera of uranium miners exposed to quartz dust and patients with possible development of systemic sclerosis (scleroderma). J Rheumatol. 1995;22(7):1286–94.
19. Kreiss K, Danilovs JA, Newman LS. Histocompatibility antigens in a population based silicosis series. Br J Ind Med. 1989;46(6):364–9.
20. Conrad K, Mehlhorn J. Diagnostic and prognostic relevance of autoantibodies in uranium miners. Int Arch Allergy Immunol. 2000;123(1):77–91.
21. Doll NJ, Stankus RP, Hughes J, Weill H, Gupta RC, Rodriguez M, et al. Immune complexes and autoantibodies in silicosis. J Allergy Clin Immunol. 1981;68(4):281–5.
22. Jones RN, Turner-Warwick M, Ziskind M, Weill H. High prevalence of antinuclear antibodies in sandblasters' silicosis. Am Rev Respir Dis. 1976;113(3):393–5.
23. Lippmann M, Eckert HL, Hahon N, Morgan WK. Circulating antinuclear and rheumatoid factors in coal miners. A prevalence study in Pennsylvania and West Virginia. Ann Intern Med. 1973;79(6):807–11.
24. Subra JF, Renier G, Reboul P, Tollis F, Boivinet R, Schwartz P, et al. Lymphopenia in occupational pulmonary silicosis with or without autoimmune disease. Clin Exp Immunol. 2001;126(3):540–4.
25. Aminian O, Sharifian SA, Mehrdad R, Haghighi KS, Mazaheri M. Antinuclear antibody and rheumatoid factor in silica-exposed workers. Arh Hig Rada Toksikol. 2009;60(2):185–90.
26. Carlsten C, de Roos AJ, Kaufman JD, Checkoway H, Wener M, Seixas N. Cell markers, cytokines, and immune parameters in cement mason apprentices. Arthritis Rheum. 2007;57 (1):147–53.
27. Sauni R, Oksa P, Lehtimaki L, Toivio P, Palmroos P, Nieminen R, et al. Increased alveolar nitric oxide and systemic inflammation markers in silica-exposed workers. Occup Environ Med. 2012;69(4):256–60.
28. Huaux F. New developments in the understanding of immunology in silicosis. Curr Opin Allergy Clin Immunol. 2007;7(2):168–73.
29. Steenland K. One agent, many diseases: exposure-response data and comparative risks of different outcomes following silica exposure. Am J Ind Med. 2005;48(1):16–23.
30. Ghahramani N. Silica nephropathy. Int J Occup Environ Med. 2010;1(3):108–15.
31. Lee S, Hayashi H, Maeda M, Chen Y, Matsuzaki H, Takei-Kumagai N, et al. Environmental factors producing autoimmune dysregulation – chronic activation of T cells caused by silica exposure. Immunobiology. 2012;217(7):743–8.

32. Otsuki T, Hayashi H, Nishimura Y, Hyodo F, Maeda M, Kumagai N, et al. Dysregulation of autoimmunity caused by silica exposure and alteration of Fas-mediated apoptosis in T lymphocytes derived from silicosis patients. Int J Immunopathol Pharmacol. 2011;24 (1 Suppl):11S–6.
33. Bernstein D, Dunnigan J, Hesterberg T, Brown R, Velasco JA, Barrera R, et al. Health risk of chrysotile revisited. Crit Rev Toxicol. 2013;43(2):154–83.
34. Liu G, Cheresh P, Kamp DW. Molecular basis of asbestos-induced lung disease. Annu Rev Pathol. 2013;8:161–87.
35. Noonan CW, Pfau JC, Larson TC, Spence MR. Nested case-control study of autoimmune disease in an asbestos-exposed population. Environ Health Perspect. 2006;114(8):1243–7.
36. Olsson AR, Skogh T, Axelson O, Wingren G. Occupations and exposures in the work environment as determinants for rheumatoid arthritis. Occup Environ Med. 2004;61 (3):233–8.
37. Miller FW, Pollard KM, Parks CG, Germolec DR, Leung PS, Selmi C, et al. Criteria for environmentally associated autoimmune diseases. J Autoimmun. 2012;39(4):253–8.
38. Miller FW, Alfredsson L, Costenbader KH, Kamen DL, Nelson LM, Norris JM, et al. Epidemiology of environmental exposures and human autoimmune diseases: findings from a National Institute of Environmental Health Sciences Expert Panel Workshop. J Autoimmun. 2012;39(4):253–8.
39. Germolec D, Kono DH, Pfau JC, Pollard KM. Animal models used to examine the role of the environment in the development of autoimmune disease: findings from an NIEHS Expert Panel Workshop. J Autoimmun. 2012;39(4):285–93.
40. Brown JM, Archer AJ, Pfau JC, Holian A. Silica accelerated systemic autoimmune disease in lupus-prone New Zealand mixed mice. Clin Exp Immunol. 2003;131(3):415–21.
41. Al-Mogairen SM. Role of sodium silicate in induction of scleroderma-related autoantibodies in brown Norway rats through oral and subcutaneous administration. Rheumatol Int. 2011;31 (5):611–5.
42. Al-Mogairen SM, Al-Arfaj AS, Meo SA, Adam M, Al-Hammad A, Gad El Rab MO. Induction of autoimmunity in Brown Norway rats by oral and parenteral administration of sodium silicate. Lupus. 2009;18(5):413–7.
43. Brown JM, Pfau JC, Holian A. Immunoglobulin and lymphocyte responses following silica exposure in New Zealand mixed mice. Inhal Toxicol. 2004;16(3):133–9.
44. Hala K, Malin G, Dietrich H, Loesch U, Boeck G, Wolf H, et al. Analysis of the initiation period of spontaneous autoimmune thyroiditis (SAT) in obese strain (OS) of chickens. J Autoimmun. 1996;9(2):129–38.
45. Nash JR, Everson NW, Wood RF, Bell PR. Effect of silica and carrageenan on the survival of islet allografts. Transplantation. 1980;29(3):206–8.
46. Wright Jr JR, Lacy PE. Silica prevents the induction of diabetes with complete Freund's adjuvant and low-dose streptozotocin in rats. Diabetes Res. 1989;11(2):51–4.
47. Amano K, Yoon JW. Studies on autoimmunity for initiation of beta-cell destruction. V. Decrease of macrophage-dependent T lymphocytes and natural killer cytotoxicity in silica-treated BB rats. Diabetes. 1990;39(5):590–6.
48. Pfau JC, Sentissi JJ, Li S, Calderon-Garciduenas L, Brown JM, Blake DJ. Asbestos-induced autoimmunity in C57BL/6 mice. J Immunotoxicol. 2008;5(2):129–37.
49. Ferro A, Zebedeo CN, Davis C, Ng KW, Pfau JC. Amphibole, but not chrysotile, asbestos induces anti-nuclear autoantibodies and IL-17 in C57BL/6 mice. J Immunotoxicol. 2014;11 (3):283–90.
50. Zebedeo CN, Davis C, Pena C, Ng KW, Pfau JC. Erionite induces production of autoantibodies and IL-17 in C57BL/6 mice. Toxicol Appl Pharmacol. 2014;275(3):257–64.
51. Salazar KD, Copeland CB, Luebke RW. Effects of Libby amphibole asbestos exposure on two models of arthritis in the Lewis rat. J Toxicol Environ Health A. 2012;75(6):351–65.

52. Salazar KD, Copeland CB, Wood CE, Schmid JE, Luebke RW. Evaluation of anti-nuclear antibodies and kidney pathology in Lewis rats following exposure to Libby amphibole asbestos. J Immunotoxicol. 2013;10(4):329–33.
53. Mahler M, Miller FW, Fritzler MJ. Idiopathic inflammatory myopathies and the anti-synthetase syndrome: a comprehensive review. Autoimmun Rev. 2014;13(4-5):367–71.
54. Lee S, Matsuzaki H, Kumagai-Takei N, Yoshitome K, Maeda M, Chen Y, et al. Silica exposure and altered regulation of autoimmunity. Environ Health Prev Med. 2014;19 (5):322–9.
55. Tomokuni A, Otsuki T, Isozaki Y, Kita S, Ueki H, Kusaka M, et al. Serum levels of soluble Fas ligand in patients with silicosis. Clin Exp Immunol. 1999;118(3):441–4.
56. Ueki A, Isozaki Y, Tomokuni A, Ueki H, Kusaka M, Tanaka S, et al. Different distribution of HLA class II alleles in anti-topoisomerase I autoantibody responders between silicosis and systemic sclerosis patients, with a common distinct amino acid sequence in the HLA-DQB1 domain. Immunobiology. 2001;204(4):458–65.
57. Otsuki T, Sakaguchi H, Tomokuni A, Aikoh T, Matsuki T, Kawakami Y, et al. Soluble Fas mRNA is dominantly expressed in cases with silicosis. Immunology. 1998;94(2):258–62.
58. Silman AJ, Pearson JE. Epidemiology and genetics of rheumatoid arthritis. Arthritis Res. 2002;4 Suppl 3:S265–72.
59. Osio-Salido E, Manapat-Reyes H. Epidemiology of systemic lupus erythematosus in Asia. Lupus. 2010;19(12):1365–73.
60. Tomokuni A, Otsuki T, Sakaguchi H, Isozaki Y, Hyodoh F, Kusaka M, et al. Detection of anti-topoisomerase I autoantibody in patients with silicosis. Environ Health Prev Med. 2002;7(1):7–10.
61. Basu D, Reveille JD. Anti-scl-70. Autoimmunity. 2005;38(1):65–72.
62. Takata-Tomokuni A, Ueki A, Shiwa M, Isozaki Y, Hatayama T, Katsuyama H, et al. Detection, epitope-mapping and function of anti-Fas autoantibody in patients with silicosis. Immunology. 2005;116(1):21–9.
63. Ueki A, Isozaki Y, Tomokuni A, Hatayama T, Ueki H, Kusaka M, et al. Intramolecular epitope spreading among anti-caspase-8 autoantibodies in patients with silicosis, systemic sclerosis and systemic lupus erythematosus, as well as in healthy individuals. Clin Exp Immunol. 2002;129(3):556–61.
64. Ueki H, Kohda M, Nobutoh T, Yamaguchi M, Omori K, Miyashita Y, et al. Antidesmoglein autoantibodies in silicosis patients with no bullous diseases. Dermatology. 2001;202 (1):16–21.
65. Parks CG, Miller FW, Pollard KM, Selmi C, Germolec D, Joyce K, et al. Expert panel workshop consensus statement on the role of the environment in the development of autoimmune disease. Int J Mol Sci. 2014;15(8):14269–97.
66. Davis GS, Leslie KO, Hemenway DR. Silicosis in mice: effects of dose, time, and genetic strain. J Environ Pathol Toxicol Oncol. 1998;17(2):81–97.
67. Callis AH, Sohnle PG, Mandel GS, Wiessner J, Mandel NS. Kinetics of inflammatory and fibrotic pulmonary changes in a murine model of silicosis. J Lab Clin Med. 1985;105 (5):547–53.
68. Ohtsuka Y, Wang XT, Saito J, Ishida T, Munakata M. Genetic linkage analysis of pulmonary fibrotic response to silica in mice. Eur Respir J. 2006;28(5):1013–9.
69. Rabolli V, Lo Re S, Uwambayinema F, Yakoub Y, Lison D, Huaux F. Lung fibrosis induced by crystalline silica particles is uncoupled from lung inflammation in NMRI mice. Toxicol Lett. 2011;203(2):127–34.
70. Foo SY, Phipps S. Regulation of inducible BALT formation and contribution to immunity and pathology. Mucosal Immunol. 2010;3(6):537–44.
71. Miller FW, Pollard KM, Parks CG, Germolec DR, Leung PS, Selmi C, et al. Criteria for environmentally associated autoimmune diseases. J Autoimmun. 2012;39(4):253–8.

72. Giordano G, van den Brule S, Lo Re S, Triqueneaux P, Uwambayinema F, Yakoub Y, et al. Type I interferon signaling contributes to chronic inflammation in a murine model of silicosis. Toxicol Sci. 2010;116(2):682–92.
73. Barbarin V, Nihoul A, Misson P, Arras M, Delos M, Leclercq I, et al. The role of pro- and anti-inflammatory responses in silica-induced lung fibrosis. Respir Res. 2005;6:112.
74. Guo J, Gu N, Chen J, Shi T, Zhou Y, Rong Y, et al. Neutralization of interleukin-1 beta attenuates silica-induced lung inflammation and fibrosis in C57BL/6 mice. Arch Toxicol. 2013;87(11):1963–73.
75. Choi M, Cho WS, Han BS, Cho M, Kim SY, Yi JY, et al. Transient pulmonary fibrogenic effect induced by intratracheal instillation of ultrafine amorphous silica in A/J mice. Toxicol Lett. 2008;182(1-3):97–101.
76. Beamer CA, Holian A. Antigen-presenting cell population dynamics during murine silicosis. Am J Respir Cell Mol Biol. 2007;37(6):729–38.
77. Davis GS, Pfeiffer LM, Hemenway DR. Interferon-gamma production by specific lung lymphocyte phenotypes in silicosis in mice. Am J Respir Cell Mol Biol. 2000;22(4):491–501.
78. Lo Re S, Dumoutier L, Couillin I, Van Vyve C, Yakoub Y, Uwambayinema F, et al. IL-17A-producing gammadelta T and Th17 lymphocytes mediate lung inflammation but not fibrosis in experimental silicosis. J Immunol. 2010;184(11):6367–77.
79. Misson P, Brombacher F, Delos M, Lison D, Huaux F. Type 2 immune response associated with silicosis is not instrumental in the development of the disease. Am J Physiol Lung Cell Mol Physiol. 2007;292(1):L107–13.
80. Maeda M, Nishimura Y, Kumagai N, Hayashi H, Hatayama T, Katoh M, et al. Dysregulation of the immune system caused by silica and asbestos. J Immunotoxicol. 2010;7(4):268–78.
81. Beamer CA, Migliaccio CT, Jessop F, Trapkus M, Yuan D, Holian A. Innate immune processes are sufficient for driving silicosis in mice. J Leukoc Biol. 2010;88(3):547–57.
82. Hamilton Jr RF, Thakur SA, Mayfair JK, Holian A. MARCO mediates silica uptake and toxicity in alveolar macrophages from C57BL/6 mice. J Biol Chem. 2006;281(45):34218–26.
83. Rabolli V, Badissi A, Devosse R, Uwambayinema F, Yakoub Y, Palmai-Pallag M, et al. The alarmin IL-1α is a master cytokine in acute lung inflammation induced by silica micro- and nanoparticles. Part Fibre Toxicol. 2014;11(1):69.
84. Hornung V, Bauernfeind F, Halle A, Samstad EO, Kono H, Rock KL, et al. Silica crystals and aluminum salts activate the NALP3 inflammasome through phagosomal destabilization. Nat Immunol. 2008;9(8):847–56.
85. Dostert C, Petrilli V, Van Bruggen R, Steele C, Mossman BT, Tschopp J. Innate immune activation through Nalp3 inflammasome sensing of asbestos and silica. Science. 2008;320 (5876):674–7.
86. Kusaka T, Nakayama M, Nakamura K, Ishimiya M, Furusawa E, Ogasawara K. Effect of silica particle size on macrophage inflammatory responses. PLoS One. 2014;9(3), e92634.
87. Harijith A, Ebenezer DL, Natarajan V. Reactive oxygen species at the crossroads of inflammasome and inflammation. Front Physiol. 2014;5:352.
88. Hari A, Zhang Y, Tu Z, Detampel P, Stenner M, Ganguly A, et al. Activation of NLRP3 inflammasome by crystalline structures via cell surface contact. Sci Rep. 2014;4:7281.
89. Li M, Gunter ME, Fukagawa NK. Differential activation of the inflammasome in THP-1 cells exposed to chrysotile asbestos and Libby "six-mix" amphiboles and subsequent activation of BEAS-2B cells. Cytokine. 2012;60(3):718–30.
90. Davis GS, Pfeiffer LM, Hemenway DR. Persistent overexpression of interleukin-1beta and tumor necrosis factor-alpha in murine silicosis. J Environ Pathol Toxicol Oncol. 1998;17 (2):99–114.
91. Hubbard AK, Timblin CR, Shukla A, Rincon M, Mossman BT. Activation of NF-kappaB-dependent gene expression by silica in lungs of luciferase reporter mice. Am J Physiol Lung Cell Mol Physiol. 2002;282(5):L968–75.

92. Ohtsuka Y, Munakata M, Ukita H, Takahashi T, Satoh A, Homma Y, et al. Increased susceptibility to silicosis and TNF-alpha production in C57BL/6J mice. Am J Respir Crit Care Med. 1995;152(6 Pt 1):2144–9.
93. Davis GS, Holmes CE, Pfeiffer LM, Hemenway DR. Lymphocytes, lymphokines, and silicosis. J Environ Pathol Toxicol Oncol. 2001;20 Suppl 1:53–65.
94. Piguet PF, Collart MA, Grau GE, Sappino AP, Vassalli P. Requirement of tumour necrosis factor for development of silica-induced pulmonary fibrosis. Nature. 1990;344(6263):245–7.
95. Kumar RK. Quantitative immunohistologic assessment of lymphocyte populations in the pulmonary inflammatory response to intratracheal silica. Am J Pathol. 1989;135(4):605–14.
96. Arras M, Huaux F, Vink A, Delos M, Coutelier JP, Many MC, et al. Interleukin-9 reduces lung fibrosis and type 2 immune polarization induced by silica particles in a murine model. Am J Respir Cell Mol Biol. 2001;24(4):368–75.
97. Barbarin V, Arras M, Misson P, Delos M, McGarry B, Phan SH, et al. Characterization of the effect of interleukin-10 on silica-induced lung fibrosis in mice. Am J Respir Cell Mol Biol. 2004;31(1):78–85.
98. Lo Re S, Lison D, Huaux F. CD4+ T lymphocytes in lung fibrosis: diverse subsets, diverse functions. J Leukoc Biol. 2013;93(4):499–510.
99. Wu P, Miura Y, Hyodoh F, Nishimura Y, Hatayama T, Hatada S, et al. Reduced function of CD4+25+ regulatory T cell fraction in silicosis patients. Int J Immunopathol Pharmacol. 2006;19(2):357–68.
100. Hayashi H, Miura Y, Maeda M, Murakami S, Kumagai N, Nishimura Y, et al. Reductive alteration of the regulatory function of the CD4(+)CD25(+) T cell fraction in silicosis patients. Int J Immunopathol Pharmacol. 2010;23(4):1099–109.
101. Hayashi H, Maeda M, Murakami S, Kumagai N, Chen Y, Hatayama T, et al. Soluble interleukin-2 receptor as an indicator of immunological disturbance found in silicosis patients. Int J Immunopathol Pharmacol. 2009;22(1):53–62.
102. Russell SE, Moore AC, Fallon PG, Walsh PT. Soluble IL-2Ralpha (sCD25) exacerbates autoimmunity and enhances the development of Th17 responses in mice. PLoS One. 2012;7 (10), e47748.
103. Weissman DN, Hubbs AF, Huang SH, Stanley CF, Rojanasakul Y, Ma JK. IgG subclass responses in experimental silicosis. J Environ Pathol Toxicol Oncol. 2001;20 Suppl 1:67–74.
104. Huang SH, Hubbs AF, Stanley CF, Vallyathan V, Schnabel PC, Rojanasakul Y, et al. Immunoglobulin responses to experimental silicosis. Toxicol Sci. 2001;59(1):108–17.
105. Kalliny MS, Bassyouni MI. Immune response due to silica exposure in Egyptian phosphate mines. J Health Care Poor Underserved. 2011;22(4 Suppl):91–109.
106. Calhoun WJ, Christman JW, Ershler WB, Graham WG, Davis GS. Raised immunoglobulin concentrations in bronchoalveolar lavage fluid of healthy granite workers. Thorax. 1986;41 (4):266–73.
107. Karnik AB, Saiyed HN, Nigam SK. Humoral immunologic dysfunction in silicosis. Indian J Med Res. 1990;92:440–2.
108. Mahler M, Bluthner M, Pollard KM. Advances in B-cell epitope analysis of autoantigens in connective tissue diseases. Clin Immunol. 2003;107(2):65–79.
109. Arbuckle MR, McClain MT, Rubertone MV, Scofield RH, Dennis GJ, James JA, et al. Development of autoantibodies before the clinical onset of systemic lupus erythematosus. N Engl J Med. 2003;349(16):1526–33.
110. Davis GS, Pfeiffer LM, Hemenway DR, Rincon M. Interleukin-12 is not essential for silicosis in mice. Part Fibre Toxicol. 2006;3:2.
111. Cassel SL, Eisenbarth SC, Iyer SS, Sadler JJ, Colegio OR, Tephly LA, et al. The Nalp3 inflammasome is essential for the development of silicosis. Proc Natl Acad Sci U S A. 2008;105(26):9035–40.
112. Biswas R, Bunderson-Schelvan M, Holian A. Potential role of the inflammasome-derived inflammatory cytokines in pulmonary fibrosis. Pulm Med. 2011;2011:105707.

113. Srivastava KD, Rom WN, Jagirdar J, Yie TA, Gordon T, Tchou-Wong KM. Crucial role of interleukin-1beta and nitric oxide synthase in silica-induced inflammation and apoptosis in mice. Am J Respir Crit Care Med. 2002;165(4):527–33.
114. Re SL, Yakoub Y, Devosse R, Uwambayinema F, Couillin I, Ryffel B, et al. Uncoupling between inflammatory and fibrotic responses to silica: evidence from MyD88 knockout mice. PLoS One. 2014;9(7), e99383.
115. Thakur SA, Beamer CA, Migliaccio CT, Holian A. Critical role of MARCO in crystalline silica-induced pulmonary inflammation. Toxicol Sci. 2009;108(2):462–71.
116. Beamer CA, Holian A. Scavenger receptor class A type I/II (CD204) null mice fail to develop fibrosis following silica exposure. Am J Physiol Lung Cell Mol Physiol. 2005;289(2): L186–95.
117. Wermeling F, Chen Y, Pikkarainen T, Scheynius A, Winqvist O, Izui S, et al. Class A scavenger receptors regulate tolerance against apoptotic cells, and autoantibodies against these receptors are predictive of systemic lupus. J Exp Med. 2007;204(10):2259–65.
118. Churchill GA, Gatti DM, Munger SC, Svenson KL. The diversity outbred mouse population. Mamm Genome. 2012;23(9–10):713–8.

Chapter 10
Asbestos Exposure and Autoimmunity

Jean C. Pfau, Kinta Serve, Linda Woods, and Curtis Noonan

Abstract Inflammation and immune dysfunction occur with inhalation exposure to fibrous (asbestiform) silicon oxide dusts. As research delves deeper, it is clear that despite some commonalities in the responses to mineral fibers, there appear to be distinct differences in the specific nature of the dysfunction elicited by various fibers that leads ultimately to fiber-specific disease outcomes. A growing body of evidence supports an association between asbestos exposure and autoimmune responses such as antinuclear antibodies (ANA). However, there is limited epidemiological support for an association between asbestos exposure and any specific autoimmune disease. While there are several possible reasons for this, recent data strongly suggests that a key factor lies in the physical chemistry of the fibers themselves, requiring comparative studies of different fiber types. In order to illustrate the importance of this premise, this chapter explores the current data comparing the autoantibody responses following amphibole exposure with those seen following chrysotile exposure. Both human and mouse data suggest that amphibole, but not chrysotile, increases the frequency of positive ANA tests and may increase the risk for systemic autoimmune diseases such as systemic lupus erythematosus. Asbestiform amphibole also drives production of pathogenic autoantibodies against mesothelial cells that appear to contribute to a severe and progressive pleural fibrosis. While occupational asbestos exposures may be decreasing, environmental exposures are on the rise as evidenced by multiple recent discoveries of naturally occurring asbestos. These findings emphasize the need for renewed efforts toward screening and understanding fiber-specific disease manifestations.

Keywords Asbestos • Amphibole • Autoantibodies • Chrysotile

J.C. Pfau, Ph.D. (✉) • L. Woods
Department of Biological Sciences, Idaho State University, 921 South 8th Ave, Stop 8007, Pocatello, ID 83209, USA
e-mail: pfaujean@isu.edu

K. Serve
Mars Hill University, Mars Hill, NC 28754, USA

C. Noonan
University of Montana, Missoula, MT 59812, USA

T. Otsuki et al. (eds.), *Biological Effects of Fibrous and Particulate Substances*, Current Topics in Environmental Health and Preventive Medicine,
DOI 10.1007/978-4-431-55732-6_10

10.1 Introduction

Animal model studies strongly support a role for environmental exposures in autoimmune diseases [1], although systemic autoimmune diseases (SAID) including systemic lupus erythematosus (SLE), systemic sclerosis (SSc), and rheumatoid arthritis (RA) clearly have complex etiologies that include gene-environment interactions [2]. Inhalation of silicate dusts, including crystalline silica and asbestos, increases the production of various autoantibodies. Although the mechanistic details remain unclear, it has been hypothesized that chronic tissue damage induced by the presence of persistent particles within the lungs contributes to autoantibody formation. In this model, apoptotic events following lung tissue injury lead to excessive cellular debris that may in turn become antigenic within the highly inflammatory environment of the injured lung [2–4]. The critical question remains regarding how much these autoantibodies contribute to disease outcomes.

While an association between crystalline silica and both increased antinuclear antibodies (ANA) and increased risk of SLE, RA, and SSc is widely accepted [3, 5, 6], such links have not been well established with asbestos exposure despite reports of immune markers that are consistent with autoimmune mechanisms [reviewed in [7]]. The limited support for an association between asbestos and autoimmune disease may be attributed to several issues, including (a) small or diffuse exposure cohorts, (b) uncertain disease latency, (c) subclinical disease manifestation or autoimmune responses that do not meet current clinical diagnostic criteria, and (d) imprecision regarding fiber types within the exposure. This latter issue refers to the term “asbestos,” which has traditionally been limited to commercially exploited mineral fibers with an aspect ratio greater than 3:1 and defined as either “serpentine” (chrysotile) or “amphibole” (tremolite, amosite, crocidolite, actinolite, anthophyllite) [8]. Broadly speaking, asbestos is known as both a carcinogen and a cause for pulmonary fibrotic disease called “asbestosis.” However, this generalization is misleading due to the distinct physicochemical properties (shape, durability in physiological fluids, surface chemistry, aerodynamic properties) of the various fibers [7, 8], distinctions that could result in very different disease outcomes.

The asbestos research community has been tasked by both the US Environmental Protection Agency and the National Institute for Environmental Health Sciences to address problems with nomenclature and dosage and to better understand the modes of action (MOA) behind asbestos-induced health effects [9, 10]. This effort has been triggered in part by the growing awareness of increasing environmental exposures to elongated mineral fibers that do not fall into the strict definition of asbestos but clearly have the potential for severe health effects. Best known among these is the mixture of amphibole fibers that contaminated the vermiculite mined outside of Libby, Montana, termed “Libby amphibole” (LA). This material has led to hundreds of deaths from cancers and fibrotic diseases in and around this small rural town. Moreover, LA-containing products have been used in homes and other buildings throughout the USA. Due to recent discoveries, asbestos exposure cannot be considered an outdated occupational exposure hazard. First, data have clearly shown that mineral fibers not meeting the strict regulatory definition of "asbestos" nevertheless have severe health consequences [11, 12]. Therefore, the current public health hazard includes asbestiform fibers such as winchite, erionite, and even novel elongated nanomaterials such as "nanotubes" that may behave similarly to asbestos [13]. Second, newly discovered rock outcroppings containing such mineral fibers occur in many parts of the USA, leading to high levels of exposure due to land development and use of the material in roads, parking lots, and recreational areas [14–16]. The severe health outcomes of these exposures include mesothelioma, pulmonary carcinoma, and a variety of fibrotic pleural diseases [16–20]. The possibility of an increased risk for systemic or local autoimmune disease by these materials adds to the public health risk from these exposures.

The Libby Epidemiology Research Program (LERP), funded by the Agency for Toxic Substances and Disease Registry (ATSDR), was designed to develop the necessary data to study relationships (a) between different fiber exposures and autoimmune responses and (b) between those autoimmune responses and pulmonary disease. This chapter reviews current data, including critical findings from the LERP that help distinguish the immunological effects of different fiber types and that may help guide future mechanistic and epidemiological studies.

10.2 Health Effects of Amphibole and Chrysotile

Chrysotile and amphibole asbestos are structurally distinct silicate fibers that cause a range of respiratory tract diseases, including malignant mesothelioma, lung cancer, and asbestosis. Nonmalignant pleural abnormalities are also associated with asbestos exposure and traditionally manifest as pleural plaques, diffuse pleural thickening, or pleural effusions. Plaques are circumscribed, acellular deposits of collagen often located on the parietal pleura and are generally asymptomatic [21]. In contrast, diffuse pleural thickening often affects the visceral pleura [22, 23] and is associated with decreased lung function indicative of restrictive pulmonary disease [24, 25].

Some researchers have suggested that amphibole fibers, including amosite, tremolite, and crocidolite, are more potent inducers of malignant and nonmalignant respiratory diseases than are chrysotile fibers [26, 27]. This increased potency may be related to longer retention of amphibole fibers in lung tissue compared to chrysotile [28–30]. Biopersistent fibers provide a source of prolonged irritation, thus inducing chronic inflammation, cellular proliferation, and collagen deposition – all hallmarks of the fibrotic disease process. However, it is possible that differences in fiber biopersistence alone do not fully explain the striking differences in nonmalignant respiratory disease incidence and progression observed between groups exposed to chrysotile or amphibole asbestos.

Libby amphibole (LA), a unique mixture of amphibole fibers including winchite, richterite, tremolite, and amosite [31], seems to be especially potent in inducing pleural disease [17, 32, 33]. Several studies of populations exposed to

LA-contaminated vermiculite mined from Libby, Montana, demonstrate increased incidence of pleural abnormalities and cancers among people working in and living near either the vermiculite mine or the processing plants [32, 34–37]. Even at the relatively low cumulative fiber exposure (CFE) of 1 fiber/cc-year, a significantly increased risk of developing pleural abnormalities has been reported [12, 36]. Additionally, pleural disease in this population is described as thin, but extensive, lamellar scarring associated with a progressive loss of pulmonary function and constitutes a significant source of morbidity and mortality [17, 19, 33], an outcome not reported for chrysotile-exposed populations. Chrysotile-associated pleural disease is primarily characterized by localized plaques with minimal disease progression [38, 39]. A better understanding of the mechanistic basis for these striking fiber-specific differences in disease presentation is essential. Data reviewed below suggest that part of the difference may be explained by differential autoimmune responses following fiber exposure.

10.3 Asbestos Exposure and Autoantibodies

The history of epidemiological studies exploring an association between asbestos exposure and autoantibody responses was recently reviewed [7]. As early as 1965, cross-sectional studies demonstrated that humoral responses, including rheumatoid factor (RF) and ANA, as well as increased serum IgG/IgA and immune complexes, were associated with asbestos exposures. Most recently, subjects exposed to LA were shown to have elevated frequency and titers of ANA compared to a reference population [40]. Among the autoantibodies detected were those that target common SLE autoantigens, including dsDNA, SSA/Ro52, and ribonuclear proteins (RNP) [40, 41].

Exposure to amphibole asbestos increases the frequency of positive ANA tests in non-autoimmune-prone mice and rats as well. Mice exposed to tremolite exhibited immune complex deposition in the kidneys and mild glomerular changes suggestive of lupus nephritis [42]. LA has also been shown to induce ANA in intratracheally exposed mice [43] and rats [44]. Amosite, a component of LA, was also shown to induce ANA in rats [44]. However, it was recently demonstrated that unlike LA, chrysotile asbestos does not induce ANA in mice [43, 45].

This interesting finding correlates with our comparisons of human cohorts exposed to LA versus chrysotile. Figure 10.1 shows ANA frequency data for a subset of the Libby cohort which is matched for age distribution with a cohort of asbestos workers exposed almost entirely to chrysotile. The latter subjects are steamfitters and pipe insulators from New York [46], and they are part of the ongoing screening of that population. Because the Libby cohort includes nearly 50 % females, while the chrysotile subjects are all male, we compared the ANA frequency among only the males in the Libby cohort and found a similar result (Fig. 10.1, Table 10.1). The ANA testing was performed both in a research laboratory with extensive experience ("in-house," J. Pfau) and a certified clinical

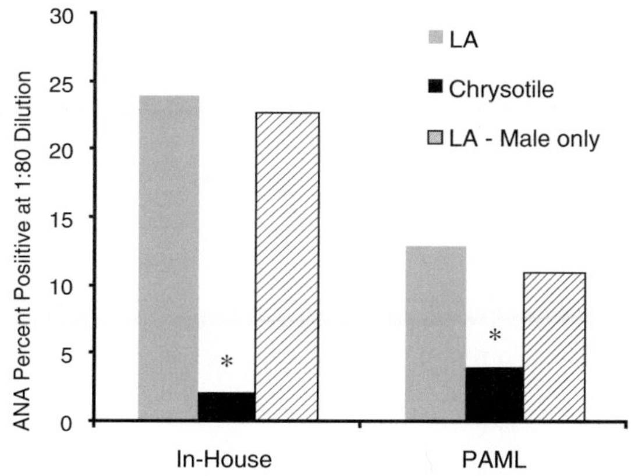

Fig. 10.1 Percent positive ANA by indirect immunofluorescence (in-house) and ELISA (PAML), comparing a set of subjects exposed to Libby amphibole (LA, n=313) or to chrysotile (n=227). The subjects are matched by age, but the LA group is 48 % female. We therefore also provide the percent positive for the males in the LA group. *=$p<0.05$ by Fisher's exact test comparing LA vs chrysotile

laboratory (Pathology Associates Medical Laboratories, PAML) in order to demonstrate that these results are consistent across assay sites. The significant difference in frequency of ANA between these cohorts exposed to different types of fibers is paralleled by a striking difference in the titers of the ANA (Table 10.1), where titers among the five ANA-positive chrysotile-exposed workers are much lower than those among the ANA-positive LA-exposed subjects. Generally, a higher titer would be considered a higher risk for autoimmune disease [47].

While the chrysotile subjects are occupationally exposed males, the LA cohort had primarily environmental exposure (homes, gardens, community) and includes males and females. These demographic differences limit our ability to confidently assign the striking differences in outcome to the fiber type. However, combined with the mouse studies mentioned above, the data appear to support the hypothesis that LA, but not chrysotile, induces systemic autoantibodies characteristic of systemic autoimmune diseases such as SLE.

10.4 Systemic Autoimmune Disease (SAID) and Asbestos

Despite the presence of autoantibodies, however, there are very few epidemiological studies that support an association between asbestos exposure and SAID. There may be several reasons to explain this, ranging from small cohort sizes, long latency for disease, asbestos-related autoimmune responses that do not fit SAID diagnostic criteria, and problems with exposure assessment [7, 48]. Among the SAIDs, rheumatoid arthritis has been most frequently associated with asbestos exposure [49–51]. Other SAIDs are so rare (prevalence estimates ranging from 4 to 24 per 100,000 subjects) that most studies of asbestos-exposed populations have insufficient statistical power to detect robust risk estimates for these outcomes. Nevertheless, an increased risk for scleroderma (SSc) deaths was described for a cohort with likely occupational exposure to asbestos [52]. A recent case-control study of self-

Table 10.1 Demographic and autoantibody data

	Libby amphibole	Chrysotile	*P* value
N (females/males)	313 (154/159)	227 (0/227)	
Mean age (SD)	60.4 (11.2)	59.3 (10.3)	0.166[a]
Females, mean age (SD)	60.3 (11.7)	NA	
Males, mean age (SD)	61.7 (10.7)	59.3 (10.3)	0.051[a]
ANA findings[b]			
No. positive (%)	81 (26 %)	5 (2 %)	<0.001[c]
No. positive among males (%)	38 (24 %)	5 (2 %)	<0.001[c]
No. ANA titer[d] ≥320 (% of ANA-positive males)	17 (45 %)	1 (20 %)	0.38[c]
MCAA findings			
No. positive (%)	97 (31 %)	41 (18 %)	<0.001[c]

[a]2-Tailed, unpaired *t*-test
[b]Pfau lab, "in-house"
[c]Fisher's exact test
[d]ANA titers were calculated by IIF using serial dilutions of ANA-positive sera. The titer is the maximal dilution at which a positive test was still detected

reported SLE patients, nested within a medically screened general population cohort in Libby, Montana, showed a more than fourfold increased risk associated with a history of greater opportunities for LA exposure via environmental pathways [50].

To our knowledge, no studies have clearly demonstrated the induction or exacerbation of SAID by asbestos exposure in animal models. Tremolite was shown to increase immune complex deposition in the kidneys of exposed mice along with autoantibodies to dsDNA, Ro52, and RNP [42], which are common in human SLE. However, these animals did not exhibit significant proteinurea or overt kidney disease. In rats, despite induction of ANA after exposure to Libby amphibole or amosite, there was little evidence of exacerbated disease in a model of induced RA other than increased proteinurea [44, 53].

Taken together, there are fairly strong human and animal data regarding induction of autoantibodies by asbestos, but the corresponding studies supporting an association between asbestos exposure and SAID are limited [7]. When focused on studies of amphibole asbestos, or mixtures with heavy amphibole content, however, recent reviews support an association between asbestos exposure and autoimmunity [7, 54]. This therefore raises the issue of the different mineralogy of these fibers and whether they have differential effects in immune dysfunction.

10.5 Autoantibodies and Pulmonary Disease

Several of the studies reporting ANA following asbestos exposure also indicated that having a positive ANA test was associated with either more severe or more rapid progression of lung disease [40, 55–58]. However, it will be very challenging to determine whether this association represents causation. The longitudinal studies by Tamura et al. argue in favor of causation since the autoantibodies were present prior to lung disease in many cases [57, 59]. However, it may be easier to demonstrate an etiological role for antibodies that are associated with localized autoimmunity rather than SAID. Autoantibodies to specific cell types have been implicated in vascular and fibrotic disorders. Anti-endothelial cell antibodies may contribute to vasculitis [60], SSc [61], and SLE [62], while anti-fibroblast antibodies (AFAs) are implicated in the pathogenesis of SSc [63–65]. Recently, investigators have explored associations between asbestos fiber exposure and such cell-specific autoantibodies. AFAs and mesothelial cell autoantibodies (MCAAs) have been demonstrated in serum of mice and humans, respectively, exposed to LA fibers [56, 66]. MCAA presence also was significantly associated with radiographic changes in the pleura. AFAs and MCAAs were shown to induce collagen production following binding to cultured fibroblasts and mesothelial cells, respectively [66, 67]. Together, these data suggest a mechanism by which asbestos-associated autoantibodies could directly increase collagen accumulation within the pleural space, contributing to the fibrotic process (Fig. 10.2).

Similar studies examining cell-specific autoantibody presence and association with pleural disease have not been reported following chrysotile exposure. As part of the LERP, researchers hypothesized that, if the MCAAs are involved in progressive pleural disease, MCAA would occur less frequently in the chrysotile-exposed cohort compared to the LA cohort. To examine MCAA frequency, a cell-based binding ELISA was performed using the Met5A cells as previously described [56]. Consistent with the hypothesis, the percent of subjects positive for MCAA was significantly higher in the LA group compared to the chrysotile group (Table 10.1). It was therefore critical to determine whether the MCAAs were associated with pleural disease in either group.

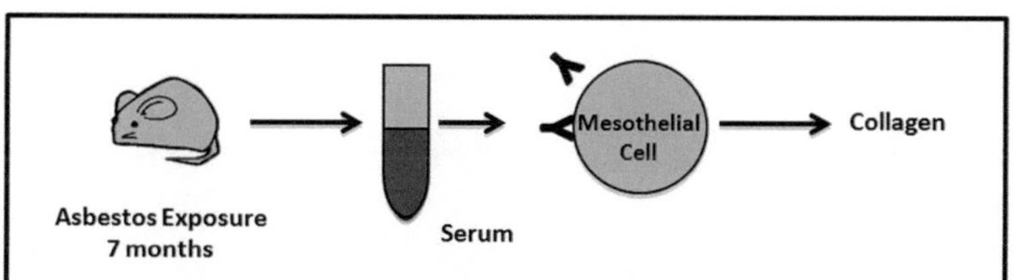

Fig. 10.2 Schematic of possible mechanism of MCAA-induced fibrosis. Exposure to asbestos leads to production of MCAA in mouse serum. MCAAs bind to mesothelial cells and induce collagen production

Subjects demonstrating any pleural change as assessed by radiographic screenings were equivalent between the two populations (58 %). However, the percentage of subjects testing positive for both MCAAs and pleural abnormalities was different between the two asbestos-exposed populations, with 44 % double positive for the LA population and only 6 % double positive for the chrysotile population. Logistic regression analysis, adjusted for age and sex, revealed no association between chrysotile MCAA and pleural disease ($p=0.17$), whereas this association was statistically significant for the Libby MCAA (0=0.04). These data suggested that the LA MCAA might be more pathogenic than the chrysotile MCAA with respect to pleural changes. Interestingly, the association between MCAA was significant for pleural, but not interstitial disease, suggesting a specific local autoimmune contribution to pleural disease [56].

10.6 MCAA and Serum Antibody Isotypes

Studies of other tissue-specific antibodies have indicated that the different IgG subtypes vary in their potential to be pathogenic [68]. For MCAA-positive samples, binding was lost upon clearance of IgG from the sera, confirming that the MCAAs are IgG-type antibodies [67]. Screening of MCAA for IgG subtypes revealed differences in subtype distribution between LA MCAA and chrysotile MCAA. LA MCAAs were comprised predominantly of a mix of subtypes IgG1 and IgG3, with no detectable levels of IgG2 or IgG4, while chrysotile MCAAs were an equal mix of subtypes 1, 3, and 4 (Fig. 10.3). Additionally, IgG1 made up a significantly larger proportion of LA MCAA compared to chrysotile MCAA, while IgG4 made up a significantly higher proportion of the chrysotile MCAA.

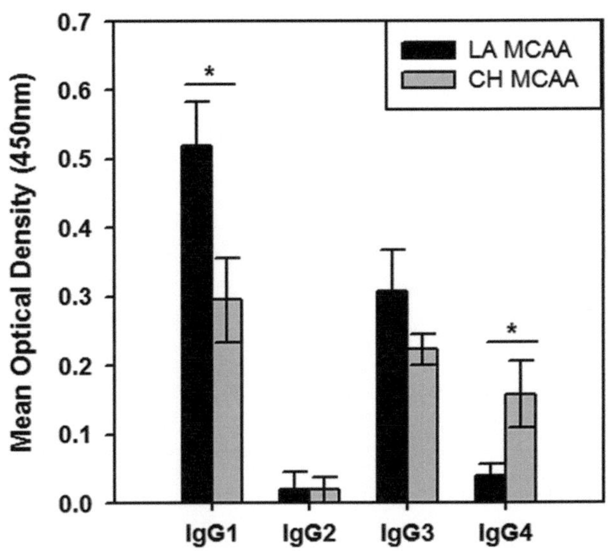

Fig. 10.3 IgG subclass distribution differed significantly among LA and chrysotile MCAAs, as assessed by cell-based ELISA. Comparison of IgG subtype distribution among LA MCAAs to chrysotile MCAAs demonstrated significantly higher proportion of IgG1 in LA MCAAs and IgG4 in chrysotile MCAAs, $*p<0.005$ by 2-tailed t-test, mean$\pm$SE, n=at least 9

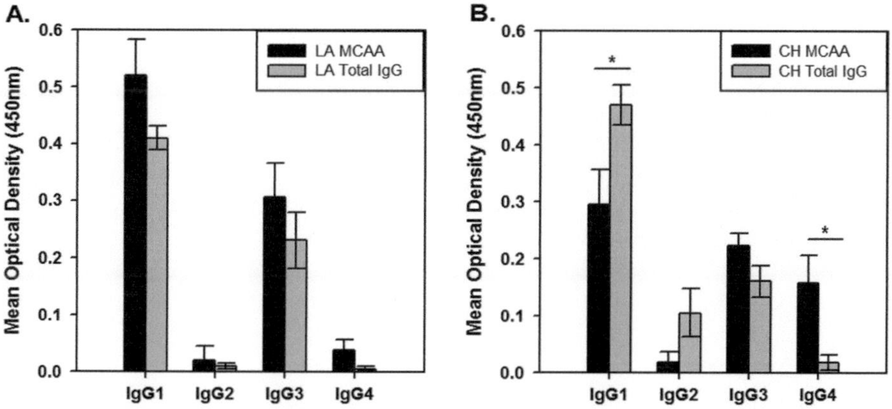

Fig. 10.4 IgG subclass distributions differed among total IgGs and MCAAs detected in sera of LA and chrysotile-exposed populations. (**a**) In sera of LA-exposed subjects, IgG1 and IgG3 were the predominant subtypes detected when distributions of total IgG were assessed, with undetectable IgG2 and IgG4 levels. (**b**) In sera of chrysotile-exposed subjects, IgG1 was the predominant subtype detected, followed by IgG3 and IgG2. Low levels of IgG4 were detected. IgG1 detection was significantly higher and IgG4 significantly lower among total sera IgG compared to MCAA-specific IgG, $*p=0.018$ by one-way ANOVA, mean $\pm$ S.E., $n \geq 9$

Normal human serum has an IgG subtype distribution where IgG1 □ IgG2 □ IgG3 > IgG4 [69]. Interestingly, IgG subtype distributions of total serum IgG also differed between the two fiber exposures (Fig. 10.4). Analysis of a representative sample of the larger population revealed a similar IgG subtype distribution among total serum IgG of LA-exposed subjects and LA MCAA, with predominantly IgG1 and IgG3 subtypes (Fig. 10.4a). In contrast, the total serum IgG subtype distribution in chrysotile-exposed subjects was quite different from their MCAA-specific distributions, with chrysotile MCAA demonstrating significantly decreased ($p<0.02$) IgG1 and increased IgG4 in a cell-based ELISA for MCAA (Fig. 10.4b). Thus, while particularly apparent with LA, both forms of asbestos shifted the total IgG subtype distribution away from IgG2 and toward IgG3. However, the most compelling difference remains the shift in the MCAA IgG distributions with LA maintaining high levels of IgG1 and IgG3, while the chrysotile MCAA shifted toward IgG4.

Although this analysis represents a subset of the entire cohort, these data provide a striking difference between the immune effects of LA compared to chrysotile asbestos. Certain IgG subclasses are considered more pathogenic and have a stronger correlation with autoimmune disease than others based on their effector functions [68]. IgG1 and IgG3 are considered inflammatory immunoglobulins due to their ability to bind Fc receptors and activate complement [70], while IgG4 is a small, noninflammatory peptide that does not bind Fc-γ receptors or activate complement [71]. Since IgG1 and IgG3 have strong complement-binding capabilities, the increased proportions of these IgG subtypes among LA MCAAs may contribute to overall autoantibody pathogenicity in vivo. In contrast, IgG4 does not activate complement, potentially providing a degree of protection against inflammation and cellular death in chrysotile-exposed subjects, thus partially attenuating pleural diseases. Additionally, it has recently been suggested that IgG4 binds to a subclass of Fc-γ receptors (IIB) with higher affinity than other IgG subtypes [72]. Since IgG binding of FcγRIIB blocks cellular activation, it is possible that the decreased association of chrysotile MCAA with pleural disease may be in part due to the inhibitory functions of IgG4.

10.7 Conclusions

Asbestos-related pleural disease is considered a hallmark of asbestos exposure and is described as localized or diffuse pleural thickening. These conditions may be associated with restrictive lung function and decreased quality of life, at least among subjects exposed to LA [19, 73]. While chrysotile asbestos has previously constituted a more significant source of human asbestos exposure due to its widespread commercial use, LA is considered a more potent inducer of nonmalignant pulmonary disease including the unique thin lamellar pleural thickening that leads to severe and progressive disease [17]. Therefore, generalization of pleural outcomes without distinguishing fiber type could be leading to mischaracterization of pleural findings that also contributes to inconsistencies in reported disease outcomes and patient management. To begin to understand what appear to be fiber-specific pathologies, it is essential to explore mechanistic hypotheses. This chapter has reviewed the background for a possible immune-based etiology wherein either systemic or tissue-specific autoantibodies contribute to the onset or progression of asbestos-induced pleural disease.

While amphibole asbestos such as LA induces ANA in mice, rats, and humans, chrysotile does not appear to do so. This differential in fiber-specific responses may help explain the limited epidemiological data linking "asbestos" in general with SAID. In addition, while both LA and chrysotile induce antibodies that target mesothelial cells, only those associated with LA exposure appear to be pathogenic and to be associated with pleural disease in humans. These data provide a critical foundation for future mechanistic studies that will determine the trigger for the autoantibodies and begin to identify potential immune-based therapeutic targets for the severe and progressive pulmonary manifestations of LA exposure.

Acknowledgments The authors gratefully acknowledge the intellectual contributions of the Libby Epidemiology Research Program (LERP): Icahn School of Medicine at Sinai including Raja Flores MD and Jaime Szeinuk MD; rheumatology consultant Roger Diegel, MD, Kalispell MT; and the Center for Asbestos Related Diseases, Brad Black MD. This work was funded in part by the LERP Grant from CDC/ATSDR TS000099-01 and by the Idaho COBRE P20 GM103408. We dedicate this work in the memory of Dr. Stephen Levin, Mount Sinai Medical Center, New York, whose insights and vision spearheaded this work.

References

1. Germolec D, Kono DH, Pfau JC, Pollard KM. Animal models used to examine the role of the environment in the development of autoimmune disease: findings from an NIEHS Expert Panel Workshop. J Autoimmun. 2012;39(4):285–93. PubMed. Pubmed Central PMCID: 3465484.
2. Cooper GS, Gilbert KM, Greidinger EL, James JA, Pfau JC, Reinlib L, et al. Recent advances and opportunities in research on lupus: environmental influences and mechanisms of disease. Environ Health Perspect. 2008;116(6):695–702. PubMed. Pubmed Central PMCID: 2430222.
3. Brown JM, Pfau JC, Pershouse MA, Holian A. Silica, apoptosis, and autoimmunity. J Immunotoxicol. 2005;1(3):117–87. PubMed.
4. Pfau JC, Brown JM, Holian A. Silica-exposed mice generate autoantibodies to apoptotic cells. Toxicology. 2004;195(2–3):167–76. PubMed.
5. Cooper GS, Wither J, Bernatsky S, Claudio JO, Clarke A, Rioux JD, et al. Occupational and environmental exposures and risk of systemic lupus erythematosus: silica, sunlight, solvents. Rheumatology. 2010;49(11):2172–80. PubMed. Pubmed Central PMCID: 2954367.
6. De Capitani EM, Schweller M, Silva CM, Metze K, Cerqueira EM, Bertolo MB. Rheumatoid pneumoconiosis (Caplan's syndrome) with a classical presentation. Jornal brasileiro de pneumologia: publicacao oficial da Sociedade Brasileira de Pneumologia e Tisilogia. 2009;35(9):942–6. PubMed.
7. Pfau JC, Serve KM, Noonan CW. Autoimmunity and asbestos exposure. Autoimmune Dis. 2014;2014:782045. PubMed Pubmed Central PMCID: 4022069.
8. Sporn TA. Mineralogy of asbestos. Recent Results Cancer Res Fortschritte der Krebsforschung Progres dans les recherches sur le cancer. 2011;189:1–11. PubMed.
9. Gwinn MR. Multiple modes of action of asbestos and related mineral fibers. J Toxicol Environ Health B Crit Rev. 2014;14(1–4):1–2. PubMed Pubmed Central PMCID: 3118491.
10. Gwinn MR, DeVoney D, Jarabek AM, Sonawane B, Wheeler J, Weissman DN, et al. Meeting report: mode(s) of action of asbestos and related mineral fibers. Environ Health Perspect. 2011;119(12):1806–10. PubMed. Pubmed Central PMCID: 3261973.
11. Carbone M, Yang H. Molecular pathways: targeting mechanisms of asbestos and erionite carcinogenesis in mesothelioma. Clin Cancer Res. 2012;18(3):598–604. PubMed. Pubmed Central PMCID: 3291331.
12. Larson TC, Antao VC, Bove FJ, Cusack C. Association between cumulative fiber exposure and respiratory outcomes among Libby vermiculite workers. J Occup Environ Med/Am College Occup Environ Med. 2012;54(1):56–63. PubMed.
13. Donaldson K, Murphy FA, Duffin R, Poland CA. Asbestos, carbon nanotubes and the pleural mesothelium: a review of the hypothesis regarding the role of long fibre retention in the parietal pleura, inflammation and mesothelioma. Part Fibre Toxicol. 2010;7:5. PubMed Pubmed Central PMCID: 2857820.
14. Buck BJ, Goossens D, Metcalf RV, McLaurin B, Ren M, Freudenberger F. Naturally occurring asbestos: potential for human exposure, Southern Nevada, USA. Soil Sci Soc Am J. 2013;77:2192–204.
15. Lee RJ, Strohmeier BR, Bunker KL, Van Orden DR. Naturally occurring asbestos: a recurring public policy challenge. J Hazard Mater. 2008;153(1–2):1–21. PubMed.
16. Van Gosen BS, Blitz TA, Plumlee GS, Meeker GP, Pierson MP. Geologic occurrences of erionite in the United States: an emerging national public health concern for respiratory disease. Environ Geochem Health. 2013;35:419–30. PubMed.
17. Black B, Szeinuk J, Whitehouse AC, Levin SM, Henschke CI, Yankelevitz DF, et al. Rapid progression of pleural disease due to exposure to Libby amphibole: "Not your grandfather's asbestos related disease". Am J Ind Med. 2014;57(11):1197–206. PubMed.
18. Emri S, Demir A, Dogan M, Akay H, Bozkurt B, Carbone M, et al. Lung diseases due to environmental exposures to erionite and asbestos in Turkey. Toxicol Lett. 2002;127(1–3):251–7. PubMed.

19. Whitehouse AC. Asbestos-related pleural disease due to tremolite associated with progressive loss of lung function: serial observations in 123 miners, family members, and residents of Libby, Montana. Am J Ind Med. 2004;46(3):219–25. PubMed.
20. Whitehouse AC, Black CB, Heppe MS, Ruckdeschel J, Levin SM. Environmental exposure to Libby Asbestos and mesotheliomas. Am J Ind Med. 2008;51(11):877–80. PubMed.
21. Nishimura SL, Broaddus VC. Asbestos-induced pleural disease. Clin Chest Med. 1998;19 (2):311–29. PubMed.
22. Broaddus VC, Everitt JI, Black B, Kane AB. Non-neoplastic and neoplastic pleural endpoints following fiber exposure. J Toxicol Environ Health B Crit Rev. 2011;14(1–4):153–78. PubMed Pubmed Central PMCID: 3118521.
23. Gevenois PA, de Maertelaer V, Madani A, Winant C, Sergent G, De Vuyst P. Asbestosis, pleural plaques and diffuse pleural thickening: three distinct benign responses to asbestos exposure. Eur Respir J. 1998;11(5):1021–7. PubMed.
24. Kee ST, Gamsu G, Blanc P. Causes of pulmonary impairment in asbestos-exposed individuals with diffuse pleural thickening. Am J Respir Crit Care Med. 1996;154(3 Pt 1):789–93. PubMed.
25. Schwartz DA, Galvin JR, Dayton CS, Stanford W, Merchant JA, Hunninghake GW. Determinants of restrictive lung function in asbestos-induced pleural fibrosis. J Appl Physiol. 1990;68(5):1932–7. PubMed.
26. McDonald JC. Mineral fibre persistence and carcinogenicity. Ind Health. 1998;36(4):372–5. PubMed.
27. Mossman BT, Bignon J, Corn M, Seaton A, Gee JB. Asbestos: scientific developments and implications for public policy. Science. 1990;247(4940):294–301. PubMed.
28. Bernstein D, Dunnigan J, Hesterberg T, Brown R, Velasco JA, Barrera R, et al. Health risk of chrysotile revisited. Crit Rev Toxicol. 2013;43(2):154–83. PubMed Pubmed Central PMCID: 3581056.
29. Bernstein DM, Donaldson K, Decker U, Gaering S, Kunzendorf P, Chevalier J, et al. A biopersistence study following exposure to chrysotile asbestos alone or in combination with fine particles. Inhal Toxicol. 2008;20(11):1009–28. PubMed Pubmed Central PMCID: 2565272.
30. McDonald JC. Epidemiological significance of mineral fiber persistence in human lung tissue. Environ Health Perspect. 1994;102 Suppl 5:221–4. PubMed Pubmed Central PMCID: 1567253.
31. Meeker GP, Bern AM, Brownfield IK, Lowers HA, Sutley SJ, Hoefen TM, et al. The composition and morphology of amphiboles from the Rainy Creek Complex, Near Libby, Montana. Am Mineral. 2003;88:1955–69.
32. Larson TC, Antao VC, Bove FJ. Vermiculite worker mortality: estimated effects of occupational exposure to Libby amphibole. J Occup Environ Med/Am College Occup Environ Med. 2010;52(5):555–60. PubMed.
33. Peipins LA, Lewin M, Campolucci S, Lybarger JA, Miller A, Middleton D, et al. Radiographic abnormalities and exposure to asbestos-contaminated vermiculite in the community of Libby, Montana, USA. Environ Health Perspect. 2003;111(14):1753–9. PubMed Pubmed Central PMCID: 1241719.
34. Alexander BH, Raleigh KK, Johnson J, Mandel JH, Adgate JL, Ramachandran G, et al. Radiographic evidence of nonoccupational asbestos exposure from processing Libby vermiculite in Minneapolis, Minnesota. Environ Health Perspect. 2012;120(1):44–9. PubMed Pubmed Central PMCID: 3261940.
35. Antao VC, Larson TC, Horton DK. Libby vermiculite exposure and risk of developing asbestos-related lung and pleural diseases. Curr Opin Pulm Med. 2012;18(2):161–7. PubMed.
36. Rohs AM, Lockey JE, Dunning KK, Shukla R, Fan H, Hilbert T, et al. Low-level fiber-induced radiographic changes caused by Libby vermiculite: a 25-year follow-up study. Am J Respir Crit Care Med. 2008;177(6):630–7. PubMed Pubmed Central PMCID: 2267337.

37. Sullivan PA. Vermiculite, respiratory disease, and asbestos exposure in Libby, Montana: update of a cohort mortality study. Environ Health Perspect. 2007;115(4):579–85. PubMed Pubmed Central PMCID: 1852671.
38. Koskinen K, Zitting A, Tossavainen A, Rinne JP, Roto P, Kivekas J, et al. Radiographic abnormalities among Finnish construction, shipyard and asbestos industry workers. Scand J Work Environ Health. 1998;24(2):109–17. PubMed.
39. Markowitz SB, Morabia A, Lilis R, Miller A, Nicholson WJ, Levin S. Clinical predictors of mortality from asbestosis in the North American Insulator Cohort, 1981 to 1991. Am J Respir Crit Care Med. 1997;156(1):101–8. PubMed.
40. Pfau JC, Sentissi JJ, Weller G, Putnam EA. Assessment of autoimmune responses associated with asbestos exposure in Libby, Montana, USA. Environ Health Perspect. 2005;113(1):25–30. PubMed Pubmed Central PMCID: 1253705.
41. Pfau JC, Blake DJ, Fritzler MJ. Autoantibody profiles of an asbestos-exposed population. In: Vogel FL, Zimmermann LF, editors. Autoimmunity: role, regulation and disorders. New York: Nova; 2009. p. 245–68.
42. Pfau JC, Sentissi JJ, Li S, Calderon-Garciduenas L, Brown JM, Blake DJ. Asbestos-induced autoimmunity in C57BL/6 mice. J Immunotoxicol. 2008;5(2):129–37. PubMed.
43. Ferro A, Zebedeo CN, Davis C, Ng KW, Pfau JC. Amphibole, but not chrysotile, asbestos induces anti-nuclear autoantibodies and IL-17 in C57BL/6 mice. J Immunotoxicol. 2013. doi:10.3109/1547691X.2013.847510. PubMed.
44. Salazar KD, Copeland CB, Wood CE, Schmid JE, Luebke RW. Evaluation of anti-nuclear antibodies and kidney pathology in Lewis rats following exposure to Libby amphibole asbestos. J Immunotoxicol. 2012;10:329–33. PubMed.
45. Zebedeo CN, Davis C, Pena C, Ng KW, Pfau JC. Erionite induces production of autoantibodies and IL-17 in C57BL/6 mice. Toxicol Appl Pharmacol. 2014;275(3):257–64. PubMed.
46. Markowitz SB, Levin SM, Miller A, Morabia A. Asbestos, asbestosis, smoking, and lung cancer. New findings from the North American insulator cohort. Am J Respir Crit Care Med. 2013;188(1):90–6. PubMed.
47. Tan EM, Feltkamp TE, Smolen JS, Butcher B, Dawkins R, Fritzler MJ, et al. Range of antinuclear antibodies in "healthy" individuals. Arthritis Rheum. 1997;40(9):1601–11. PubMed.
48. Noonan CW, Pfau JC. Asbestos exposure and autoimmune disease. In: Nriagu J, editor. Encyclopedia of environmental health, vol. 1. New York: Elsevier; 2011. p. 193–203.
49. Greaves IA. Rheumatoid "pneumoconiosis" (Caplan's syndrome) in an asbestos worker: a 17 years' follow-up. Thorax. 1979;34(3):404–5. PubMed Pubmed Central PMCID: 471084.
50. Noonan CW, Pfau JC, Larson TC, Spence MR. Nested case-control study of autoimmune disease in an asbestos-exposed population. Environ Health Perspect. 2006;114(8):1243–7. PubMed Pubmed Central PMCID: 1551997.
51. Olsson AR, Skogh T, Axelson O, Wingren G. Occupations exposures in the work environment as determinants for rheumatoid arthritis. Occup Environ Med. 2004;61(3):233–8. PubMed Pubmed Central PMCID: 1740725.
52. Gold LS, Ward MH, Dosemeci M, De Roos AJ. Systemic autoimmune disease mortality and occupational exposures. Arthritis Rheum. 2007;56(10):3189–201. PubMed.
53. Salazar KD, Copeland CB, Luebke RW. Effects of Libby amphibole asbestos exposure on two models of arthritis in the Lewis rat. J Toxicol Environ Health A. 2012;75(6):351–65. PubMed.
54. Bunderson-Schelvan M, Pfau JC, Crouch E, Holian A. Nonpulmonary outcomes of asbestos exposure. J Toxicol Environ Health B Crit Rev. 2011;14(1–4):122–52. PubMed Pubmed Central PMCID: 3118539.
55. Gregor A, Parkes RW, du Bois R, Turner-Warwick M. Radiographic progression of asbestosis: preliminary report. Ann N Y Acad Sci. 1979;330:147–56. PubMed.
56. Marchand LS, St-Hilaire S, Putnam EA, Serve KM, Pfau JC. Mesothelial cell and anti-nuclear autoantibodies associated with pleural abnormalities in an asbestos exposed population of Libby MT. Toxicol Lett. 2012;208(2):168–73. PubMed Pubmed Central PMCID: 3241886.

57. Tamura M, Tokuyama T, Kasuga H, Yoneda T, Miyazaki R, Narita N. [Study on correlation between chest X-P course findings and change in antinuclear antibody in asbestos plant employees]. Sangyo Eiseigaku Zasshi J Occup Health. 1996;38(3):138–41. PubMed.
58. Turner-Warwick M. Immunology and asbestosis. Proc R Soc Med. 1973;66(9):927–30. PubMed Pubmed Central PMCID: 1645453.
59. Tamura M, Liang D, Tokuyama T, Yoneda T, Kasuga H, Narita N, et al. [Study on the relationship between appearance of autoantibodies and chest X-ray findings of asbestos plant employees]. Sangyo igaku Japanese J Ind Health. 1993;35(5):406–12. PubMed.
60. del Papa N, Meroni PL, Barcellini W, Sinico A, Radice A, Tincani A, et al. Antibodies to endothelial cells in primary vasculitides mediate in vitro endothelial cytotoxicity in the presence of normal peripheral blood mononuclear cells. Clin Immunol Immunopathol. 1992;63(3):267–74. PubMed.
61. Ihn H, Sato S, Fujimoto M, Igarashi A, Yazawa N, Kubo M, et al. Characterization of autoantibodies to endothelial cells in systemic sclerosis (SSc): association with pulmonary fibrosis. Clin Exp Immunol. 2000;119(1):203–9. PubMed Pubmed Central PMCID: 1905540.
62. Renaudineau Y, Dugue C, Dueymes M, Youinou P. Antiendothelial cell antibodies in systemic lupus erythematosus. Autoimmun Rev. 2002;1(6):365–72. PubMed.
63. Chizzolini C, Raschi E, Rezzonico R, Testoni C, Mallone R, Gabrielli A, et al. Autoantibodies to fibroblasts induce a proadhesive and proinflammatory fibroblast phenotype in patients with systemic sclerosis. Arthritis Rheum. 2002;46(6):1602–13. PubMed.
64. Fineschi S, Goffin L, Rezzonico R, Cozzi F, Dayer JM, Meroni PL, et al. Antifibroblast antibodies in systemic sclerosis induce fibroblasts to produce profibrotic chemokines, with partial exploitation of toll-like receptor 4. Arthritis Rheum. 2008;58(12):3913–23. PubMed.
65. Ronda N, Raschi E, Testoni C, Borghi MO, Gatti R, Dayer JM, et al. Anti-fibroblast antibodies in systemic sclerosis. Isr Med Assoc J IMAJ. 2002;4(11 Suppl):858–64. PubMed.
66. Pfau JC, Li S, Holland S, Sentissi JJ. Alteration of fibroblast phenotype by asbestos-induced autoantibodies. J Immunotoxicol. 2011;8(2):159–69. PubMed Pubmed Central PMCID: 3201780.
67. Serve KM, Black B, Szeinuk J, Pfau JC. Asbestos-associated mesothelial cell autoantibodies promote collagen deposition in vitro. Inhal Toxicol. 2013;25(14):774–84. PubMed.
68. Zouali M, Jefferis R, Eyquem A. IgG subclass distribution of autoantibodies to DNA and to nuclear ribonucleoproteins in autoimmune diseases. Immunology. 1984;51(3):595–600. PubMed Pubmed Central PMCID: 1454452.
69. Morell A, Skvaril F, Steinberg AG, Van Loghem E, Terry WD. Correlations between the concentrations of the four sub-classes of IgG and Gm Allotypes in normal human sera. J Immunol. 1972;108(1):195–206. PubMed.
70. Jean WC, Dalmau J, Ho A, Posner JB. Analysis of the IgG subclass distribution and inflammatory infiltrates in patients with anti-Hu-associated paraneoplastic encephalomyelitis. Neurology. 1994;44(1):140–7. PubMed.
71. van der Neut KM, Schuurman J, Losen M, Bleeker WK, Martinez-Martinez P, Vermeulen E, et al. Anti-inflammatory activity of human IgG4 antibodies by dynamic Fab arm exchange. Science. 2007;317(5844):1554–7. PubMed.
72. Bruhns P, Iannascoli B, England P, Mancardi DA, Fernandez N, Jorieux S, et al. Specificity and affinity of human Fcgamma receptors and their polymorphic variants for human IgG subclasses. Blood. 2009;113(16):3716–25. PubMed.
73. Winters CA, Hill WG, Rowse K, Black B, Kuntz SW, Weinert C. Descriptive analysis of the respiratory health status of persons exposed to Libby amphibole asbestos. BMJ Open. 2012;2 (6):1–9. PubMed Pubmed Central PMCID: 3532993.

Chapter 11
T Cell Alteration Caused by Exposure to Asbestos

Megumi Maeda, Shoko Yamamoto, Tamayo Hatayama, Hidenori Matsuzaki, Suni Lee, Naoko Kumagai-Takei, Kei Yoshitome, Yasumitsu Nishimura, Yoshinobu Kimura, and Takemi Otsuki

Abstract A model to examine the effects of continuous exposure to asbestos on human T cells was established to interpret experimental findings for clinical utilization. Although transient exposure causes apoptosis in the human polyclonal cell line MT-2, continuous and relatively low-dose exposure resulted in resistance against asbestos-induced apoptosis with a higher production of TGF-β and IL-10 and subsequent resistance to TGF-β-induced growth inhibition and activation of STAT3 and Bcl-2. These alterations caused by continuous exposure to chrysotile asbestos were also observed in a subline exposed continuously to crocidolite and included resistance to apoptosis, changes of cytokine production, and demonstration of the importance of Bcl-2 for resistance against apoptosis. In addition, analysis of protein expression among the MT-2 original cell line, which was never exposed to asbestos, and the continuously exposed subline showed the phosphorylation of β-actin and the increasing level of cytoskeletal molecules. These findings indicate the importance of the cytoskeleton as the initial contact site between cells and asbestos fibers, particularly fibers that cannot move into the inside of cells because of their physical features. Finally, the CXCR3 chemokine receptor and related antitumor cytokine IFN-γ were assayed in these sublines continuously exposed to asbestos, as well as in vitro stimulated freshly isolated peripheral CD4+ T cells derived from healthy donors and exposed to asbestos fibers. The CXCR3 expression and production capacity for IFN-γ were reduced by asbestos exposure, and these findings were also confirmed for peripheral CD4+ T cells derived from patients with pleural plaque and malignant mesothelioma. The overall findings observed in continuously exposed human T cell models will contribute towards the early

M. Maeda • Y. Kimura
Department of Biofunctional Chemistry, Division of Bioscience, Graduate School of Natural Science and Technology, Okayama University, Okayama 700-8530, Japan

S. Yamamoto • T. Hatayama • H. Matsuzaki • S. Lee • N. Kumagai-Takei • K. Yoshitome • Y. Nishimura • T. Otsuki, M.D., Ph.D. (✉)
Department of Hygiene, Kawasaki Medical School, 577 Matsushima, Kurashiki, Okayama 701-0192, Japan
e-mail: takemi@med.kawasaki-m.ac.jp

T. Otsuki et al. (eds.), *Biological Effects of Fibrous and Particulate Substances*, Current Topics in Environmental Health and Preventive Medicine,
DOI 10.1007/978-4-431-55732-6_11

detection of asbestos exposure and occurrence of mesothelioma using peripheral blood and will improve the immune status (reducing antitumor immunity in asbestos-exposed patients) through the use of certain physiological substances derived from plants, foods, and microorganisms.

Keywords Asbestos • T cell • Apoptosis • Continuous exposure • β-actin • CXCR3

11.1 Local Immunological Effects of Asbestos Fibers

Asbestos exposure causes lung fibrosis (asbestosis) and various forms of cancer such as lung cancer and malignant mesothelioma (MM) [1–5]. Basically, asbestos fibers are inhaled through the airway, and the initial portal of entry is the lung. Asbestos fibers possess an aspect ratio of more than 3:1, usually ranging from 20:1 to 100:1 or higher (>5 μm in length). As a consequence, not all fibers reach the end of the respiratory tracts such as the alveolar space, and fibers may straggle towards the small bronchus when moving to alveolar spaces [1–5].

The first component that meets and attempts to handle the asbestos fibers comprises the alveolar macrophages (AM) [1–6]. Once AM recognize these fibers, the activation of inflammasomes occurs. The discovery of inflammasomes led to a better understanding of the cellular and molecular events that occur after certain danger signals are recognized as foreign bodies that enter through the cell surface [7–10]. These danger signals vary from extracellular substances such as silica particles, aluminum, bacterial toxins, as well as asbestos fibers and intracorporeal crystals such as uric acid and amyloid. All of these ligands/foreign bodies activate the intracytoplasmic NALP3 (NOD-like receptor family, pyrin domain containing 3) receptor. NALP3, which contains a pyrin domain, a nucleotide-binding site (NBS) domain, and a leucine-rich repeat (LRR) motif, forms the inflammasome with an adaptor protein called ASC (apoptosis-associated speck-like protein containing a CARD, caspase recruitment domain) at the site of its pyrin domain (PYD) and pro-forms of caspases 1 and 5 [7–10]. The NALP3-inflammasome formed by these cascades truncates and activates interleukin (IL)-1β and IL-18 to trigger the inflammation and immune responses. The danger signals possessing crystalline structures activate the NLRP3 inflammasome in macrophages, leading to the production of IL-1β. Thus, the initial biological reactions unfolded when AM initially meets asbestos fibers resulting in the attraction of fibroblasts into the surrounding areas where AM is located by the action of secreted IL-1β [7–10].

The progression of these danger signals towards lung fibrosis is known as pneumoconiosis, as represented by silicosis and asbestosis, and involves important roles played by reactive oxygen species (ROS) and reactive nitrogen species (RNS) and inflammatory cytokines such as tumor necrosis factor (TNF)-α, transforming growth factor (TGF)-β, IL-6, as well as IL-1β secreted from AM as activated by asbestos fibers [11–14]. We previously reported details of these cytokine reactions following asbestos exposure and emphasized the crucial role of the long-surviving AM with higher production of TGF-β [6].

The abovementioned reactions begin to affect the human body after asbestos fibers are inhaled and start the development of lung fibrosis and/or other cancers.

11.2 Immunological Effects of Asbestos

11.2.1 Bi-Views of General Immunological Effects Caused by Asbestos

As mentioned above, we are beginning to obtain a better understanding of the initial local reactions occurring when asbestos is inhaled into the respiratory systems in regard to immunological reactions [7–10]. However, most of the fibers remain in the human body at the lung spaces, as well as the local lymph nodes, and continuously meet with circulating immune cells. These direct effects may therefore affect the asbestos-induced health impairments. Although researchers maintain there is inadequate regulation of autoimmunity that causes various autoimmune diseases in asbestos-exposed patients [15–18], we have been investigating this issue by focusing on silicosis patients [19–24] because of the incidence of complicated autoimmune diseases such as rheumatoid arthritis, systemic sclerosis, and antineutrophil cytoplasmic antibody-related vasculitis/nephritis [25–28]. Silica particles induce an unbalance between CD4+25+ regulatory T cells (Treg: positive for FOXP3 (forkhead box P3) gene) [29–31] and responder T cells to form reduction of Treg and the long survival of responder T cells. Details of these investigations have been described elsewhere [22–24].

A consideration of the occurrences of cancers may reveal that asbestos-exposed patients have reduced antitumor immunity and that this might be the reason why asbestos-related cancers show a long-term latency period of 30–40 years [1–5]. We therefore focused on the immunological investigation of the effects of asbestos on immune cells.

11.2.2 Immunological Effects of Asbestos on Natural Killer (NK) Cells and Cytotoxic T Lymphocytes (CTL)

We have been investigating the cellular and molecular effects of asbestos fibers on various immune cells. The effects of NK cells have been summarized previously [32–34]. Asbestos exposure causes impaired cytotoxicity of NK cells with reduction in the expression of activating receptors. Among such receptors, the NKp46 receptor was particularly crucial. We conducted experiments in which a human NK cell line and freshly isolated human NK cells derived from healthy donors

(HD) activated in vitro were cultured with chrysotile fibers [32–34]. Results showed that the cell line exhibited a reduction of NKG2D and 2B4 receptors, with a diminishing level of extracellular signal-regulated kinase (ERK) phosphorylation to signal the release of cytotoxic granules such as perforin and granzymes [32–34]. The in vitro activated NK cells showed decreased expression of NKG2D or NKp46, but not 2B4. Since the expression of some activating receptors was reduced as a whole, we analyzed the status of these receptors in asbestos-exposed patients such as those exhibiting pleural plaque (PP) and MM. Our results revealed that the reduced expression of NKp46 was clearly correlated with NK cell cytotoxicity in these patients and in healthy donors. These findings indicated that asbestos causes impairment of NK cell activity and may induce the unencumbered progression of transformed mesothelioma cells [32–34].

The effects of asbestos fibers on CTL and CD8+ T cells as naïve CTL is described in another chapter of this book [35]. Experiments involving in vitro exposure of chrysotile asbestos onto a mixed lymphocyte reaction (MLR) assay to estimate clonal expansion (proliferation and differentiation) of CD8+ T cells revealed the inhibition of both proliferation and differentiation [36]. These results should be interpreted as the impairment of CTL differentiation in the lymph nodes where asbestos fibers are located continuously in asbestos-exposed people. In addition, analyses of cellular functions in asbestos-exposed patients with pleural plaque (PP) and malignant mesothelioma (MM) are discussed. PP patients showed an increase in effector memory CD8+ T cells compared to healthy donors or MM patients [37]. Furthermore, MM patients showed a decrease in perforin-expressing CD8+ T cells. These results indicated that although asbestos-exposed individuals are ready to respond with transformed cells, CTLs may lose their function once mesothelioma progresses [35–37].

11.2.3 Effects of Asbestos Fibers on T Cells

11.2.3.1 Establishment of an Asbestos Exposure Cell-Line Model (Fig. 11.1)

There are numerous studies of the effects of asbestos fibers on alveolar epithelial cells and pleural mesothelial cells by transient and relatively high (as a means to cause cellular toxicity) doses of asbestos [38–47]. Most of these reports showed the importance of ROS/RNS in causing DNA damage and activation of the mitochondrial apoptotic pathway to cause cell death. It was then suggested that certain molecular changes trigger escape from the apoptotic pathway with persistent DNA damage during long-term, chronic, and recurrent exposure following the continuous presence of asbestos fibers in the body. This could be interpreted as carcinogenesis. The carcinogenic effects of asbestos fibers are regarded as (a) ROS/RNS mainly produced by iron contained in fibers, (b) physiological damage of

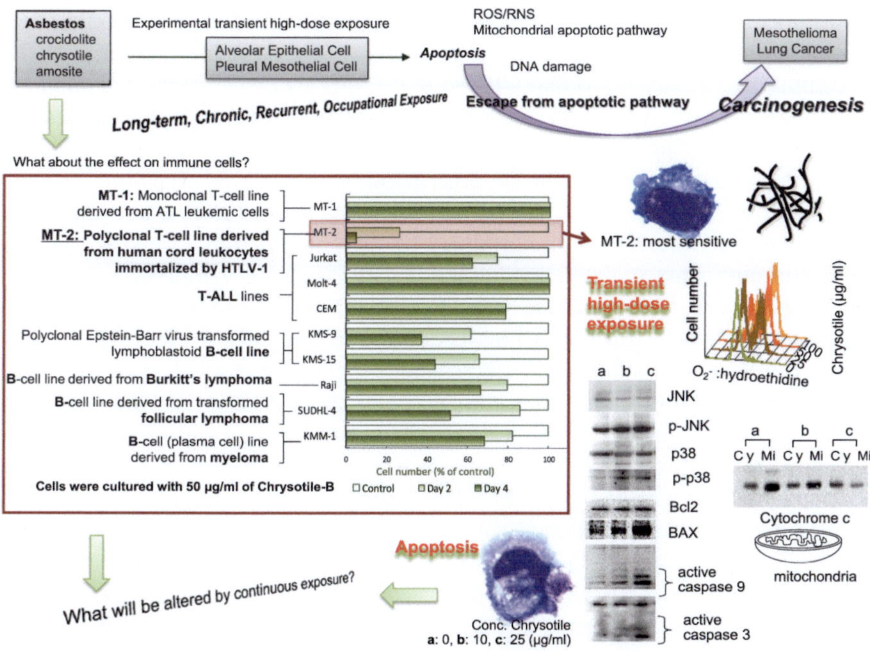

Fig. 11.1 Schematic model showing the effects of asbestos fibers on alveolar epithelial and pleural mesothelial cells, on which production of ROS/RNS causes DNA damage, and the appearance of induced apoptosis and escape from these cellular changes as recognized steps of asbestos-induced carcinogenesis and their effects on human immune cells. The initial experiments were designed to examine the growth inhibitory effects of chrysotile asbestos on various human cell lines, including transformed B or T cell lines and virus-immortalized B or T cell lines. Our findings led us to select MT-2 as the candidate cell line for an analysis of the effects of asbestos on T cells. The transient and high-dose exposure of chrysotile on MT-2 cells causes production of ROS, activation of mitochondrial apoptotic pathways including proapoptotic activation of MAP kinase signaling, and subsequent apoptosis

cellular chromatins and genes by fiber tangling, and (c) adsorption of other carcinogenic agents around the fiber bodies [48–50].

We attempted to establish a continuous and long-term exposure model of asbestos exposure on human T cells to investigate the chronic alteration of T cells caused by fibers as shown in Fig. 11.1. After first determining to use the candidate cell lines including those derived from T cells and B cells (listed in Fig. 11.1), we performed experiments using an initial transient and high-dose (as a means of causing certain toxic effects such as cell damage and cell death caused by fibers) exposure for several culture days [51]. Chrysotile B asbestos was initially selected because of its common usage (more than 90% of utilized asbestos) worldwide. Furthermore, we investigated whether iron-containing fibers such as crocidolite and amosite induce dominant cellular effects on cells due to the presence of iron [1–5].

Results revealed that most of the cell lines from malignant cells, including those derived from T and B cells, were not sensitive to 50 μg/ml of chrysotile B. The concentration was similar to that utilized in the various abovementioned published experiments that used alveolar and mesothelial cells while changing "$\mu g/cm^2$" in culture dishes to "μg/ml" because of the difference between adhered cells and floating hematological cells. On the other hand, we employed virus-immortalized cell lines such as KMS-9 and KMS-15, which are our own established lymphoblastoid B cell lines immortalized by the Epstein-Barr virus [52], and the MT-2 cell line immortalized by human T cell leukemia/lymphoma virus type 1 (HTLV-1). The Mt-2 cell line was most sensitive to asbestos-induced growth inhibition. The MT-2 cell line, which is derived from CD4+ T cells [53, 54], was therefore selected for subsequent studies since the T cell is much more important for antitumor immunity and immortalized cells show greater resemblance to the human immune counterparts rather than cells in transformed cell lines.

Growth retardation of MT-2 by asbestos exposure was analyzed. Cells that died by apoptosis were verified by a TUNEL assay and morphological observations. Cellular and molecular changes were then investigated. The production of O_2- (hydroethidine), phosphorylation of JNK (c-Jun N-terminal kinases) and p38 signaling molecule-mediated proapoptotic MAPK (mitogen-activated protein kinases), release of cytochrome c from mitochondria, increase of the BAX/Bcl-2 expression ratio, and activation of caspases 9 and 3 were found in a dose-dependent manner relative to the added chrysotile concentrations [51].

These results indicated that the human T cell model MT-2 exhibited asbestos-induced apoptosis similar to that reported for alveolar and mesothelial cells. The next task was to determine changes caused by the continuous and long-term exposure to chrysotile in MT-2.

11.2.3.2 Cellular Features of Continuously Exposed Sublines (Fig. 11.2)

The MT-2 cell line (original cell line: ORG) was exposed continuously to 5 or 10 μg/ml of chrysotile. These concentrations were determined through trials in which less than half of the cells died from the induced apoptosis [55]. After the chrysotile fibers were removed from the culture and cultured without fibers, the MT-2 continuously exposed subline cells (MT-2CE) were examined every month and the level of apoptosis following exposure to 0–50 μg/ml of chrysotile was determined and compared to that of MT-2ORG cells. MT-2CE cells showed a significantly lower level of apoptosis after eight months, indicating that the cells of this subline acquired resistance to the asbestos-induced apoptosis [55]. Cellular and molecular characterizations were then made, which revealed that the MT-2CE cells showed (a) enhanced production of IL-10 and TGF-β, (b) excess phosphorylation of STAT3 located downstream of IL-10 (autocrine usage of IL-10), (c) upregulation of Bcl-2 and downregulation of BAX, (d) acquisition of resistance to TGFβ-induced growth inhibition, and (e) increased p38 phosphorylation located downstream of TGF-β signaling (Fig. 11.2) [55, 56].

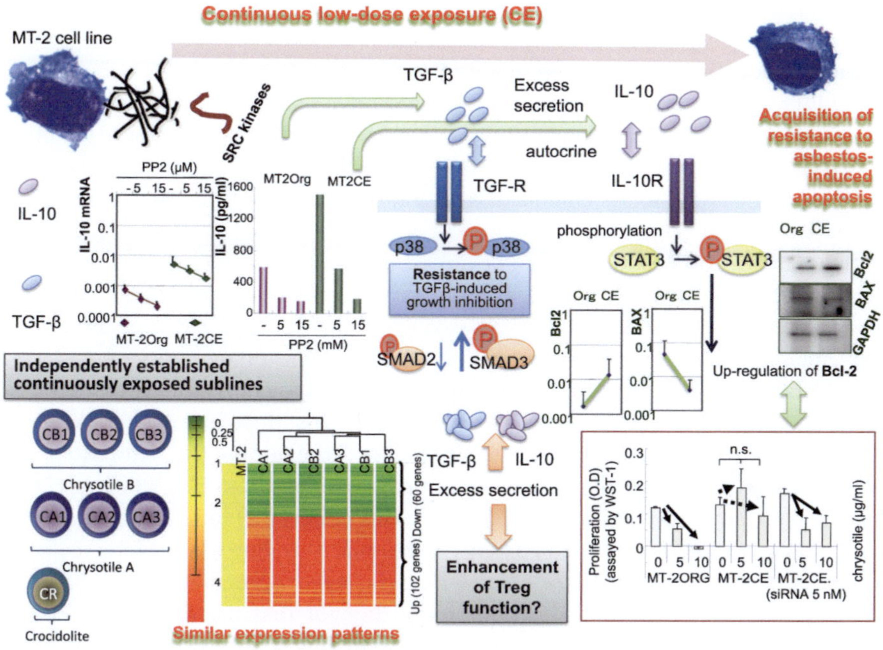

Fig. 11.2 Establishment of MT-2 sublines continuously exposed to asbestos (CB1–3, CA1-3, and CR). The continuous and low-dose exposure of chrysotile onto the MT-2 cell line yielded a subline that exhibited resistance to asbestos-induced apoptosis and was designated MT-2CE. This subline was later named CB1 after another six sublines were established independently. The MT-2CE subline exhibited excess production of TGF-β following p38 phosphorylation and resistance to TGF-β-induced growth inhibition. Furthermore, this subline showed excess production of IL-10 causing phosphorylation of STAT3 and upregulation of Bcl-2. The importance of Bcl-2 for the acquisition of resistance to asbestos-induced apoptosis was confirmed using siRNA for Bcl-2 in the subline. The six independently established chrysotile-exposed sublines showed similar mRNA expression patterns when assayed by cDNA microarrays

Regarding the IL-10 to Bcl-2 scenario, the importance of Src kinases was verified by an assay using the Src-kinase-specific inhibitor PP2. This inhibitor reduced mRNA expression and secretion of IL-10 in both MT-2ORG and MT-2CE cells. In addition, the crucial role of Bcl-2 was assayed using siRNA for Bcl-2. The Bcl-2 silenced clones of the MT-2CE subline revealed significant growth inhibition due to re-coculture with chrysotile fibers [55].

For the TGF-β-scenario, MT-2CE cells showed excess production of TGF-β and a reduced growth inhibitory property with reduced expression of TGF receptor 2. As already mentioned above, the MAPK signaling molecules such as ERK2, p38, and JNK were phosphorylated when MT-2ORG was exposed to chrysotile, and MT-2CE cells maintained only p38 phosphorylation which was canceled in the TGF-β knockdown MT-2CE clones. In addition, MT-2CE cells showed a decrease of phosphorylation of SMAD2 and increase of phosphorylation of SMAD3, and both of these molecules are also signaling molecules located downstream of TGF-β.

However, these SMAD2/3 changes were not altered in TGF-β knockdown MT-2CE clones [55, 56].

Furthermore, excess secretion of both IL-10 and TGF-β suggested an interesting possibility because both cytokines are typical soluble factors of Treg [29–31]. Thus, an evaluation of Treg function as altered by continuous exposure to asbestos fibers is needed since Treg plays an important role in antitumor immunity, and if its numbers and/or function is enhanced by some factors, the antitumor immunity has to be reduced [29–31].

Since these observations were performed using only the MT-2CE subline, we tried to establish other continuously exposed sublines. We established two more independently established sublines exposed to chrysotile B (the first one used in the abovementioned experiments was called CB1, and the other two sublines were called CB2 and CB3) and three other sublines exposed to chrysotile A (called CA1, CA2, and CA3) [57]. Chrysotile A and B show tiny differences in which iron contents are slightly higher in chrysotile B [58]. To examine the similarities and differences among these six sublines continuously exposed to chrysotile, a cDNA microarray assay was performed [57]. The results (Fig. 11.2) indicated that most of the upregulated and downregulated genes were similar among the six sublines when compared with the MT-2ORG line. 84 genes were upregulated and 55 were downregulated. In addition, it is commonly thought that the carcinogenicity of crocidolite is approximately 500 times higher than that of chrysotile because of the difference in iron contents and physical properties [1–5]. The usage of these continuously exposed sublines may indicate changes in T cells of asbestos-exposed patients such as PP and MM. Therefore, the cellular and molecular characterizations of these sublines were analyzed and compared with MT-2ORG, which has never been exposed to asbestos fibers [55, 57].

11.2.3.3 Cellular Effects of Chrysotile and Crocidolite on T Cell and Protein Expression (Fig. 11.3)

Since most of the asbestos fibers used in the world are those of chrysotile, a serpentine material, this fiber was initially used for observations of its immunological effects on T cells, although we should not ignore the amphibole forms of asbestos such as amosite and crocidolite [59]. As mentioned above, carcinogenicity is thought to be significantly higher for amphibole than chrysotile. We therefore compared differences and similarities of cellular alterations between MT-2ORG cells exposed to chrysotile and those exposed to crocidolite. For the transient exposure experiments, the degrees of growth inhibition and appearance of apoptosis (assayed by staining with annexin V on Day 2, detection of active caspase 3 on Day 3, and TUNEL staining on Day 4) were much higher when MT-2ORG cells were exposed to chrysotile rather than crocidolite. Although the production of ROS was higher in cells exposed to crocidolite rather than chrysotile, the overall level of apoptosis and observed mechanisms were similar between cells exposed to the two asbestos fibers [59].

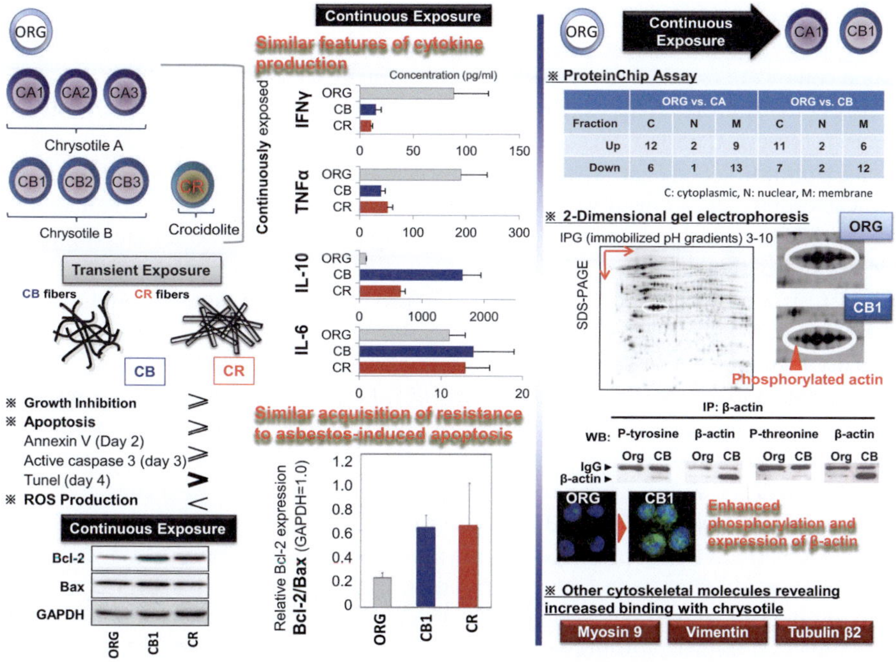

Fig. 11.3 The acquisition of resistance to asbestos-induced apoptosis was also verified in the subline MT-2CR, which was continuously exposed to crocidolite (CR) asbestos for more than one year. The transient exposure caused growth inhibition and apoptosis with production of ROS. The degrees of these changes differed slightly between chrysotile B (CB) and CR exposures, whereas the tendencies of cellular changes were similar. In addition, cytokine profile levels and activation of Bcl-2 were also observed changes in MT-2CB1 and MT-2CR sublines when compared with MT2ORG cells, which were never exposed to asbestos fibers. In addition to the cDNA microarray analysis, the differences and similarities among MT-2ORG, MT-2CBa, and CA1 sublines were examined. The ProteinChip assay revealed that up- and downregulated proteins in the cytoplasmic, nuclear, and membrane fractions of the CA1 and CB1 sublines were similar to those of the MT-2ORG line. A 2-dimensional gel electrophoresis assay revealed enhanced phosphorylation of β-actin in the CB1 subline in comparison to the MT-2ORG line. Moreover, various cytoskeletal molecules were also upregulated in the continuously exposed subline. The overall findings indicate the importance of cytoskeletal molecules for initiation of the cellular and molecular alterations

A subline of MT-2 exposed continuously was then established and named the CR subline, as mentioned above. As with the sublines continuously exposed to chrysotile, the acquisition of resistance to asbestos-induced apoptosis was monitored monthly, and the continuously exposed subline was then examined after more than one year [59]. Some properties of the continuously exposed sublines in the CB series were then examined (Fig. 11.3). Cytokine production showed a similar tendency between CB1 and CR sublines. The cytokine profile showed reduced secretion of interferon (IFN)-γ and TNF-α, markedly increased production of IL-10 (although CB was producing this cytokine to a high level), and no change of IL-6 [59]. Furthermore, upregulation of the Bcl-2/BAX expression ratio was also observed in the MT-2CR subline. The overall results indicate that the effects of crocidolite on the human T cell CD4+ were similar to those caused by chrysotile when cells were exposed to asbestos fibers continuously with a relatively low dose. Data of cDNA arrays (Org vs. CB1 and Org vs. CR) showed that commonly altered genes represented 650 of 2,074 total genes uniquely altered in the first set and 1,970 genes from the second set. In addition, network analyses using a cDNA array assay indicated both sets showed very similar transcription factors in which the numbers of expressed molecules, including alternative splice variants, were ranked highly, i.e., HNF4-α (hepatocyte nuclear factor 4α), SP1 (specificity protein 1), c-Myc, ESR1 (estrogen receptor 1 (α)), CREB1 (CAMP-responsive element-binding protein), and others [59].

The differences and similarities of protein expression between CB1 and CA1 were assayed using the ProteinChip assay [60]. Figure 11.3 shows that the tendencies of up- and downregulated proteins were almost similar to those of the MT-2ORG line, and as mentioned above, the differences between chrysotile A and B were very slight. These results therefore seemed to be reasonable [60]. An attempt to identify some altered protein in the CB1 subline in comparison to the ORG line yielded a single change as shown by the spot in the figure. This alteration was then identified as excess phosphorylation of β-actin, as well as higher expression of β-actin in protein and mRNA levels [60]. This may be explained by assuming that the asbestos fibers were not incorporated into the intracellular spaces, and the change in cellular and molecular functions was supposedly caused by the initial and recurrent and continuous and chronic attachments between fibers and cell surface molecules. Therefore, modification of cytoskeletal molecules is the most considerable change occurring in continuously exposed sublines [60]. In response to these considerations, a cell-free binding assay was performed on extracted proteins derived from ORG and CB1 cells exposed to the chrysotile fibers. Results showed increased levels of several cytoskeletal molecules such as myosin 9, vimentin, and tubulin β2. The assays analyzing alteration of proteins indicated that cytoskeletal molecules may be the initial and continuous targets of the effects of asbestos that induce the cellular and molecular changes of cell functions [60].

11.2.3.4 Reduced Expression of CXCR3 Caused by Asbestos Exposure in T Cells

Pathway and network analyses using data from the cDNA microarray shown in Fig. 11.2 reveal the interesting reduction of CXCR3 (C-X-C chemokine receptor type 3) expression in sublines continuously exposed to asbestos in comparison to MT-2ORG cells [57, 61]. We then analyzed the importance of the role played by the expression of CXCR3 and its related cytokine IFN-γ in antitumor immunity. The mRNA and protein levels of CXCR3 expression were again confirmed by real-time RT-PCR, a flow cytometric assay, and immunohistochemical analysis and compared with those of MT-2ORG cells [57, 61]. All six sublines continuously exposed to chrysotile showed reduced expression of CXCR3 (Fig. 11.4). In addition, IFN-γ

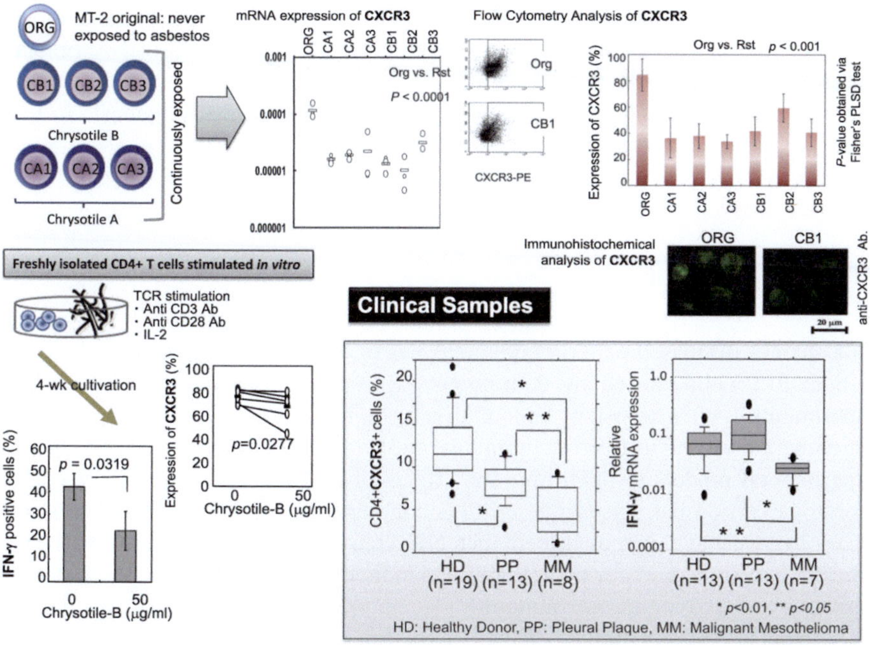

Fig. 11.4 Pathway and network analyses using data from the cDNA microarrays shown in Fig. 11.2 show the interesting reduction of CXCR3 (C-X-C chemokine receptor type 3) expression in sublines continuously exposed to asbestos when compared to MT-2ORG cells. All sublines exhibited reduction of XCXR3 expression at mRNA and protein levels. Furthermore, freshly isolated peripheral CD4+ cells stimulated in vitro also showed reduction of CXCR3 and IFN-γ. Finally, these findings were confirmed when using freshly isolated peripheral CD4+ cells derived from asbestos-exposed patients with PP and MM. These results indicated that our continuously exposed model is suitable for the observation of cellular and molecular alterations caused by continuous exposure to asbestos fibers and that it can be utilized for effective clinical implementations for the early detection of exposed patients and improvement of diminished antitumor immunity in asbestos-exposed patients for the prevention of cancers

production in the culture supernatants also decreased in the six sublines compared to that of the MT-2ORG line. The changes were then examined in freshly isolated peripheral blood CD4+ T cells derived from HD stimulated with anti-CD3 and CD28 monoclonal antibodies and IL-2 for 4 weeks with or without chrysotile fibers. Results showed that the reduction of CXCR3 surface expression and intracellular IFN-γ positive cells decreased significantly when cells were cultured with chrysotile (Fig. 11.4) [57, 61]. The CXCR3 expression of peripheral blood CD4+ cells from asbestos-exposed patients such as PP and MM was then analyzed. Our findings revealed that CD4+CXCR3+ cells in CD4+ cells were significantly reduced in PP compared with HD and in MM compared with HD and PP. In addition, the relative IFN-γ-mRNA expression in these cells decreased in MM compared with PP and HD. These results indicated that our established MT-2 sublines that were continuously exposed to asbestos exhibited altered cellular characteristics in peripheral blood T cells caused by asbestos exposure [57, 61]. These observations and the abovementioned impairment of NK cells and CTL cell functions indicated that antitumor immunity in asbestos-exposed patients was reduced, and this may be part of the factors causing carcinogenesis in these patients with a very long latency period [62–65].

11.3 Conclusion

This chapter discussed experimental analyses of cellular and molecular alterations in human T cells caused by continuous exposure to asbestos. Instead of using experiments with a transient and relatively high-dose exposure to asbestos, our experimental setting utilized a continuous and relatively low-dose exposure to yield experimental models to determine the effects of asbestos on peripheral T cells in asbestos-exposed patients. Although this chapter presented details of T cell modifications, we have demonstrated that NK cells and CTL were also altered by asbestos exposure, and our overall findings indicated that asbestos-exposed patients possess a reduced antitumor immunity [34, 35, 62–64].

A clinical implementation of these experimental findings would be to extract modified cytokines, proteins, and genes altered by chronic, continuous, and recurrent asbestos exposure in peripheral blood immune cells for the development of an early detection screening device for asbestos exposure and the occurrence of malignant tumors in these patients. This will support screening for people who reside or have resided near asbestos-handling manufacturers, as well as building demolition workers or laborers handling rubble resulting from an earthquake or other disasters. Another approach would be to recover reduced antitumor immunity in immune cells caused by asbestos exposure using certain physiologically active substances derived from plants, foods, or other structural components of microorganisms.

Future investigations will examine the effects of asbestos on other immune cells such as dendritic, Th17, and NKT cells in order to understand the whole status of antitumor immunity. A comprehensive understanding of the immunological effects of asbestos will then follow and form the basis of effective clinical implementations and investigations of other fibrous and particulate substances such as silica, nanoparticles, and nanotubes.

Acknowledgements The authors thank Ms. Tamayo Hatayama, Minako Katoh, and Naomi Miyahara for their technical assistance. All the experimental findings performed in the Department of Hygiene, Kawasaki Medical School, were supported by Special Coordination Funds for Promoting Science and Technology grant H18-1-3-3-1; JPSS KAKENHI grants 19790411 and 22700933; Kawasaki Medical School Project grants 18-209T, 19-205Y, 20-210O, 21–201, and 22-A58; the Kawasaki Foundation for Medical Science and Medical Welfare (2007); the Science Research Promotion Fund (2010); and the Ryobi Teien Memorial Foundation (2008).

References

1. Oury TD, Thomas A, Sporn TA, Roggli VL, editors. Pathology of asbestos-associated diseases. 3rd ed. New York: Springer; 2014.
2. Soto A, Salazar G, editors. Asbestos: risks, environment and impact, Environmental health – physical chemical and biological factors series. New York: Nova Science Pub Inc; 2009.
3. Institute of Medicine (U. S.), Committee on Asbestos: Selected Health Effects. Asbestos: selected cancers. Washington, DC: National Academy Press; 2006.
4. Dodson RF, Samuel P, Hammar SP, editors. Asbestos: risk assessment, epidemiology, and health effects. 2nd ed. Boca Raton: CRC Press; 2011.
5. Craighead JE, Gibbs AR, editors. Asbestos and its diseases. New York: Oxford University Press; 2008.
6. Nishimura Y, Nishiike-Wada T, Wada Y, Miura Y, Otsuki T, Iguchi H. Long-lasting production of TGF-beta1 by alveolar macrophages exposed to low doses of asbestos without apoptosis. Int J Immunopathol Pharmacol. 2007;20:661–71.
7. Agostini L, Martinon F, Burns K, McDermott MF, Hawkins PN, Tschopp J. NALP3 forms an IL-1beta-processing inflammasome with increased activity in Muckle-Wells autoinflammatory disorder. Immunity. 2004;20:319–25.
8. Dostert C, Pétrilli V, Van Bruggen R, Steele C, Mossman BT, Tschopp J. Innate immune activation through Nalp3 inflammasome sensing of asbestos and silica. Science. 2008;320:674–7. doi:10.1126/science.1156995.
9. Cassel SL, Eisenbarth SC, Iyer SS, Sadler JJ, Colegio OR, Tephly LA, Carter AB, Rothman PB, Flavell RA, Sutterwala FS. The Nalp3 inflammasome is essential for the development of silicosis. Proc Natl Acad Sci U S A. 2008;105:9035–40. doi:10.1073/pnas.0803933105.
10. Pétrilli V, Dostert C, Muruve DA, Tschopp J. The inflammasome: a danger sensing complex triggering innate immunity. Curr Opin Immunol. 2007;19:615–22.
11. Shukla A, Gulumian M, Hei TK, Kamp D, Rahman Q, Mossman BT. Multiple roles of oxidants in the pathogenesis of asbestos-induced diseases. Free Radic Biol Med. 2003;34:1117–29.
12. Upadhyay D, Kamp DW. Asbestos-induced pulmonary toxicity: role of DNA damage and apoptosis. Exp Biol Med (Maywood). 2003;228:650–9.
13. Fubini B, Hubbard A. Reactive oxygen species (ROS) and reactive nitrogen species (RNS) generation by silica in inflammation and fibrosis. Free Radic Biol Med. 2003;34:1507–16.
14. Valavanidis A, Vlachogianni T, Fiotakis K, Loridas S. Pulmonary oxidative stress, inflammation and cancer: respirable particulate matter, fibrous dusts and ozone as major causes of lung carcinogenesis through reactive oxygen species mechanisms. Int J Environ Res Public Health. 2013;10:3886–907. doi:10.3390/ijerph10093886.
15. Rosenthal GJ, Simeonova P, Corsini E. Asbestos toxicity: an immunologic perspective. Rev Environ Health. 1999;14:11–20.
16. Pfau JC, Sentissi JJ, Weller G, Putnam EA. Assessment of autoimmune responses associated with asbestos exposure in Libby, Montana, USA. Environ Health Perspect. 2005;113:25–30.
17. Noonan CW, Pfau JC, Larson TC, Spence MR. Nested case–control study of autoimmune disease in an asbestos-exposed population. Environ Health Perspect. 2006;114:1243–7.
18. Pfau JC, Serve KM, Noonan CW. Autoimmunity and asbestos exposure. Autoimmune Dis. 2014;2014:782045. doi:10.1155/2014/782045.
19. Otsuki T, Miura Y, Nishimura Y, Hyodoh F, Takata A, Kusaka M, Katsuyama H, Tomita M, Ueki A, Kishimoto T. Alterations of Fas and Fas-related molecules in patients with silicosis. Exp Biol Med (Maywood). 2006;231:522–33.
20. Wu P, Miura Y, Hyodoh F, Nishimura Y, Hatayama T, Hatada S, Sakaguchi H, Kusaka M, Katsuyama H, Tomita M, Otsuki T. Reduced function of CD4+25+ regulatory T cell fraction in silicosis patients. Int J Immunopathol Pharmacol. 2006;19(2):357–68.

21. Hayashi H, Maeda M, Murakami S, Kumagai N, Chen Y, Hatayama T, Katoh M, Miyahara N, Yamamoto S, Yoshida Y, Nishimura Y, Kusaka M, Fujimoto W, Otsuki T. Soluble interleukin-2 receptor as an indicator of immunological disturbance found in silicosis patients. Int J Immunopathol Pharmacol. 2009;22:53–62.
22. Hayashi H, Miura Y, Maeda M, Murakami S, Kumagai N, Nishimura Y, Kusaka M, Urakami K, Fujimoto W, Otsuki T. Reductive alteration of the regulatory function of the CD4(+)CD25(+) T cell fraction in silicosis patients. Int J Immunopathol Pharmacol. 2010;23:1099–109.
23. Lee S, Hayashi H, Maeda M, Chen Y, Matsuzaki H, Takei-Kumagai N, Nishimura Y, Fujimoto W, Otsuki T. Environmental factors producing autoimmune dysregulation–chronic activation of T cells caused by silica exposure. Immunobiology. 2012;217:743–8. doi:10.1016/j.imbio.2011.12.009.
24. Lee S, Matsuzaki H, Kumagai-Takei N, Yoshitome K, Maeda M, Chen Y, Kusaka M, Urakami K, Hayashi H, Fujimoto W, Nishimura Y, Otsuki T. Silica exposure and altered regulation of autoimmunity. Environ Health Prev Med. 2014;19:322–9. doi:10.1007/s12199-014-0403-9.
25. Benedek TG. Rheumatoid pneumoconiosis. Documentation of onset and pathogenic considerations. Am J Med. 1973;55:515–24.
26. Uber CL, McReynolds RA. Immunotoxicology of silica. Crit Rev Toxicol. 1982;10:303–19.
27. Steenland K, Goldsmith DF. Silica exposure and autoimmune diseases. Am J Ind Med. 1995;28:603–8.
28. Shanklin DR, Smalley DL. The immunopathology of siliconosis. History, clinical presentation, and relation to silicosis and the chemistry of silicon and silicone. Immunol Res. 1998;18:125–73.
29. Fehérvari Z, Sakaguchi S. Development and function of CD25+CD4+ regulatory T cells. Curr Opin Immunol. 2004;16(2):203–8.
30. Hori S, Sakaguchi S. Foxp3: a critical regulator of the development and function of regulatory T cells. Microbes Infect. 2004;6:745–51.
31. Thompson C, Powrie F. Regulatory T cells. Curr Opin Pharmacol. 2004;4:408–14.
32. Nishimura Y, Miura Y, Maeda M, Kumagai N, Murakami S, Hayashi H, Fukuoka K, Nakano T, Otsuki T. Impairment in cytotoxicity and expression of NK cell- activating receptors on human NK cells following exposure to asbestos fibers. Int J Immunopathol Pharmacol. 2009;22:579–90.
33. Nishimura Y, Maeda M, Kumagai N, Hayashi H, Miura Y, Otsuki T. Decrease in phosphorylation of ERK following decreased expression of NK cell-activating receptors in human NK cell line exposed to asbestos. Int J Immunopathol Pharmacol. 2009;22:879–88.
34. Nishimura Y, Maeda M, Kumagai-Takei N, Lee S, Matsuzaki H, Wada Y, Nishiike-Wada T, Iguchi H, Otsuki T. Altered functions of alveolar macrophages and NK cells involved in asbestos-related diseases. Environ Health Prev Med. 2013;18:198–204. doi:10.1007/s12199-013-0333-y.
35. Kumagai-Takei N, Nishimura Y, Matsuzaki H, Maeda M, Lee S, Yoshitome K, Otsuki T. Effects of asbestos fibers on human cytotoxic T cells. In: Otsuki T, Holian A, Yoshioka Y, editors. Biological effects of fibrous and particulate substances. Tokyo: Springer; 2015. doi:10.1007/978-4-431-55732-6_12.
36. Kumagai-Takei N, Nishimura Y, Maeda M, Hayashi H, Matsuzaki H, Lee S, Hiratsuka J, Otsuki T. Effect of asbestos exposure on differentiation of cytotoxic T lymphocytes in mixed lymphocyte reaction of human peripheral blood mononuclear cells. Am J Respir Cell Mol Biol. 2013;49:28–36. doi:10.1165/rcmb.2012-0134OC.
37. Kumagai-Takei N, Nishimura Y, Maeda M, Hayashi H, Matsuzaki H, Lee S, Kishimoto T, Fukuoka K, Nakano T, Otsuki T. Functional properties of CD8(+) lymphocytes in patients with pleural plaque and malignant mesothelioma. J Immunol Res. 2014;2014:670140. doi:10.1155/2014/670140.

38. Kamp DW, Graceffa P, Pryor WA, Weitzman SA. The role of free radicals in asbestos-induced diseases. Free Radic Biol Med. 1992;12:293–315.
39. Jung M, Davis WP, Taatjes DJ, Churg A, Mossman BT. Asbestos and cigarette smoke cause increased DNA strand breaks and necrosis in bronchiolar epithelial cells in vivo. Free Radic Biol Med. 2000;28:1295–9.
40. Aljandali A, Pollack H, Yeldandi A, Li Y, Weitzman SA, Kamp DW. Asbestos causes apoptosis in alveolar epithelial cells: role of iron-induced free radicals. J Lab Clin Med. 2001;137:330–9.
41. Riganti C, Aldieri E, Bergandi L, Fenoglio I, Costamagna C, Fubini B, Bosia A, Ghigo D. Crocidolite asbestos inhibits pentose phosphate oxidative pathway and glucose 6-phosphate dehydrogenase activity in human lung epithelial cells. Free Radic Biol Med. 2002;32:938–49.
42. Panduri V, Weitzman SA, Chandel N, Kamp DW. The mitochondria-regulated death pathway mediates asbestos-induced alveolar epithelial cell apoptosis. Am J Respir Cell Mol Biol. 2003;28:241–8.
43. Kamp DW, Panduri VA, Weitzman SA, Chandel N. Asbestos-induced alveolar epithelial cell apoptosis: role of mitochondrial dysfunction caused by iron-derived free radicals. Mol Cell Biochem. 2002;234–235:153–60.
44. Yang H, Rivera Z, Jube S, Nasu M, Bertino P, Goparaju C, Franzoso G, Lotze MT, Krausz T, Pass HI, Bianchi ME, Carbone M. Programmed necrosis induced by asbestos in human mesothelial cells causes high-mobility group box 1 protein release and resultant inflammation. Proc Natl Acad Sci U S A. 2010;107:12611–6. doi:10.1073/pnas.1006542107.
45. Poser I, Rahman Q, Lohani M, Yadav S, Becker HH, Weiss DG, Schiffmann D, Dopp E. Modulation of genotoxic effects in asbestos-exposed primary human mesothelial cells by radical scavengers, metal chelators and a glutathione precursor. Mutat Res. 2004;559:19–27.
46. Aung W, Hasegawa S, Furukawa T, Saga T. Potential role of ferritin heavy chain in oxidative stress and apoptosis in human mesothelial and mesothelioma cells: implications for asbestos-induced oncogenesis. Carcinogenesis. 2007;28:2047–52.
47. Pacurari M, Yin XJ, Zhao J, Ding M, Leonard SS, Schwegler-Berry D, Ducatman BS, Sbarra D, Hoover MD, Castranova V, Vallyathan V. Raw single-wall carbon nanotubes induce oxidative stress and activate MAPKs, AP-1, NF-kappaB, and Akt in normal and malignant human mesothelial cells. Environ Health Perspect. 2008;116:1211–7. doi:10.1289/ehp.10924.
48. Toyokuni S. Role of iron in carcinogenesis: cancer as a ferrotoxic disease. Cancer Sci. 2009;100:9–16. doi:10.1111/j.1349-7006.2008.01001.x.
49. Toyokuni S. Iron overload as a major targetable pathogenesis of asbestos-induced mesothelial carcinogenesis. Redox Rep. 2014;19:1–7. doi:10.1179/1351000213Y.0000000075.
50. Toyokuni S. Mechanisms of asbestos-induced carcinogenesis. Nagoya J Med Sci. 2009;71:1–10.
51. Hyodoh F, Takata-Tomokuni A, Miura Y, Sakaguchi H, Hatayama T, Hatada S, Katsuyama H, Matsuo Y, Otsuki T. Inhibitory effects of anti-oxidants on apoptosis of a human polyclonal T cell line, MT-2, induced by an asbestos, chrysotile-A. Scand J Immunol. 2005;61:442–8.
52. Otsuki T, Yata K, Takata-Tomokuni A, Hyodoh F, Miura Y, Sakaguchi H, Hatayama T, Hatada S, Tsujioka T, Sato Y, Murakami H, Sadahira Y, Sugihara T. Expression of protein gene product 9.5 (PGP9.5)/ubiquitin-C-terminal hydrolase 1 (UCHL-1) in human myeloma cells. Br J Haematol. 2004;127:292–8.
53. Miyoshi I, Kubonishi I, Yoshimoto S, Shiraishi Y. A T cell line derived from normal human cord leukocytes by co-culturing with human leukemic T cells. Gan. 1981;72:978–81.
54. Miyoshi I, Kubonishi I, Yoshimoto S, Akagi T, Ohtsuki Y, Shiraishi Y, Nagata K, Hinuma Y. Type C virus particles in a cord T cell line derived by co-cultivating normal human cord leukocytes and human leukaemic T cells. Nature. 1981;294:770–1.

55. Miura Y, Nishimura Y, Katsuyama H, Maeda M, Hayashi H, Dong M, Hyodoh F, Tomita M, Matsuo Y, Uesaka A, Kuribayashi K, Nakano T, Kishimoto T, Otsuki T. Involvement of IL-10 and Bcl-2 in resistance against an asbestos-induced apoptosis of T cells. Apoptosis. 2006;11:1825–35.
56. Maeda M, Chen Y, Hayashi H, Kumagai-Takei N, Matsuzaki H, Lee S, Nishimura Y, Otsuki T. Chronic exposure to asbestos enhances TGF-β1 production in the human adult T cell leukemia virus-immortalized T cell line MT-2. Int J Oncol. 2014;45:2522–32. doi:10.3892/ijo.2014.2682.
57. Maeda M, Nishimura Y, Hayashi H, Kumagai N, Chen Y, Murakami S, Miura Y, Hiratsuka J, Kishimoto T, Otsuki T. Reduction of CXC chemokine receptor 3 in an in vitro model of continuous exposure to asbestos in a human T cell line, MT-2. Am J Respir Cell Mol Biol. 2011;45:470–9. doi:10.1165/rcmb.2010-0213OC.
58. Kohyama N, Shinohara Y, Suzuki Y. Mineral phases and some reexamined characteristics of the International Union against cancer standard asbestos samples. Am J Ind Med. 1996;30:515–28.
59. Maeda M, Yamamoto S, Chen Y, Kumagai-Takei N, Hayashi H, Matsuzaki H, Lee S, Hatayama T, Miyahara N, Katoh M, Hiratsuka J, Nishimura Y, Otsuki T. Resistance to asbestos-induced apoptosis with continuous exposure to crocidolite on a human T cell. Sci Total Environ. 2012;429:174–82. doi:10.1016/j.scitotenv.2012.04.043.
60. Maeda M, Chen Y, Kumagai-Takei N, Hayashi H, Matsuzaki H, Lee S, Hiratsuka J, Nishimura Y, Kimura Y, Otsuki T. Alteration of cytoskeletal molecules in a human T cell line caused by continuous exposure to chrysotile asbestos. Immunobiology. 2013;218:1184–91. doi:10.1016/j.imbio.2013.04.007.
61. Maeda M, Nishimura Y, Hayashi H, Kumagai N, Chen Y, Murakami S, Miura Y, Hiratsuka J, Kishimoto T, Otsuki T. Decreased CXCR3 expression in CD4+ T cells exposed to asbestos or derived from asbestosexposed patients. Am J Respir Cell Mol Biol. 2011;45:795–803. doi:10.1165/rcmb.2010-0435OC.
62. Otsuki T, Maeda M, Murakami S, Hayashi H, Miura Y, Kusaka M, Nakano T, Fukuoka K, Kishimoto T, Hyodoh F, Ueki A, Nishimura Y. Immunological effects of silica and asbestos. Cell Mol Immunol. 2007;4:261–8.
63. Maeda M, Nishimura Y, Kumagai N, Hayashi H, Hatayama T, Katoh M, Miyahara N, Yamamoto S, Hirastuka J, Otsuki T. Dysregulation of the immune system caused by silica and asbestos. J Immunotoxicol. 2010;7:268–78. doi:10.3109/1547691X.2010.512579.
64. Kumagai-Takei N, Maeda M, Chen Y, Matsuzaki H, Lee S, Nishimura Y, Hiratsuka J, Otsuki T. Asbestos induces reduction of tumor immunity. Clin Dev Immunol. 2011;2011:481439. doi:10.1155/2011/481439.
65. Matsuzaki H, Maeda M, Lee S, Nishimura Y, Kumagai-Takei N, Hayashi H, Yamamoto S, Hatayama T, Kojima Y, Tabata R, Kishimoto T, Hiratsuka J, Otsuki T. Asbestos-induced cellular and molecular alteration of immunocompetent cells and their relationship with chronic inflammation and carcinogenesis. J Biomed Biotechnol. 2012;2012:492608. doi:10.1155/2012/492608.

Chapter 12
Effects of Asbestos Fibers on Human Cytotoxic T Cells

Naoko Kumagai-Takei, Yasumitsu Nishimura, Hidenori Matsuzaki, Megumi Maeda, Suni Lee, Kei Yoshitome, and Takemi Otsuki

Abstract The immunological effects of asbestos have been demonstrated and include reduction of antitumor immunity such as the reduction of natural killer (NK) cell activity with decreased expression of NK cell-activating receptor, NKp46, as well as reduced expression of CXCR3, chemokine receptor, and interferon (IFN)-γ in CD4+ T cells. In this review, the effects of asbestos as demonstrated by our investigations on the cellular characteristics and functions of cytotoxic T lymphocytes (CTLs) differentiated from CD8+ T cells are shown and discussed. Experiments involving in vitro exposure of chrysotile asbestos onto a mixed lymphocyte reaction (MLR) assay to estimate clonal expansion (proliferation and differentiation) of CD8+ T cells revealed the inhibition of both proliferation and differentiation. These results should be interpreted as the impairment of CTL differentiation in the lymph nodes, where asbestos fibers are located continuously in asbestos-exposed people. In addition, analyses of cellular functions in asbestos-exposed patients with pleural plaque (PP) and malignant mesothelioma (MM) are discussed. PP patients showed an increase in effector memory CD8+ T cells compared to healthy donors or MM patients. Furthermore, MM patients showed a decrease in perforin-expressing CD8+ T cells. These results indicated that although asbestos-exposed individuals are ready to respond with transformed cells, CTLs may lose their function once mesothelioma progresses.

Keywords Asbestos • CTL (cytotoxic T cell) • Perforin • Interferon γ • Pleural plaque • Malignant mesothelioma

N. Kumagai-Takei • Y. Nishimura • H. Matsuzaki • S. Lee • K. Yoshitome •
T. Otsuki, M.D., Ph.D. (✉)
Department of Hygiene, Kawasaki Medical School, 577 Matsushima, Kurashiki, Okayama 701-0192, Japan
e-mail: takemi@med.kawasaki-m.ac.jp

M. Maeda
Department of Biofunctional Chemistry, Division of Bioscience, Graduate School of Natural Science and Technology, Okayama University, Okayama, Japan

T. Otsuki et al. (eds.), *Biological Effects of Fibrous and Particulate Substances*, Current Topics in Environmental Health and Preventive Medicine,
DOI 10.1007/978-4-431-55732-6_12

12.1 Asbestos and Antitumor Immunity

The cellular and molecular biological effects of asbestos fibers are usually considered in regard to fibrogenesis and carcinogenesis [1–3], since people who have been exposed suffer from lung fibrosis known as asbestosis [4–6], one of the typical forms of pneumoconiosis, as well as malignancies such as malignant mesothelioma (MM) and lung cancer [7–9]. In addition, several reports have shown that people exposed to asbestos show increased incidences of other malignancies such as those involving the larynx, gastrointestinal tracts, and ovary [10–12]. A consideration of these facts might suggest that these people possess reduced antitumor immunity caused by asbestos exposure as evidenced by the occurrence of the abovementioned tumors and the long-term latent period of 30–40 years since the initial exposure.

Based on these considerations, issues regarding asbestos remain an important concern globally, particularly problems related to asbestos-causing malignancies [13, 14]. The occurrence of MM is expected to total 300,000 people worldwide. In response to these concerns, the asbestos issue in Japan was explored in the summer of 2005 [15–17]. The media as represented by broadcasts and newspapers announced details of patients who developed MM without any history of direct exposure, but who lived near asbestos-handling factories. Awareness of the dangers associated with environmental exposure to asbestos created social and political problems, especially since these patients were not compensated by any common worker compensation policy, and the lack of responsibility of companies and government was highlighted. Eight months later, a new law for compensation of work-unrelated MM patients had been enacted, and people in Japan became aware of the many problems associated with asbestos exposure, such as the types of health impairments created; the steps involved in the diagnosis, treatment, and prognosis of these diseases; and how they can apply and benefit from the compensation law. However, it is very difficult to identify the low-dose exposure history in individual cases [15–17]. Furthermore, earlier diagnosis of MM is not easy, and the prognosis is still poor, even though various therapies have been introduced involving advances in surgical methods, molecular targeting therapies, and immunotherapies [18–20].

There are few investigations regarding the general immunological effects of asbestos [21, 22], except for recent advances in the recognition of inflammasomes [23–25]. It was considered that asbestos may affect human immune cells because silica (SiO_2), which represents the core atomic elements of asbestos, acts on the human immune system and causes autoimmune diseases in silicosis patients [26, 27]. We have been studying the mechanisms of silica-induced dysregulation of autoimmunity [28–31], although silica-induced impairment of autoimmunity was considered to be an adjuvant mechanism. Our findings indicated that silica particles activate both responder/effector T cells (Tresp) and regulatory T cells (Treg). Tresp produces acquired resistance for CD95/Fas-mediated apoptosis due to excess production of soluble Fas (sFas), as well as decoy receptor 3 (DcR3) and other alternative spliced variants, which function in a manner similar to sFas by inhibiting

CD95/Fas-mediated apoptosis and enabling Tresp to survive for a longer period. Treg is also activated by exposure to silica particles and expresses CD95/Fas at excessive levels to cause early apoptotic cell death [32]. Both induce an unbalance of the Tresp/Treg population that results in less Treg and the development of autoimmune diseases [28–31].

A physical aspect of asbestos is its fibrous property, which is completely different from that of silica particles. These differences may affect human immune cells and cause reduction of antitumor immunity as indicated by the occurrence of malignant tumors in asbestos-exposed people. Our investigations in regard to these considerations have shown that natural killer (NK) cells have impaired cytotoxic function following asbestos exposure and reduced expression of the NK cell-activating receptor, NKp46. We also found reduction of signal transduction located downstream from NKp46 and decreased cytotoxic granules such as granzymes and perforin [26–33], as well as reduction of CXCR3, a chemokine receptor, on the cell surface of CD4+ T cells, including reduced secretion of interferon (IFN)-γ [37–40].

In this review, the effects of asbestos on CD8+ cytotoxic lymphocytes (CTLs) are presented and discussed.

12.2 The Role of CTLs in Antitumor Immunity

CTLs and NK cells play an important role in antitumor immunity through recognition of tumor antigens and the direct attack and killing of target tumor cells [41–43]. Although NK cells do not express antigen-specific receptors, they have various activating and inhibitory receptors that produce cytotoxicity against target tumor cells. In contrast, since CTLs possess T cell receptors specific to a tumor antigen, CTLs attack tumor cells through MHC (major histocompatibility complex) class I antigen at the tumor-cell surface. After activation of naïve CD8+ cells that recognize the tumor antigens, it is important to process clonal expansion with cell proliferation and differentiation in order to possess the killing activity in a tumor antigen-specific manner [41–43]. The differentiated CTLs store the lytic granules, including granzyme B, and perforin induces apoptosis of target tumor cells by secreting these molecules by degranulation after recognizing the tumor antigen [44, 45]. The lytic granule is composed of a lipid bilayer including lysosome-associated membrane glycoprotein-1 (LAMP1/CD107a) and is known to expose CD107a transiently on the cell surface of CTLs at degranulation [46]. In addition, CTLs secret tumor-killing cytokines such as IFN-γ and tumor necrosis factor-α [41–43].

12.2.1 Effects of Asbestos Exposure on CTL Differentiation

To investigate the effects of asbestos exposure on CTL differentiation, a mixed lymphocyte reaction (MLR) system using human peripheral blood mononuclear

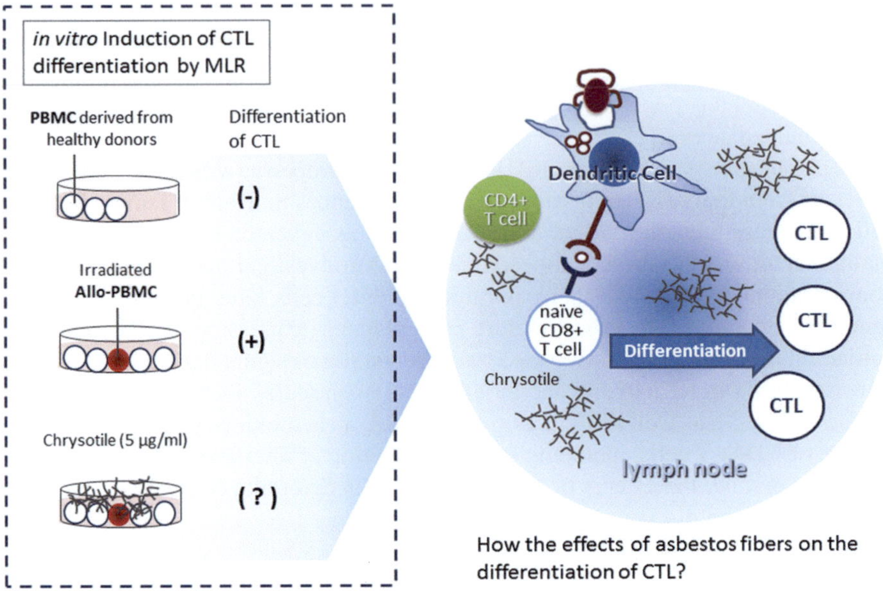

Fig. 12.1 The in vitro induction of cytotoxic T lymphocyte (CTL) differentiation by the mixed lymphocyte reaction (MLR) using peripheral blood mononuclear cells (PBMCs) derived from healthy donors with or without irradiated allo-PBMC, as well as with or without chrysotile B asbestos fibers, is used to estimate the effects of asbestos fibers on differentiation of CD8+ T cells into CTLs at the lymph node (LN) and in asbestos-exposed people

cells (PBMC) was applied for easy and effective estimation. After incubation with irradiated allo-PBMC in MLR, naïve CD8+ T cells differentiate to CTLs specific to the alloantigen. Thus, MLR using PBMCs derived from healthy donors (HD) and healthy allo-donors was performed with or without the addition of 5 μg/ml of chrysotile B for seven days. In our system, seven days is a suitable period to observe differentiation of alloantigen-specific CTLs with proliferation as clonal expansion from naïve CD8+ cells. As a control for induction of differentiation, a PBMC culture without allo-PBMC was utilized as shown in Fig. 12.1 [47].

In the allo-stimulated PBMC culture, an increase of CD3+ CD8+ cells was observed compared to the no stimulation culture, whereas an allo-stimulated culture with chrysotile did not show this increase, resulting in chrysotile fibers inhibiting the proliferation of naïve CD8+ cells. A cell killing assay was then performed using retrieved CD8+ cells from the PBMCs of MLR as effector cells and fluorescent-labeled allo-PBMC as target cells. Since the effector cells from MLR without chrysotile B caused an increase of dead target cells, it is thought that alloantigen-specific CTLs existed in the PBMC population following MLR without chrysotile fibers. However, the number of dead target cells was lower when PBMCs from MLR with chrysotile were used as the effector cells. This suggested that chrysotile fibers inhibited the differentiation of CTLs against the specific alloantigen [47].

It was thought that the reduction of cytotoxicity observed in PBMCs from MLR with chrysotile may depend on the decrease of total CD8+ cells, since proliferation was also inhibited as mentioned above. Thus, CD8+ lymphocytes were used as the effectors instead of whole PBMCs, and their cytotoxicity was examined. Results showed that CD8+ cells from MLR with chrysotile showed decreased cytotoxicity when compared to cells from MLR without chrysotile. This indicated that the function of cell killing in CD8+ CTLs was reduced in individual cells [47].

It is well known that granzyme B secreted from CTLs is important for the cytotoxicity shown by CTLs. Granzyme B is one of the proteases and induces apoptosis of target cells through activation of caspase 3. In addition, IFN-γ produced by CTLs also functions to cause inhibition of proliferation and cell death against the tumor cells. In our experimental model, the levels of both IFN-γ and granzyme B+ cells in CD8+ lymphocytes following MLR with chrysotile were lower than those following MLR without chrysotile [47].

The differentiation of CTLs can also be examined by cell surface markers such as CD45RA for the naïve type, CD25 for the activated type, and CD45RO for the effector/memory type. MLR without chrysotile revealed a decrease of CD45RA and an increase of CD25 and CD45RO, indicating allo-PBMC stimulation caused the differentiation from naïve to effector/memory CTLs. In contrast, MLR with chrysotile inhibited the above changes. A consideration of these findings, as well as inhibition of the IFN-γ+ and granzyme B+ cell population, reveals that exposure to chrysotile in MLR induced inhibition of the differentiation from CD8+ lymphocytes to CTLs [47].

We next examined whether the chrysotile-induced inhibition of proliferation in CD8+ lymphocytes is dependent on the static or apoptotic effects of chrysotile. Although the number of CD8+ lymphocytes in MLR showed a drastic increase from day 6 to 7, MLR with chrysotile did not show this change. In addition, annexin V + apoptotic cells, the so-called activation-induced cell death (AICD), in MLR without chrysotile were found at certain levels, and MLR with chrysotile also showed similar levels. Thus, apoptosis was not related to inhibition of proliferation in CD8+ lymphocytes and chrysotile-induced growth static effects on these cells [47].

Regarding cytokines, IFN-γ and TNF-α are known to induce CTL differentiation, whereas interleukin (IL)-10 inhibits this differentiation. IL-2 is essential for proliferation of CD8+ lymphocytes. The cytokine concentrations in culture supernatants at day 7 of MLR with chrysotile showed decreases of IFN-γ, TNF-α, and IL-10, whereas no change of IL-2 was observed for MLR without chrysotile. These findings indicated that the inhibition of CTL differentiation was due not to IL-10 but to the decrease of IFN-γ and TNF-α [47].

12.2.2 Significance of Experimental Findings

Naïve CD8+ lymphocytes differentiate to CTLs at lymph nodes [48]. In addition, it was reported that the number of chrysotile fibers in lymph nodes was higher than that in lung parenchyma in five asbestos-exposed cases and four of six patients with pleural plaque (PP) [49, 50]. These findings indicate that lymph nodes contain amounts of asbestos fibers similar to those of lung parenchyma and plaque, resulting in differentiation to CTLs in asbestos-exposed cases [49, 50].

It is difficult to compare the actual number of chrysotile fibers in the lymph nodes of asbestos-exposed cases and the abovementioned experimental conditions. However, we used 5 μg/ml of chrysotile in our investigations, which was lower than the level used in our other experiments to investigate the effects of these fibers on CD4+ T and NK cells [33–40]. In addition, another research group used 5–25 μg/ml of fibers to investigate the biological effects of asbestos on human mesothelial cells [51]. Considering our findings in which 5 μg/ml of chrysotile did not induce apoptosis of CD8+ lymphocytes, the overall data indicate that the experimental concentrations of chrysotile are sufficient to cause alteration of CTL differentiation, but did not produce acute toxicity.

Since we exposed chrysotile onto PBMCs derived from HD during MLR for CTL differentiation, the various findings can be interpreted to elucidate the effects of asbestos on the differentiation of naïve CD8+ lymphocytes, which have had no contact with asbestos, into CTLs at lymph nodes (Fig. 12.1) [47].

12.2.3 Functional Assays of CD8+ Lymphocytes in PP and MM Patients

The biological function of CD8+ lymphocytes derived from PP and MM patients was compared with that of cells derived from healthy volunteers. Although the population of CD3+/CD8+ lymphocytes and IFN-γ + cells in CD8+ lymphocytes did not differ, the CD45RA-negative population in PP and MM was higher than that in HD [52].

In addition, although the granzyme B+ population in CD8+ lymphocytes did not show any differences among the three groups, it was higher in PP after stimulation of CD8+ lymphocytes by phorbol 12-myristate 13-acetate (PMA) and ionomycin. A comparison of reduced values of granzyme B+ cells in CD8+ lymphocytes before and after stimulation revealed that they were higher in PP than in MM or HD [52].

The level of perforin + cells in CD8+ lymphocytes of PP and MM groups was higher than that of the HD group, whereas the level after stimulation was higher only in the PP group. In particular, the level in the MM group showed a significant reduction compared with that of the HD group. To determine whether this reduction was caused by excess degranulation of perforin in CD8+ lymphocytes of the MM group, evaluation of degranulation (expression of CD107a) did not show differences among the three groups. In addition, the individual samples which showed drastic reduction of perforin expression after stimulation did not show higher expression levels of CD107a. Thus, the reduction of perforin in CD8+ lymphocytes derived from MM patients was not due to the excess degranulation [52].

12.2.4 Insights into the Function of Peripheral CD8+ Lymphocytes from Asbestos-Exposed Patients

Among the asbestos-exposed groups, MM patients showed a lower level of perforin + cells after in vitro stimulation on CD8+ lymphocytes than PP patients. The level of perforin + cells before stimulation is interpreted as a certain level of perforin in peripherally circulating CD8+ lymphocytes. Furthermore, if the individual values of perforin + cells are higher after simulation, the cytotoxicity in whole CD8+ lymphocytes is enhanced by stimulation in individual patients. Thus, the whole cytotoxicity that resulted was reduced in MM patients. Moreover, the alteration of perforin levels in CD8+ lymphocytes after stimulation may be an indicator of the occurrence of MM in the asbestos-exposed population (Fig. 12.2) [52].

It was revealed that the increase of perforin + cells and decrease of CD45RA-negative cells were the same features of CD8+ lymphocytes in PP and MM groups. These findings indicate elevation of CTLs possessing cytotoxic function in the peripheral blood of those patients and, particularly, in PP patients who do not carry malignant tumors. It is interesting that there are immune reactions against non-self cells and cancerous cells caused by the carcinogenicity of asbestos in PP patients. In addition, since the perforin present is limited in effector memory CD8+ T cells and not in central memory cells, the asbestos-exposed patients with or without malignant tumors showed a higher effector memory population in their CD8+ lymphocytes. On the other hand, since MM patients showed persistent reduction of cytotoxicity, the maintenance of adequate antitumor immunity in asbestos-exposed patients is a key factor for the occurrence of cancers [52].

We initially assumed a reduction of non-naïve CT8+ cells in PP patients from the results of CTL differentiation using MLR. However, CD8+ lymphocytes from PP revealed an increase of perforin + and CDRA-negative populations in CD8+ lymphocytes, as well as an increase of the perforin + and granzyme B + fractions after in vitro stimulation. The differences may be explained by noting that the MLR assay indicates the direct effects of asbestos fibers on differentiation into CTLs, whereas the functional assay in CD8+ lymphocytes derived from PP patients examines not only the immunological effects of asbestos fibers but also the complicated biological reactions in the whole body of asbestos-exposed patients. Thus, it would be better to distinguish these results when they are interpreted in clinical situations. It is noteworthy that there was an apparent difference in functional assays of CD8+ lymphocytes between PP and MM. The capacity of antitumor

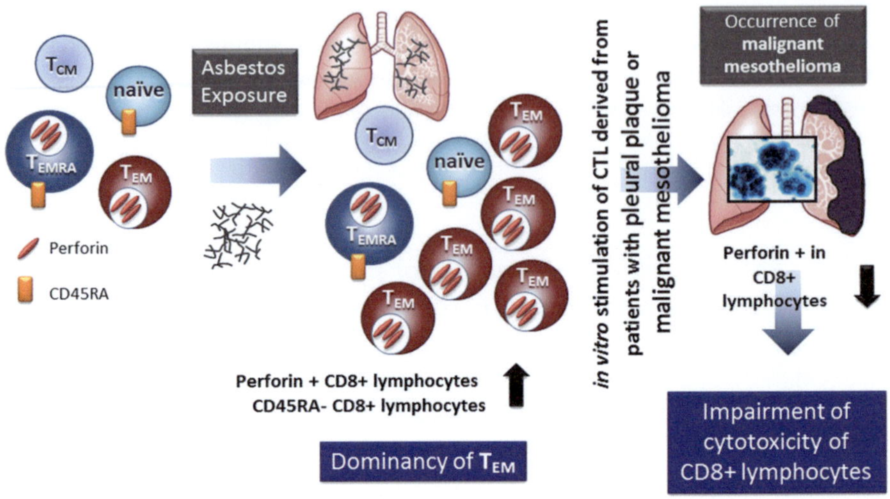

Fig. 12.2 Functional assays using CD8+ lymphocytes derived from asbestos-exposed patients with pleural plaque (PP) and malignant mesothelioma (MM). The CD8+ lymphocytes showed an increase of perforin+ and CD45RA-negative CD8+ lymphocytes. These results indicated that CD8+ lymphocytes showed a predominance of effector memory cells in asbestos-exposed patients. In addition, MM showed a reduction in the population of the perforin+ fraction after in vitro stimulation with PMA and ionomycin, whereas this was not observed for PP. This suggests that MM patients have impaired cytotoxicity of CD8+ lymphocytes

immunity, at least which induced by CTLs, may be bifurcation of the occurrence of cancerous diseases in asbestos-exposed patients [52].

12.3 Conclusion

In this chapter, the effects of chrysotile fibers on CD8+ lymphocytes were presented and discussed [47, 52]. A consideration of all the data and our other findings regarding the effects of asbestos on CD4+ T cells and NK cells suggests that asbestos-exposed patients progress toward a reduction of antitumor immunity. Regarding CD8+ lymphocytes, there are many other factors and cells such as dendritic cells and CD4+ helper T cells that can affect the differentiation of CTLs. Thus, future investigations to examine the effects of asbestos on these cells and analyze unified immune responses are required for a better understanding of the immunological effects of asbestos fibers and to utilize these findings for the development of new clinical devices for the early diagnosis and prevention of asbestos-induced malignancies.

Acknowledgements The authors thank Ms. Tamayo Hatayama, Minako Katoh, Naomi Miyahara, and Shoko Yamamoto for their technical assistance. All the experimental findings performed in the Department of Hygiene, Kawasaki Medical School were supported by Special Coordination Funds for Promoting Science and Technology grant H18-1-3-3-1; JPSS KAKENHI grants 20890270, 20390178, 1965153, and 21,659,161; Kawasaki Medical School Project grants 21–107, 22-A29, 20-411I, and 21–401, the Kawasaki Foundation for Medical Science and Medical Welfare (2009), and the Ryobi Teien Memorial Foundation (2009).

References

1. Robledo R, Mossman B. Cellular and molecular mechanisms of asbestos-induced fibrosis. J Cell Physiol. 1999;180:158–66.
2. Toyokuni S. Iron overload as a major targetable pathogenesis of asbestos-induced mesothelial carcinogenesis. Redox Rep. 2014;19:1–7. doi:10.1179/1351000213Y.0000000075.
3. Mossman BT, Kamp DW, Weitzman SA. Mechanisms of carcinogenesis and clinical features of asbestos-associated cancers. Cancer Invest. 1996;14:466–80.
4. Lazarus A, Massoumi A, Hostler J, Hostler DC. Asbestos-related pleuropulmonary diseases: benign and malignant. Postgrad Med. 2012;124:116–30. doi:10.3810/pgm.2012.05.2555.
5. Jamrozik E, de Klerk N, Musk AW. Asbestos-related disease. Int Med J. 2011;41:372–80. doi:10.1111/j.1445-5994.2011.02451.x.
6. Lazarus AA, Philip A. Asbestosis. Dis Mon. 2011;57(1):14–26. doi:10.1016/j.disamonth.2010.11.004.
7. Moolgavkar SH, Anderson EL, Chang ET, Lau EC, Turnham P, Hoel DG. A review and critique of U.S. EPA's risk assessments for asbestos. Crit Rev Toxicol. 2014;44:499–522. doi:10.3109/10408444.2014.902423.
8. Bayram M, Bakan ND. Environmental exposure to asbestos: from geology to mesothelioma. Curr Opin Pulm Med. 2014;20:301–7. doi:10.1097/MCP.0000000000000053.
9. Goswami E, Craven V, Dahlstrom DL, Alexander D, Mowat F. Domestic asbestos exposure: a review of epidemiologic and exposure data. Int J Environ Res Pub Health. 2013;10:5629–70. doi:10.3390/ijerph10115629.
10. Edelman DA. Laryngeal cancer and occupational exposure to asbestos. Int Arch Occup Environ Health. 1989;61:223–7.
11. Weiss W. Asbestos and colorectal cancer. Gastroenterology. 1990;99:876–84.
12. Bunderson-Schelvan M, Pfau JC, Crouch R, Holian A. Nonpulmonary outcomes of asbestos exposure. J Toxicol Environ Health B Critic Rev. 2011;14:122–52. doi:10.1080/10937404.2011.556048.
13. Robinson BW, Lake RA. Advances in malignant mesothelioma. N Engl J Med. 2005;353:1591–603.
14. Powell CA, Halmos B, Nana-Sinkam SP. Update in lung cancer and mesothelioma 2012. Am J Respir Crit Care Med. 2013;188:157–66. doi:10.1164/rccm.201304-0716UP.
15. Kumagai S, Kurumatani N, Tsuda T, Yorifuji T, Suzuki E. Increased risk of lung cancer mortality among residents near an asbestos product manufacturing plant. Int J Occup Environ Health. 2010;16:268–78.
16. Kumagai S, Kurumatani N. Asbestos fiber concentration in the area surrounding a former asbestos cement plant and excess mesothelioma deaths in residents. Am J Ind Med. 2009;52:790–8. doi:10.1002/ajim.20743.
17. Kurumatani N, Kumagai S. Mapping the risk of mesothelioma due to neighborhood asbestos exposure. Am J Respir Crit Care Med. 2008;178:624–9. doi:10.1164/rccm.200801-063OC.
18. Papaspyros S, Papaspyros S. Surgical management of malignant pleural mesothelioma: impact of surgery on survival and quality of life-relation to chemotherapy, radiotherapy, and alternative therapies. ISRN Surg. 2014;2014:817203. doi:10.1155/2014/817203.

19. Wong RM, Ianculescu I, Sharma S, Gage DL, Olevsky OM, Kotova S, Kostic MN, Grundfest WS, Hou D, Cameron RB. Immunotherapy for malignant pleural mesothelioma. Current status and future prospects. Am J Respir Cell Mol Biol. 2014;50:870–5. doi:10.1165/rcmb.2013-0472TR.
20. Christoph DC, Eberhardt WE. Systemic treatment of malignant pleural mesothelioma: new agents in clinical trials raise hope of relevant improvements. Curr Opin Oncol. 2014;26:171–81. doi:10.1097/CCO.0000000000000053.
21. Doll NJ, Stankus RP, Barkman HW. Immunopathogenesis of asbestosis, silicosis, and coal workers' pneumoconiosis. Clin Chest Med. 1983;4:3–14.
22. Rosenthal GJ, Simeonova P, Corsini E. Asbestos toxicity: an immunologic perspective. Rev Environ Health. 1999;14:11–20.
23. Rastrick J, Birrell M. The role of the inflammasome in fibrotic respiratory diseases. Minerva Med. 2014;105:9–23.
24. Kukkonen MK, Vehmas T, Piirilä P, Hirvonen A. Genes involved in innate immunity associated with asbestos-related fibrotic changes. Occup Environ Med. 2014;71:48–54. doi:10.1136/oemed-2013-101555.
25. Hillegass JM, Miller JM, MacPherson MB, Westbom CM, Sayan M, Thompson JK, Macura SL, Perkins TN, Beuschel SL, Alexeeva V, Pass HI, Steele C, Mossman BT, Shukla A. Asbestos and erionite prime and activate the NLRP3 inflammasome that stimulates autocrine cytokine release in human mesothelial cells. Part Fibre Toxicol. 2013;10:39. doi:10.1186/1743-8977-10-39.
26. Steenland K, Goldsmith DF. Silica exposure and autoimmune diseases. Am J Ind Med. 1995;28:603–8.
27. Shanklin DR, Smalley DL. The immunopathology of siliconosis. History, clinical presentation, and relation to silicosis and the chemistry of silicon and silicone. Immunol Res. 1998;18(3):125–73.
28. Lee S, Hayashi H, Maeda M, Chen Y, Matsuzaki H, Takei-Kumagai N, Nishimura Y, Fujimoto W, Otsuki T. Environmental factors producing autoimmune dysregulation–chronic activation of T cells caused by silica exposure. Immunobiology. 2012;217:743–8. doi:10.1016/j.imbio.2011.12.009.
29. Otsuki T, Miura Y, Nishimura Y, Hyodoh F, Takata A, Kusaka M, Katsuyama H, Tomita M, Ueki A, Kishimoto T. Alterations of Fas and Fas-related molecules in patients with silicosis. Exp Biol Med (Maywood). 2006;231:522–33.
30. Kumagai N, Hayashi H, Maeda M, Miura Y, Nishimura Y, Matsuzaki H, Lee S, Fujimoto W, Otsuki T. Immunological effects of silica and related dysregulation of autoimmunity. In: Mavragani CO, editor. Autoimmune disorders – pathogenetic aspects. Rijeka: InTech Open Access Publisher; 2011. p. 157–74. doi:10.5772/19218.
31. Hayashi H, Nishimura Y, Hyodo F, Maeda M, Kumagai N, Miura Y, Kusaka M, Uragami K, Otsuki T. Dysregulation of autoimmunity caused by silica exposure: Fas-mediated apoptosis in T lymphocytes derived from silicosis patients. In: Petro ME, editor. Autoimmune disorders: symptoms, diagnosis and treatment. Hauppauge: Nova Science Publishers Inc; 2011. p. 293–301.
32. Hayashi H, Miura Y, Maeda M, Murakami S, Kumagai N, Nishimura Y, Kusaka M, Urakami K, Fujimoto W, Otsuki T. Reductive alteration of the regulatory function of the CD4(+)CD25(+) T cell fraction in silicosis patients. Int J Immunopathol Pharmacol. 2010;23:1099–109.
33. Nishimura Y, Maeda M, Kumagai-Takei N, Lee S, Matsuzaki H, Wada Y, Nishiike-Wada T, Iguchi H, Otsuki T. Altered functions of alveolar macrophages and NK cells involved in asbestos-related diseases. Environ Health Prev Med. 2013;18:198–204. doi:10.1007/s12199-013-0333-y.
34. Nishimura Y, Kumagai N, Maeda M, Hayashi H, Fukuoka K, Nakano T, Miura Y, Hiratsuka J, Otsuki T. Suppressive effect of asbestos on cytotoxicity of human NK cells. Int J Immunopathol Pharmacol. 2011;24(1 Suppl):5S–10.

35. Nishimura Y, Maeda M, Kumagai N, Hayashi H, Miura Y, Otsuki T. Decrease in phosphorylation of ERK following decreased expression of NK cell-activating receptors in human NK cell line exposed to asbestos. Int J Immunopathol Pharmacol. 2009;22:879–88.
36. Nishimura Y, Miura Y, Maeda M, Kumagai N, Murakami S, Hayashi H, Fukuoka K, Nakano T, Otsuki T. Impairment in cytotoxicity and expression of NK cell- activating receptors on human NK cells following exposure to asbestos fibers. Int J Immunopathol Pharmacol. 2009;22:579–90.
37. Maeda M, Chen Y, Kumagai-Takei N, Hayashi H, Matsuzaki H, Lee S, Hiratsuka J, Nishimura Y, Kimura Y, Otsuki T. Alteration of cytoskeletal molecules in a human T cell line caused by continuous exposure to chrysotile asbestos. Immunobiology. 2013;218:1184–91. doi:10.1016/j.imbio.2013.04.007.
38. Maeda M, Yamamoto S, Chen Y, Kumagai-Takei N, Hayashi H, Matsuzaki H, Lee S, Hatayama T, Miyahara N, Katoh M, Hiratsuka J, Nishimura Y, Otsuki T. Resistance to asbestos-induced apoptosis with continuous exposure to crocidolite on a human T cell. Sci Total Environ. 2012;429:174–82. doi:10.1016/j.scitotenv.2012.04.043.
39. Maeda M, Nishimura Y, Hayashi H, Kumagai N, Chen Y, Murakami S, Miura Y, Hiratsuka J, Kishimoto T, Otsuki T. Decreased CXCR3 expression in CD4+ T cells exposed to asbestos or derived from asbestos-exposed patients. Am J Respir Cell Mol Biol. 2011;45:795–803. doi:10.1165/rcmb.2010-0435OC.
40. Maeda M, Nishimura Y, Hayashi H, Kumagai N, Chen Y, Murakami S, Miura Y, Hiratsuka J, Kishimoto T, Otsuki T. Reduction of CXC chemokine receptor 3 in an in vitro model of continuous exposure to asbestos in a human T cell line, MT-2. Am J Respir Cell Mol Biol. 2011;45:470–9. doi:10.1165/rcmb.2010-0213OC.
41. Doherty PC. Cell-mediated cytotoxicity. Cell. 1993;75:607–12.
42. Müllbacher A, Flynn K. Aspects of cytotoxic T cell memory. Immunol Rev. 1996;150:113–27.
43. Maher J, Davies ET. Targeting cytotoxic T lymphocytes for cancer immunotherapy. Br J Cancer. 2004;91:817–21.
44. Berke G. The CTL's kiss of death. Cell. 1995;81:9–12.
45. Pham CT, Ley TJ. The role of granzyme B cluster proteases in cell-mediated cytotoxicity. Semin Immunol. 1997;9:127–33.
46. Zaritskaya L, Shurin MR, Sayers TJ, Malyguine AM. New flow cytometric assays for monitoring cell-mediated cytotoxicity. Expert Rev Vaccines. 2010;9:601–16. doi:10.1586/erv.10.49.
47. Kumagai-Takei N, Nishimura Y, Maeda M, Hayashi H, Matsuzaki H, Lee S, Hiratsuka J, Otsuki T. Effect of asbestos exposure on differentiation of cytotoxic T lymphocytes in mixed lymphocyte reaction of human peripheral blood mononuclear cells. Am J Respir Cell Mol Biol. 2013;49:28–36. doi:10.1165/rcmb.2012-0134OC.
48. Heath WR, Carbone FR. Cross-presentation in viral immunity and self-tolerance. Nat Rev Immunol. 2001;1:126–34.
49. Dodson RF, Williams Jr MG, Corn CJ, Brollo A, Bianchi C. A comparison of asbestos burden in lung parenchyma, lymph nodes, and plaques. Ann N Y Acad Sci. 1991;643:53–60.
50. Dodson RF, Williams Jr MG, Corn CJ, Brollo A, Bianchi C. Asbestos content of lung tissue, lymph nodes, and pleural plaques from former shipyard workers. Am Rev Respir Dis. 1990;142:843–7.
51. Griffith DE, Miller EJ, Gray LD, Idell S, Johnson AR. Interleukin-1-mediated release of interleukin-8 by asbestos-stimulated human pleural mesothelial cells. Am J Respir Cell Mol Biol. 1994;10:245–52.
52. Kumagai-Takei N, Nishimura Y, Maeda M, Hayashi H, Matsuzaki H, Lee S, Kishimoto T, Fukuoka K, Nakano T, Otsuki T. Functional properties of CD8(+) lymphocytes in patients with pleural plaque and malignant mesothelioma. J Immunol Res. 2014;2014:670140. doi:10.1155/2014/670140.

MIX
Papier aus verantwortungsvollen Quellen
Paper from responsible sources
FSC® C105338

If you have any concerns about our products,
you can contact us on
ProductSafety@springernature.com

In case Publisher is established outside the EU,
the EU authorized representative is:
Springer Nature Customer Service Center GmbH
Europaplatz 3, 69115 Heidelberg, Germany

Printed by Libri Plureos GmbH
in Hamburg, Germany